PHARMACEUTICAL CARE PRACTICE

NOTICE

Medicine is an ever-changing science. As new research and clinical experience broaden our knowledge, changes in treatment and drug therapy are required. The authors and the publisher of this work have checked with sources believed to be reliable in their efforts to provide information that is complete and generally in accord with the standards accepted at the time of publication. However, in view of the possibility of human error or changes in medical sciences, neither the authors nor the publisher nor any other party who has been involved in the preparation or publication of this work warrants that the information contained herein is in every respect accurate or complete, and they are not responsible for any errors or omissions or for the result obtained from use of such information. Readers are encouraged to confirm the information contained herein with other sources. For example and in particular, readers are advised to check the product information sheet included in the package of each drug they plan to administer to be certain that the information contained in this book is accurate and that changes have not been made in the recommended dose or in the contraindications for administration. This recommendation is of particular importance in connection with new or infrequently used drugs.

PHARMACEUTICAL CARE PRACTICE

ROBERT J. CIPOLLE, Pharm.D., F.C.C.P.

University of Minnesota
College of Pharmacy
Minneapolis, Minnesota

LINDA M. STRAND, Pharm.D., Ph.D.

University of Minnesota
College of Pharmacy
Minneapolis, Minnesota

PETER C. MORLEY, Ph.D.

University of Minnesota
College of Pharmacy
Minneapolis, Minnesota

McGraw-Hill
Health Professions Division

New York St. Louis San Francisco Auckland Bogotá Caracas
Lisbon London Madrid Mexico City Milan Montreal New Delhi
San Juan Singapore Sydney Tokyo Toronto

McGraw-Hill

*A Division of The **McGraw·Hill** Companies*

PHARMACEUTICAL CARE PRACTICE

Copyright © 1998 by *The **McGraw-Hill** Companies, Inc.* All right reserved. Printed in the United States of America. Except as permitted under the United States Copyright Act of 1976, no part of this publication may be reproduced or distributed in any form or by any means, or stored in a data base or retrieval system, without the prior written permission of the publisher.

234567890 DOCDOC 99

ISBN 0-07-012046-3

This book was set in Adobe Caslon by Better Graphics, Inc.
The editors were Stephen Zollo and Muza Navrozov.
The production supervisor was Catherine H. Saggese.
The cover and text were designed by James Sullivan/RepoCat Graphics
    and Editorial Services.
The index was prepared by Maria Coughlin.
R. R. Donnelley & Sons was printer and binder.

This book is printed on recycled, acid-free paper.

Library of Congress Cataloging-in-Publication Data

Cipolle, Robert J.
    Pharmaceutical care practice / Robert J. Cipolle, Linda M. Strand,
Peter C. Morley.
        p.   cm.
    Includes bibliographical references and index.
    ISBN 0-07-012046-3
    1. Pharmacy—Practice.   I. Strand, Linda M.   II. Morley, Peter C.
III. Title.
    [DNLM: 1. Pharmacology.   2. Professional Practice.   3. Drug
Therapy.   QV 21 C577p   1998]
RS122.5.C56   1998
615'.1'068—dc21
DNLM/DLC
for Library of Congress

To the memory of

Bette Cipolle
May 27, 1964—August 9, 1985

"Multiply life by the power of two"
Emily Saliers

Clarence E. Morley
1917—1996

"O quam cito transit gloria mundi!"
Thomas à Kempis
1379–1471

Contents

ACKNOWLEDGMENTS

Many people over many years have contributed to the work presented in this book; some of them directly, many of them indirectly. To name them all would result in a directory worthy of separate publication. Indeed, they know who they are, and they know that they share this work with us.

While our intellectual debts are manifold, we are especially grateful to Doug Hepler, Don Alexander, Don Perrier, Lyle Bootman, Don Uden, Steve Schondelmeyer, Mike Frakes, and Doug Simpson. An endless thank-you goes to Dean Emeritus Lawrence C. Weaver of the College of Pharmacy, University of Minnesota, the greatest mentor any group with ideas could ever have. His moral support, wonderful vision, and constant enthusiasm have kept us focused for two decades.

We are also greatly indebted to our many colleagues in Canada, Australia, Scotland, England, New Zealand, South Africa, Singapore, Malaysia, Korea, The Netherlands, Sweden, and Spain. Sustained critical dialogue with our friends in these far away places has sharpened our focus and expanded our ideas.

We received significant financial contributions to our efforts over the years. Glaxo Wellcome, The Merck Company, The Upjohn Company, Aetna, Blue Cross/Blue Shield of Minnesota, Medica, Diversified Pharmaceutical Services (DPS), PCS Health Systems, and the Pew Foundation, all provided direct support. However, all of them contributed much more than funding. They provided us with colleagues who were able to engage in intellectual discourse, who were willing to take chances and risk exposure to the critical reflection of old ideas and challenges to time-honored paradigms. In doing so, they permitted us to engage in unfettered inquiry with a view to change a profession and its entire modus operandi. For this act we are most grateful.

A special acknowledgment is due the Peters family for granting an endowment to the Peters Institute of Pharmaceutical Care. This endowment supports educational endeavors, such as the preparation of this text, to further the practice of pharmaceutical care.

At McGraw-Hill, we are grateful to Steve Zollo, who commissioned the book, and to those whose editorial eyes transformed our often painful prose into a readable text. We would also like to thank Karen Meyers of the Peters Institute of Pharmaceutical Care, who worked diligently to see that the manuscript was completed and pryed from our hands to start its long journey.

There are other groups of individuals whose contributions to our work cannot go unmentioned. The community pharmacists with whom we worked closely, state pharmacy association representatives, university colleagues, and patients—those who make such a challenge worthwhile. We thank all of you for your commitment, your trust, and your patience.

All who have contributed to this work have demonstrated their commitment to patient care. Realistically, at the "end of the day," it is the quality of care received by patients that will legitimize this book and establish its social and ethical value.

PREFACE

Health care systems everywhere are currently experiencing unprecedented transformations of one kind or another. In some cases the degree of change can only be described as "revolutionary," while in others "evolutionary" may be a more appropriate depiction. Either way, structural and organizational changes are not difficult to find in any contemporary health care system. This is particularly true in the United States, where managed care and the values of the marketplace increasingly define and direct health care to those who can afford it.

These are indeed turbulent times characterized by cost-containment pressures, conflicting financial incentives, increasing gaps in health insurance coverage with limited access to health care, and a general, pervasive anxiety about the sustainability of a system replete with inadequacies. The public and health care professionals alike are engaged in serious critical examination of needs, expectations, values, and ethics. Health care professionals in particular are questioning their traditional roles and responsibilities, and once clearly delineated professional boundaries are becoming increasingly blurred. Indeed, in some cases the very idea of a unique and clearly defined professional identity is frequently called into question.

Pharmacy is no different from other health care professions in that it currently seeks to reorient itself to meet the challenges presented by the myriad of complexities and conflicts that permeate the contemporary health care system.

It is within this dynamic context that the profession accepted pharmaceutical care as its mandate for the future. This practice is focused on ensuring appropriate, effective, safe, and convenient drug therapy for patients. Pharmaceutical care is specifically designed to meet the patient's drug-related needs, whatever they may be. Such a practice must be comprehensive in scope and committed to the reduction and prevention of drug-related morbidity and mortality. To this end, pharmaceutical care is a systematic, rational, comprehensive approach to drug therapy decisions. Pharmaceutical care offers the pharmacist a patient-centered philosophy of practice that makes the identification, resolution, and prevention of drug therapy problems the primary responsibility of each practitioner.

This volume defines and delineates this pharmaceutical care practice in detail. Moving from a brief discussion of contemporary issues in health care, we introduce the reader to the nature and magnitude of drug therapy problems and present the case for pharmaceutical care practices as a socially and clinically valuable solution to what can only be described as a profoundly significant health issue, that of drug-related morbidity and mortality. We introduce this new practice philosophy, a patient care process, and the practice management system in a thorough and systematic manner. Additionally, we introduce the practitioner to what is required to build a practice of pharmaceutical care and discuss what is necessary to teach the practitioner and the student to provide this service to patients. Throughout this volume, the collaborative relationship between patient and practitioner is to be seen as central to the pharmaceutical care enterprise.

The problem of drug-related morbidity and mortality is unquestionably of a magnitude that requires urgent attention. Moreover, we are convinced that a very large part of the solution is to be found through the implementation of pharmaceutical care. Pharmacists are preeminently prepared to make a significant contribution to the resolution of this serious public health problem. Their education, preparation, and availability place them in the best possible position to identify, resolve, and prevent life-threatening drug therapy problems. It is our fervent desire to optimize the pharmacist's role as a health care practitioner, and it is to this end that the present volume is dedicated. The concept and practice of pharmaceutical care are empowering. Pharmaceutical care is now in the hands of those committed to improving patient outcomes by assuming responsibility for appropriate, effective, safe, and convenient drug therapy.

CHAPTER ONE

A NEW PROFESSIONAL PRACTICE

PHARMACEUTICAL CARE IN CONTEXT

Health care systems around the world are in a state of flux. Change is everywhere, and each day presents different priorities and expectations, complete with a "new" set of acronyms to be learned. Many find the present state of health care in the United States and elsewhere quite troubling; talk of reform is widespread and, in many situations, acrimonious.

Problems, their complexity and lack of solutions, can be seen everywhere. On one general issue there is agreement: we are in a state of crisis! But what does this mean in real terms? What issues justify claims to crisis? Such questions and their answers tend to fall into three categories: access, cost, and quality.

ACCESS, COST, AND QUALITY OF HEALTH CARE

Within the context of most health care debates, public discourse begins with critical reflections on access or the lack thereof. We are constantly reminded that approximately 40 million Americans lack health insurance and are not eligible for Medicare or Medicaid. Data also indicate that these same individuals do not have any private insurance plans and most likely lack the financial resources necessary to pay "out of pocket." In short, while total estimates of numbers may vary, we do know that, by any stretch of one's "ethical imagination," there are far too many Americans remaining outside of the health care system, with little or no chance of gaining access for remedy of their particular maladies. Children and young adults are particularly visible in the demographics of the excluded.

The human and economic costs of drug-related mortality and morbidity can no longer be ignored.

Recently we have seen a proliferation of alternative or complementary health care providers. "New Age" solutions to sickness are presently receiving widespread attention. Indeed, it would be correct to consider present developments in nonallopathic paradigms as a "growth industry." Also, significant moves toward self-care and an increasingly empowered consumer culture suggest a number of other changes in health-seeking behavior.

While access to health care is a problem for far too many Americans, the general issue of cost is the driving force behind most discourse on health reform. Rising health care costs—outright inflation if you will—are seen as a major threat to the long-term survival of any health care system and perhaps pose a threat *writ large* to the soundness of the economy. Identifiable causes are many: an increasingly elderly population; malpractice premiums; an out-of-control administrative overhead; expensive technology; questionable therapy; defensive medicine; escalating salaries among medical specialists, hospital administrators, and insurance CEOs; and the rising cost of pharmaceuticals. This list is by no means exhaustive. We could, for example, add a large number of socioeconomic factors, such as poverty, crime, and violence, all of which have many complex health consequences. Similarly, the impact of many diseases of epidemic proportion (e.g., AIDS) places great economic pressures on a health system that, in the view of many economists, threatens to collapse under the weight of its growing financial burden. While controversy rages over how much each of these and more contributes to the overall economic malaise, there is general agreement that the problem of rising costs must be solved and brought under control.[1]

Attempts to control costs have generated a significant growth (some might say an industry) of programs, consultants, managers, organizational frameworks, administrative structures, health economics "experts," accountants, educational programs and degrees, and other measures all dedicated to cost containment. In a real sense there is an irony in all of this activity. Attempts to find solutions to rising costs have in themselves added to the costs of health care. Indeed, we are beginning to realize that the numerous attempts to micromanage the economics of health care services are very expensive and increasingly devour financial resources, thereby moving them away from actual health care delivery and increasing administrative costs. Clearly, this is a perplexing problem that must be addressed.[1]

More recently, considerable attention has focused on the economic cost of drug-related morbidity and mortality. It would appear that this level of discourse has most certainly caught the attention of assorted politicians, who appear to have less difficulty deconstructing economic considerations than they have when confronted with the "softer," "sentimental," and qualitative dimensions of the human condition in sickness and suffering. Anyway, the economic costs are quite staggering and certainly require serious, critical scrutiny.[1]

Johnson and Bootman have presented an alarming account of the high cost of drug-related morbidity and mortality.[2,3] Estimates of personal health expenditures for prescription drugs in 1994 exceeded $73 billion. The authors also note recent research indicating that the costs associated with inappropriate drug use "may even exceed these initial expenditures for drug therapy."[2] Moreover, costs of drug-related morbidity and mortality could reach $136.8 billion![3]

Economic costs, then, are very high indeed. When combined with human costs, these figures present us with a challenge that cannot be ignored. Johnson and Bootman have developed a model that estimates the cost of drug-related morbidity and mortality, and they have also produced a probability-pathway model that estimates "the degree to which pharmaceutical care could minimize negative therapeutic outcomes."[3] Their conclusions are encouraging:

> According to the model, with the reductions in negative therapeutic outcomes that would result if all ambulatory care pharmacy settings provided pharmaceutical care, nearly 84% of patients would achieve optimal therapeutic outcomes due to drug therapy. According to our previous estimate, if pharmacists were available to provide only a dispensing function in typical ambulatory care settings, less than 60% of patients receiving medication would have an absence of a problem. Thus, the provision of pharmaceutical care would lead to an increase in optimal therapeutic outcomes of more than 40%.[3]

In summary, the level of drug-related morbidity and mortality in this country is significant, and the costs associated with it are almost unimaginable. Therefore, something must be done to control both the suffering and the expenditure of resources associated with the problem.

The provision of pharmaceutical care improves patient outcomes.

Discourse on quality abounds. Numerous books and articles in scholarly journals proudly proclaim that American medicine is "the best in the world." At technical levels, such a view is plausible. However, there are also signs of decline, as cost cutting and downsizing reduce services. Hospital stays are increasingly shortened, and journalists daily report "drive-by" delivery of babies. The even more extreme same-day surgeries, such as mastectomies, raise the ire of the American public. Interestingly, Congress feels compelled to pass legislation controlling these acts; in so doing, it judges them inappropriate and most certainly not representative of "quality care."

At the level of personnel management, it is clear that there is also cause for alarm. Morale among physicians, nurses, pharmacists, and others is widely reported to be low. All health care professionals face cutbacks, reclassification, and redundancy. Moreover, educational standards, which have risen over the years, are now being lowered in the interest of cost cutting. Technicians and others with minimal educational preparation are now filling positions previously held by practitioners holding advanced degrees. There is considerable evidence that standards and the quality of care are being driven more by economic determinants than by a moral vision or a commitment to more humane values.[1]

The U.S. health care system is marked by controversy, conflict, and rapid change. Indeed, it is a milieu of collective angst and multiple directions. The good, prodigious accomplishments of technical medicine continue to grow, but—paradoxically—they recede into the background as organizational and administrative conflicts increasingly shape our values and expectations. Practices, professional identities, and the discursive nature of rules, roles, and responsibilities are constantly challenged. The alienated health care practitioner is more than ever the norm rather than an exceptional case of a marginal character.

It is within this context of change and challenge to traditional roles and responsibilities that we focus on a particular portion of the health care dilemma, that of drug therapy.

DRUG THERAPY IN HEALTH CARE

One frequently discussed aspect of health care is that of drug therapy, particularly with reference to its high cost. Although drug products consume approximately 8 percent of the total health care budget, this item is singled out and discussed endlessly for many reasons. First, drug therapy represents the most common form of treatment in contemporary health care, meaning that drug therapy is everywhere. Second, drug products are easy to isolate in the accounting of costs, since they are tangible entities and easily identified. Third, patients are frequently called upon to pay for drugs "out of pocket," making the costs more noticeable than other health care expenditures. Fourth, drug costs are constantly on the rise, and new, highly visible brand-name products have had high "price tags" associated with them, and the public has noticed. These are simply a few of the reasons why drug costs are so widely discussed.

There are other explanations for the high cost of drug therapy. While drug development has increasingly produced numerous therapeutic agents, often at a rate frequently referred to as "explosive," not all of these have been new drug classes but rather are new brands in "old" classes. Also, the picture is more complicated when we consider the vast number of "copycat" or "me-too" drugs produced by companies intent on acquiring their market share of a highly lucrative drug product that is a "hot item" in the treatment of major diseases. Indeed, as particular morbidity patterns are identified and potential markets defined, competition between pharmaceutical companies becomes intense, with each one struggling to produce "the drug of choice" in the treatment of a particular type of disease. With billions of dollars at stake it is hardly surprising to see such intense competition. However, contrary to the received wisdom of economists, such competition does not drive prices down. On the contrary, in many cases drugs have become more expensive in spite of "market forces," and the conventional wisdom of the economist has been seriously challenged.

While it is not within our purview to focus in-depth attention on economic factors associated with drug therapy, it is useful to reflect briefly on measures taken to bring pharmaceutical costs under control. Prescribers, who are expected to become cost-conscious, are increasingly working with restrictive formularies. That is to say, hospitals, managed care, and all other forms of health care organization are implementing restrictive lists of drugs that address both therapeutic and economic criteria. Such measures have been found in hospitals for a very long time. Currently, formularies are under review and development on an unprecedented scale, and the enforcement of guidelines is similarly receiving widespread attention.

Consistent with the logic of formularies is the general idea of generic substitution. Pharmacists are permitted by law (in most states) to substitute a less expensive generic for a more costly brand name drug. This mechanism of cost control is not altogether new but is now a clearly articulated "policy position"; that is, it is no longer merely the more discretionary approach that has traditionally met with variable interest and enthusiasm. In many attempts to control drug costs, the pharmacist is in the forefront of the action, sometimes willingly and often by default, since the pharmacist (or his or her agent) is the person who has contact with the patient at the time the prescription—and frequently the nonprescription—drug product is purchased. The potential impact pharmacists can have on the control of drug costs is well documented; however, the actual impact varies considerably, since physicians have for the most part maintained control over the prescription. The prescription represents the initial decision made about drug use. It is the quality of the drug used that we wish to address next.

In the United States, the quality of a drug product is seldom called into question. Although every now and then tainted products do appear on the store shelves as a result of criminal conduct or errors in production, and periodically reference is made to human error in administering the drug product or to a miscalculation of the dosage for a given formulation (concentration and quantity of the formulation). However, the standards successfully applied by the Food and Drug Administration (FDA) in the United States are exemplary.

Discussions of quality surrounding drug use usually do not refer to the quality of the drug product, but to the quality of decisions as to whether and how a drug should be used. We call these "drug therapy decisions." Although frequently such decisions lead to positive outcomes, all too often they lead to hospitalization, additional physician visits, and at least inconvenience for the patient. So whether drug therapy is cheap or expensive is related to more than the cost of the product itself. For example, if the drug prescribed or recommended is unnecessary or is the wrong drug for the patient and the patient's disease, then that drug product would be expensive at any cost. On the other hand, if the drug prescribed or recommended is necessary but prescribed in the wrong dose, so as to cause toxicity, subtherapeutic responses, or adverse reactions (and subsequent visits to the physician or the hospital), then the drug is expensive regardless of the price of the product itself.

One fifth of hospitalized patients experience drug therapy problems, even in the most advanced medical institutions.

When we review the success (or failure) of drug use decisions in this country, we find a very troubling picture. Up to 20 percent of hospitalizations in the United States are related to drug therapy that in one way or another went wrong.[4] Inappropriate drug therapy has a high human cost in addition to the economics of error.

These statistics, according to Johnson and Bootman, lead to a cost of drug-related morbidity and mortality in this country of $76 billion.[3] If we were able to control the costs associated with inappropriate drug use, we could give away free all the prescription drug products used in this country!

These figures are staggering. We should be concerned not only with the cost of drug products but also with the costs of inappropriate drug use. And our concerns should go beyond cost, as a significant amount (50 percent is estimated) of the drug-related morbidity and mortality that patients suffer is preventable.[3] The nature and magnitude of this problem is developed in detail in Chap. 2.

APPROACHES TO THE MANAGEMENT OF DRUG USE

Although collectively those in the health care arena have been slow to recognize the magnitude and scope of the problems associated with drug use, numerous attempts have been made to influence the use of drug therapy positively. For example, politicians have tried to influence drug use positively through legislative control. They have tried to control the nonmedical use of drugs (illicit drug use) as well as the medical use of drugs (prescription/nonprescription designations). Politicians have legislated the information patients receive about drug therapy from the pharmacist [Omnibus Budget Reconciliation Act (OBRA) 1990, mandatory patient counseling], as well as the information contained on packaging, through the regulatory power of the FDA. Control at this level has brought attention to the problems associated with drug use. However, the success of such intervention is certainly debatable.

The pharmaceutical industry has traditionally influenced physicians and the drug products they prescribe through direct physician advertising, promotions, and the use of "detail people." Most recently this industry has reached the patient through direct advertising of drug products to the "consumer." There is much information to be obtained through the advertising process, but—given the commercial nature of the information—the patient is not always certain that all he or she needs to know is communicated.

Managed care organizations are currently using the concept of *disease management* to control the amounts and types of drugs used in their organizations. Disease management has, in contemporary terms, been used by the pharmaceutical industry as a marketing technique. In this framework, the industry develops drug entities, markets the product, and advertises it within a particular disease domain so that the value of the product can be managed relative to other entities treating the same disease. Managed care organizations have converted this concept to a cost-accounting system, wherein the costs of the drug entity can be understood relative to other treatments for a particular disease. Now, in a cost-accounting context, this concept is being used to control the amounts and types of drugs used in managed care organizations. This approach provides the prescriber and the patient with a means of comparing drug therapies. But patients seldom have a single disease, and treating the disease instead of the patient is associated with many limitations.

Hospitals as well as managed care organizations have attempted to manage their drug costs—and the use of drug therapy—through pharmacy and therapeutics committees, also known as P&T committees. The method most commonly used by these decision-making bodies has been the formulary system. The formulary is a list of drug products available for use in the institution, prepared by the committee members after reviewing the drug products based on their therapeutic characteristics. This process has brought attention to the need to limit available alternatives, attend to cost issues, consider therapeutic duplication, and understand how decisions are made to use drug therapy. However, the pharmaceutical industry and its pricing structure have had so much influence on the decision making of these groups that the formulary is now known more often than not to represent cost-accounting, and not drug-use decisions.

More recently the decision-making bodies in managed care organizations and hospitals have focused on developing protocols for the use of drug therapy by physicians and other health care professionals prescribing drug therapy. Protocol development is based on the "best practice" standards available in the literature or developed by a group of practitioners. The protocols are meant to represent guidelines used for decision making in situations where drug therapy is indicated. Again, this process brought to our attention the need to standardize the decisions concerning drug therapy. Their use is limited to those situations appropriate for the specific patient being treated—the protocol makes it difficult to manage patient-specific variations. In addition, practitioners in this country are not entirely comfortable with decision rules for drug therapy. This may be the case, since in none of the educational programs for prescribers is a rational, systematic decision process taught. Therefore the protocol, by definition, interferes with and does not complement the practitioner's decision-making processes for drug therapy decisions.

Pharmacists in management positions in hospitals, managed care organizations, and nursing homes have implemented drug use evaluations (DUEs) and drug utilization reviews (DURs) to influence drug use in their respective organizations. These evaluations are usually made retrospectively in response to a problem of prescribing identified in the institution. The DURs and DUEs provide a framework for critically evaluating the use of drugs. However, the results lack timeliness and have quite limited impact. These activities have been part of the clinical pharmacy movement, which influenced drug use in hospitals through the development of specialty clinics (e.g., warfarin dosing, diabetes education, refill clinics) and clinical services (e.g., pharmacokinetic dosing services, total parenteral nutrition services). The clinical pharmacy service movement had significant impact on those patients receiving the services. However, after 30 years of development, only a very small percentage of patients receive very limited assistance from these services, and this is almost exclusively in hospital settings.

All of the approaches just described have been ongoing for the past two to three decades, yet in 1995 the cost of drug-related morbidity and mortality reached $76 billion in the United States alone. As stated earlier, up to 20 percent of all hospitalizations are related to drug misadventures. Between 45 and 65 percent of patients take their drug therapy differently than suggested, with completely unpredictable consequences.[5]

No matter how you define the problem, its magnitude is significant. We are certain that there are many different reasons why the approaches described above have had a limited impact on managing the problems associated with the use of drug therapy. However, one reasonable explanation may be that these approaches have primarily been developed, implemented, and operationalized on the basis of population, political, or economic considerations, not on the basis of patient-specific care.

Drug-taking behavior is determined and acted upon at an individual patient level. Therefore, the most significant impact on that behavior will result from practitioner decisions made on the basis of patient-specific care.

DRUG USE RESPONSIBILITY

Who will accept the responsibility for appropriate drug use?

A logical question to ask about drug-related morbidity and mortality is: Who is responsible for appropriate drug use? The physician has traditionally been held responsible for a patient's drug therapy. However, the evolution of health care systems worldwide and the diverse nature of consumer lifestyles make it extremely difficult or impossible for any single physician to undertake this increasingly complex duty. Clearly, physicians are able to spend less and less time with patients, so the amount of time necessary to cope with actual or potential drug problems adequately is also shrinking. To complicate things further, let us not forget that patients frequently turn to numerous physicians, thereby creating a multiplicative factor in the "equation." However, of particular importance is the almost exponential growth in pharmaceutical knowledge. Indeed voluminous and highly complex, it will more than likely continue to move in this direction. Mastering both the complex knowledge base required for effective diagnosis and that circumscribing therapeutic decisions may very well prove to be beyond the scope of any single physician. In any event, it may be argued that to expect such accomplishment is, at the very least, unreasonable.

The physician, who traditionally has assumed this role, requires help to manage all of the increased complexities of drug use. The pharmacist is the logical choice. This individual is now educated for 6 years of higher education in the areas of medicinal chemistry, pharmaceutics, therapeutics, pathophysiology, and clinical pharmacology, to list just a few of the subjects studied in detail. In addition, the community-based location of the pharmacist means that he or she has daily and open access to the patient. However, for the pharmacist to play an active, positive role in managing a patient's drug therapy, many changes are required. The most important of these is also the most controversial—a manifesto for a new pharmacy practitioner. Indeed, we call for a reinventing of pharmacy as a health care profession, a re-visioning of purpose and collective responsibility.[6]

Pharmacists generally have a wealth of empirical knowledge, knowledge that, to a large extent, is underutilized. This pronouncement is surely less controversial than the first. The question is: What can be done to more fully utilize highly important pharmaceutical knowledge, and those who make legitimate claim to it? Attempting to answer this important question brings us squarely back to controversy. This controversy, such as it is, appears to be a direct consequence of the discursive and uncertain nature of the profession itself.

Pharmacy, as profession, is presently fragmented into differentiated academic degrees, "practices" defined by location, assorted commercial enterprises, specializations, and other "interest groups." Complicating matters further are the seemingly inescapable tensions and conflicts between "hospital" and "community" pharmacists. In short, there is very little that constitutes a unifying framework for the organization and identification of professional pharmacy activities and responsibilities. While many may well disagree as to the specifics of

Pharmaceutical care must become the organizing force for the profession of pharmacy.

conflicts presently afflicting the profession of pharmacy, surely none can claim that the profession has a secure, certain, united front. Indeed, recent discourse, at all levels of professional associations and among "the rank and file," point to disunity and despair as individuals reflect on possible futures.

The largely unmet need to address drug-related morbidity and mortality, identified earlier, and its epidemiology, as reviewed in Chap. 2, offers a simple yet profound answer to the question of purpose and responsibility. The profession of pharmacy is quite capable of uniting its members and directing its vast talents and energies toward the reduction of drug-related morbidity and mortality. All pharmacists can adopt an ethic of responsibility for, and commitment to, patient care. Our major concern is that pharmacy *writ large* must make a *collective* public commitment to this end and demonstrate its social value through its actions. Obligation, responsibility, and duty to patients in need of drug-related care will redefine pharmacy and identify pharmacists as health care providers/practitioners.

We remain convinced that pharmacy is up to the task. The pharmacoepidemiology of "drug misadventuring" provides a compelling statement of social need.[7] And, as we stated earlier, the pharmacist is the logical choice to address this major problem area. Pharmaceutical care, as we conceptualize it, provides a comprehensive framework for much-needed action. Moreover, united by a common understanding and acceptance of a systematic, rigorous approach to practice, pharmacists will provide a highly valuable service with the best of public interest in mind. We now turn our attention to the possibilities and promises of pharmaceutical care as constitutive of the new pharmacy.

ENTER PHARMACEUTICAL CARE

Pharmaceutical care was first defined by Mikeal et al.[8] in 1975 as "the care that a given patient requires and receives which assures safe and rational drug usage." Although the term has been used a number of times since its introduction, elaboration was not substantially forthcoming until Brodie et al.[9] suggested that pharmaceutical care includes the determination of the drug needs for a given individual and the provision not only of required drugs but also of the services necessary (before, during, and after treatment) to ensure optimally safe and effective therapy. The conceptualization of Brodie et al.[9] includes the idea of a feedback mechanism as a means of facilitating continuity of care by those who provide it. Thus, this work contributed to furthering the cause of safe and effective drug use and paved the way toward heightened consciousness and greater public/professional discourse. However, the changes that occurred subsequent to his work focused primarily on controlling the availability and distribution of the drug product and not specifically on patient need within identifiable clinical parameters.

In 1988, Hepler[10] in a more philosophical vein described pharmaceutical care as "a covenantal relationship between a patient and a pharmacist in which the pharmacist performs drug use control functions (with appropriate knowledge and skill) governed by the awareness of and commitment to the patient's interest." Hepler and Strand published a paper in 1990 which further developed pharmaceutical care by making the connection between the philosophy previously presented by Hepler and practice concepts which had been previously developed by Strand, Cipolle, and Morley. This paper provided a conceptualization of pharmaceutical care that stimulated widespread debate and ultimately produced broad-based agreement within the profession of pharmacy. A more detailed account of this history is provided by Posey.[12] It is the following definition that best characterizes Hepler and Strand's foundational conceptualization: "Pharmaceutical care is that component of pharmacy practice which entails the direct interaction of the pharmacist with the patient for the purpose of caring for the patient's drug-related needs."[11]

Hepler and Strand emphasized that two activities must occur for pharmaceutical care to be delivered. First, the practitioner takes time to determine the patient's specific wishes, preferences, and needs concerning his or her health and illness. Second, the practitioner makes a commitment to continue care once it is initiated. From this fundamental premise it follows that "pharmaceutical care is the responsible provision of drug therapy for the purpose of achieving definite outcomes that improve a patient's quality of life."[11] This cannot be overemphasized.

Hepler and Strand also placed considerable emphasis on the adoption of a strong patient focus and the development of a therapeutic relationship in which both patient and practitioner work together to resolve complex issues. Moreover, "Pharmaceutical care is a necessary element of health care, and should be integrated with other elements. Pharmaceutical care is, however, provided for the direct benefit of the patient, and the pharmacist is responsible directly to the patient for the quality of that care. The fundamental relationship in pharmaceutical care is a mutually beneficial exchange in which the patient grants the authority to the provider and the provider gives competence and commitment (accepts responsibility) to the patient."[11]

The concept of pharmaceutical care as enunciated by Hepler and Strand has received widespread acknowledgment as the foundational mandate for the profession of pharmacy. In this sense, *the profession has been redefined as a practice profession* with a direct and manifest responsibility for patient care.

> Pharmaceutical care is direct interaction with a patient.

Although the concept was accepted by the profession as early as 1990, efforts to develop a practice consistent with the concept did not occur until 1992.

In 1992 Strand, Cipolle, and Morley initiated a 3-year project to critically examine the relationship between the emerging theory of pharmaceutical care and practice. This was carried out within the context of community pharmacy practice. This project, known as the Minnesota Pharmaceutical Care Project, serves as the foundation for a significant portion of what has become the practice of pharmaceutical care. In essence, this project has its intellectual roots firmly grounded in work initiated almost twenty years ago by Strand. Strand's work began in 1978, when she began to look for a rational, systematic approach to decisions made in drug use. None was to be found in the literature at that time, and research conducted with physicians who were choosing drugs for the treatment of essential hypertension failed to produce empirical evidence of a rational approach. Therefore Strand, with the assistance of Cipolle (beginning in 1978) and Morley (beginning in 1983), worked on the development of an intellectual process in which the drug-related needs of patients could be approached systematically and comprehensively. These efforts resulted in the creation of a problem-solving process applied to the use of drugs. It was presented initially as a means to document drug therapy decisions and was called the Pharmacist's Workup of Drug Therapy.[13] This workup, which has undergone continuous revision since its inception, has proven effective in structuring and framing drug-use decisions. It became the cognitive map for the patient care process within pharmaceutical care.

This systematic problem-solving approach allowed Strand, Cipolle, and Morley to further focus their efforts on the clear definition of the responsibilities of a practitioner dealing with a patient's drug therapy. It became clear that such a practitioner had to assume two sets of responsibilities: (1) to assure that *all* of a patient's drug therapy was appropriate, the most effective possible, the safest available, and convenient enough to be taken as indicated and (2) to identify, resolve, and—most importantly—prevent any drug therapy problems that interfered with accomplishing the first set of responsibilities. These responsibilities were defined in 1990 and became the foundation for the responsibilities in pharmaceutical care practice.[14]

With the responsibilities of the pharmacist defined and a systematic, cognitive process with which to facilitate these responsibilities, Strand, Cipolle, and Morley set out to determine if the concept of pharmaceutical care could be introduced and developed as a practice in the community pharmacy setting. This became the primary objective of the Minnesota Pharmaceutical Care Project, which commenced in 1992. This research focused on 20 different pharmacies, with 54 different pharmacists, and relied on the truly unique collaboration of academics, practitioners, regulators, the pharmaceutical industry, managed care, and organized pharmacy to develop the practice described here. This project is described in detail in Chap. 6.

PHARMACEUTICAL CARE DEFINED

Pharmaceutical care is a practice in which the practitioner takes responsibility for a patient's drug-related needs and is held accountable for this commitment.[6] In the course of this practice, responsible drug therapy is provided for the purpose of achieving positive patient outcomes.

Pharmaceutical care is a new professional practice that has evolved from many years of research and practice in the profession of pharmacy. This new professional practice is not intended to replace the role of the physician or any other practitioner but rather to meet a need in the health care system that has arisen because of multiple prescribers of medications for a single patient, the explosion of drug products and drug information presently on the market, the increased complexity of drug therapy, the significant level of drug-related morbidity and mortality associated with drug use, and the high human and financial cost of drug misadventuring.

Pharmaceutical care will be discussed largely in terms of a professional practice. But while this practice was developed within the context of the profession of pharmacy and certainly contributes to the reformulation of this profession, the central messages and concerns are highly relevant to all health care disciplines that, in any way, involve themselves in making decisions about drug therapy for patients. Thus, while we believe that the future of pharmacy as a profession rests squarely on the acceptance of responsibility for pharmaceutical care, this position does not exclude other practitioners from a knowledge base and a comprehensive process that ultimately is of benefit to all patients. In simple terms, it is the patient who must at all times come first, and our understanding of ethical imperatives leads us to conclude that practitioners of any stripe who participate in drug-related action/practice must do everything possible to improve the patient's quality of care. This, we assert, means that all participants should adopt a systematic, comprehensive, sustained approach to therapeutics, thereby eliminating the present fragmentation all too often found in daily practice. Indeed, we will use the term *pharmacist* to refer to the practitioner who provides pharmaceutical care; in essence, however, we refer to a "new breed" of practitioner who is removed from old dispensing models, whether retail- or hospital-based. Moreover, we believe that traditional dispensing roles as the raison d'être of pharmacy practice are moving toward extinction.

Doubtless, such dire prognostication will raise a few eyebrows and more than a little angst, but we suggest that numerous indicators point

Pharmaceutical care is a PRACTICE in which the practitioner takes RESPONSIBILITY for a patient's drug-related needs, and is held ACCOUNTABLE for this COMMITMENT.

to the technician or robotic systems assuming the more technical dimensions of dispensing, thereby leaving the pharmacist with even more insecurity and loss of purpose. Assuming new roles and responsibilities requires a unique preparation, new, highly refined skills, and a value system that is foundational to the development of a total patient-centered pharmaceutical care practice. However, for the foreseeable future this means that pharmacists trained for more traditional roles will have to be reeducated and the skills of technicians will have to be improved. It is our hope that this volume will contribute to the necessary educational movement of all practitioners who, at some point, assume the responsibility and are willing to be held accountable for resolving complex pharmacological issues, thereby making the practice of pharmaceutical care a reality. Therefore, we are, in essence, concerned with the preparation of a new practitioner who will engage in a new practice to offer the patient a new service—that of pharmaceutical care. This text is dedicated to that end.

CHARACTERISTICS OF A PRACTICE

Pharmaceutical care meets a set of unique health care needs not currently met.

Pharmaceutical care is to be seen as a professional *practice*, much like those of medicine, nursing, and dentistry, where the practitioner is responsible for satisfying unique health care needs of a patient.

However, because it is a *new* professional practice—new to practitioners, new to patients, and new to the health care system—we believe that it is necessary to begin with the basic question: What is a professional practice? This question is especially challenging, since other health care practices have existed for such a long time and have changed in such relatively small ways that we tend to take for granted what a health care practice is and how it functions. We are also likely to assume that the internal logic and processes of practices (such as medicine, nursing, and dentistry) have been clearly defined and systematically studied. This has not been the case. However, over time, these professions have evolved with a reasonably well understood conceptualization of what it means to "practice" their responsibilities. Thus, almost every physician, for example, tacitly understands his or her roles and responsibilities and the rules that define practice.

In contrast, pharmacists have not arrived at this tacit understanding. This may help to explain why most states do not consider the pharmacist to be a health care practitioner, why the federal government has not recognized the pharmacist by establishing individual provider numbers for them, why there is an absence of any routine reimbursement of the pharmacist for patient care services, and why the pharmacist is absent from most health care practitioner teams focused on patient care. Although explanations for all this are beyond the scope of this text, there is one aspect of this situation which is very relevant to our discussion.

Pharmacy as a profession has created its own unique set of rules. Members of the profession have knowingly, or unknowingly, isolated themselves from the rest of the health care system under the guise of being "different." This isolation has allowed pharmacists to create their own vocabulary, establish their own standards of practice, and determine their own set of rules. Unfortunately, this behavior has led to two significant negative results. First, the behavior is so unique to pharmacy, and pharmacists communicate so infrequently with those outside of pharmacy, that the rest of the health care system has had difficulty understanding what pharmacy is, exactly how it functions, what it wants, and where it "fits." Second, keeping itself so isolated has kept the profession from learning the set of rules which apply to all other health care professions. Consequently, with the health care system changing so dramatically, pharmacy has found itself without a commonly understood vocabulary, with no respected, disciplined practice, and without a clearly differentiated role with which to sustain itself. For these reasons, the new professional practice of pharmaceutical care is of extreme importance to the profession of pharmacy.

A practice may be seen as the creative application of knowledge, guided by a commonly held philosophy and purpose, to the resolution of specific problems requiring the special knowledge held by a practitioner, in a manner and of a standard accepted by both professional review and social approbation. Moreover, a practice comprises the experiences a practitioner encounters during the process of caring for a patient.

In the present discussion, we will refer only to health care practices and not other common practices such as law. We will be discussing those professional practices offering services that are designed to meet the primary health care needs of patients. All patients have different health care needs, and a particular patient may have different health care needs at any given time; in general, however, practices can be fairly accurately represented by the variations in categories of health care needs a patient may have. A sample of these needs, representing the different health care professions, is displayed in Fig. 1-1. Although the different health care professions address unique health care needs, all of the professions have a philosophy of practice, a patient care process, and a practice management system. Each of these practice components will be discussed for the practice of pharmaceutical care.

TOWARD A PHILOSOPHY OF PHARMACEUTICAL CARE PRACTICE

A philosophy of practice is a set of values that guides behaviors associated with certain acts; in this case, those of pharmaceutical care. A philosophy defines the rules, roles, relationships, and responsibilities of the practitioner. Any philosophy of practice that is to be taken seriously must reflect the functions and activities of the practitioner—both eso-

A practice philosophy defines rules, roles, relationships, and responsibilities.

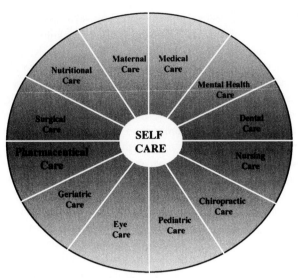

•**Figure 1-1** Health care needs of a patient.

teric and common, appropriate and questionable—and also critically provide direction toward the formation of a consistent practice. How a practitioner practices from day to day should reflect a philosophy of practice.

A philosophy of practice helps a practitioner make decisions, determine what is important, and set priorities over the course of the day. Ethical dilemmas, management issues, and clinical judgments are all resolved with the assistance of a practitioner's philosophy of practice. This is why the philosophy of practice must be well understood and clearly articulated, so it is explicit and relied on in the face of difficult problems.

A philosophy of practice is specific to a practice, not to the practitioner. This is very different from an individual's philosophy of life, which is usually whatever the individual chooses it to be. When a practitioner takes an oath to practice a profession, it is the philosophy of practice the practitioner is promising to uphold. Therefore, all practitioners who purport to be engaged in a specific professional practice will hold the same philosophy of practice. This uniformity of philosophy, and therefore standardization of behaviors, can then result in consistently high-quality services and expectations from patients, which then leads to a new demand for the service. Additionally, the philosophy must be applied to all patients in that practice and not applied selectively depending on convenience, time availability, or personal preferences. The philosophy of practice is the "prescriptive" component of a practice as it defines *what should be done*. A practice philosophy is "time-

A philosophy of practice is specific to a practice, not a practitioner.

A philosophy of practice defines what SHOULD be done.

	PHILOSOPHY OF PRACTICE	PATIENT- CARE PROCESS	PR MAN
TABLE 1-1 PRACTICE COMPONENTS AND THEIR CHARACTERIS			
Purpose	Prescriptive	Descriptive	Predic
Those influenced	All practitioners, all patients	Individual practitioner Individual patient	A gr A group o
Relevant time frame	Continuous	Present	Future

less" in that it does not change on a daily basis, nor is it different among and between practitioners. This is not to say that the philosophy is dogmatic and unchanging, but rather that it is to be seen as a set of ideals, principles, concepts, values, and axioms held in common by "all practitioners" who draw upon this framework to define the nature of their practice. The major characteristics of a philosophy of practice are summarized in Table 1-1.

The philosophy of practice specific to pharmaceutical care describes a patient-centered approach that allows us to meet the social need to manage drug-related morbidity and mortality, with an explicit objective to care for a patient's drug-related needs by making it the practitioner's responsibility to ensure that all of a patient's drug therapy is appropriate, the most effective available, the safest possible, and is used as indicated. This is accomplished by identifying, resolving, and preventing drug therapy problems that can or could interfere with successfully meeting a patient's drug therapy goals and producing positive patient outcomes.

This philosophy of practice remains only "wishful thinking," or abstract, until a therapeutic relationship is built with the patient, and the pharmacist engages in the patient care process to provide a service. There is always a tendency to want to "get on with the practice" when one is learning about pharmaceutical care. However, because everything about the practice emanates from the philosophy and reflexively returns to "push against" it, we need to understand the philosophy of pharmaceutical care in some detail.

THE PHILOSOPHY OF PHARMACEUTICAL CARE

The philosophy of pharmaceutical care practice consists of a number of elements. It begins with a statement of social need; it continues with a patient-centered approach to meeting this need, has at its core the caring of and for another through the development and maintenance of a therapeutic relationship, and ends with a description of the practitioner's specific responsibilities.

MEETING A SOCIAL NEED

First, in order to justify their position and privileges in society, all professions must meet a unique social need, and this should be at the heart of their philosophy of practice.

Professional activities are rewarded only when they meet a unique social need by applying specialized knowledge and skills to provide a service to address "client" problems. In the case of health care professionals, these unique needs are health-related. And, although all health care professionals are first and foremost in the business of keeping patients healthy, they usually do so by preventing, identifying, and resolving a unique set of health-related problems. Meeting a unique social need balances the benefits realized by professionals. For example, society supports an extensive education for the professional student through public taxes. Society provides the professional with an exclusive right to earn a relatively high income, grants him or her an elevated status in the community, and generally accepts the autonomy with which professions govern themselves. Such privileges come with certain social responsibilities and are frequently the subject of controversy. This is particularly true in the area of accountability.

In the case of pharmaceutical care practice, the practitioner minimizes drug-related morbidity and mortality. The practitioner meets this social need by attending to the needs of patients, *one at a time*. Individuals requiring drug therapy need assurance that this will be appropriate, effective, and safe. Traditionally, we have assumed that physicians provide such assurance, sometimes nurses take on a portion of this responsibility, and sometimes pharmacists contribute to this goal. It is this fragmentation of responsibility, along with an ever-expanding range of new, more complex drug products, that has created the dilemma of drug misadventuring.[7] Drug-related morbidity and mortality has now reached such a magnitude in our society that it is necessary for a specific professional to be designated to correct this openly and comprehensively, since only then can a specific individual be held accountable for its management. Only when such a person is "in place" will the level of drug-related morbidity and mortality experienced in society be minimized and the cost to society of drug-related illness managed. Therefore we emphasize that the first premise of the philosophy of pharmaceutical care is that the pharmacist's essential responsibility is to contribute to meeting society's need for appropriate, effective, safe, and convenient drug therapy.

A PATIENT-CENTERED APPROACH

To effectively meet the social need described above, it is necessary for the practitioner of pharmaceutical care to use a patient-centered approach to practice. This approach considers the patient as a whole individual whose health care needs generally and drug-related needs specifically are the primary concern of the practitioner. The patient is seen as an individual with rights, knowledge, and experience, all of which are necessary for the practitioner to fulfill his or her responsibilities. This approach requires that the practitioner treat the patient as a partner in care planning and always as the ultimate decision maker, since the patient experiences the ultimate consequences of drug therapy. Most importantly, this approach prevents the patient from being seen as a repository for drugs to be studied and evaluated. It also prevents the individual from being defined as a conglomerate of organ systems and drug reactions. Such objectification is not acceptable to the pharmaceutical care practitioner.

A patient-centered approach means that *all* of the patient's drug-related needs are seen as the responsibility of the practitioner, not just those needs representing a specific drug category or a specific disease state. This means that all of the patient's concerns, expectations, and understanding of his or her illness—and associated drug therapy—become the practitioner's responsibilities. In addition, the patient-centered approach insists that the patient's needs, not the practitioner's preferences, "drive" the practice of pharmaceutical care. In a pragmatic sense, this means that the practitioner will start with the patient's needs and provide care until all of these needs are met. This means that the practitioner will do whatever is necessary to meet the drug-related needs of the patient.

> Choosing to focus on a particular disease or drug category is not patient-centered.

CARING THROUGH A THERAPEUTIC RELATIONSHIP

For many, the concept of care is "soft" and vague. In a world of "hard" facts and empirical pronouncements, care is frequently seen as "out of place." Moreover, it is a concept that to date has received very little philosophical reflection among pharmacy educators or practitioners. Medicine[15] and nursing[16] have celebrated many years of intense and often acrimonious discourse on the nature of caring and, to a large extent, accept this as an integral part of defining who they are. This is not to say that these professions have all the answers. Clearly, they do not. Rather, we contend that important questions are being asked and that there is a particular urgency in the present health care context for pharmacy to participate in this important discourse. Here, while we do

The therapeutic relationship is required to care for another's drug therapy needs.

not intend to provide an exhaustive account of the idea of care, we will draw attention to the importance and centrality of an ethic of care, for in our view, this is foundational to our conceptualization of pharmaceutical care.

Within the context of health care, discourse on the idea of care generally derives from two different but complementary concerns:

1. The technical dimensions of taking care of patients
2. Caring for or about a particular patient, thereby demonstrating a concern for the well-being of another person[17]

The first of these is reasonably well understood. Indeed, some may very well argue that it is too well "understood" and is reflected in our national preoccupation with "high-tech" solutions to all manner of health problems. Certainly, pharmacy is in general agreement on such matters as these manifest themselves in the empirically driven utilization of pharmaceutical agents—the usual emphasis being on the actual therapeutic agent in question at any given time.

It is the second concern that provides pharmaceutical care with the most puzzles, perplexities, and problems. Here the focus is on the "softer" side of practitioner purpose. To use a somewhat well-worn distinction, the first exemplifies the *science* of pharmacy at work, the second plumbs the depths of the *art* of practice.

The philosophy of pharmaceutical care includes (1) the recognition of a social need, (2) the patient-centered approach, (3) caring as a modus operandi, and (4) specific responsibilities to identify, resolve, and prevent drug therapy problems.

Drugs don't have doses . . . people have doses.

Within the context of pharmaceutical care, the emphasis/focus moves from product to person—from pharmaceutical agent to patient. We emphasize that this does not diminish the importance of pharmaceutical knowledge! But, it does refocus attention on the recipient of such technical knowledge. We begin with the understanding that "drugs don't have doses—people have doses."[18] Thus, the patient becomes the central focus for our interventions. Such a change of focus involves very serious cognitive, conceptual, and—some would add—emotional, shifts on the part of those committed to giving and receiving pharmaceutical care. Conventional boundaries, tracing their legitimacy to disciplines and professionally arrogated authority, must be critically examined and practitioners intending to practice pharmaceutical care should be prepared to ground technical knowledge within a broader philosophical and sociocultural context. Facts and values must both be examined as these affect persons who are more than biological specimens or organ systems. In essence, the practitioner of pharmaceutical care will welcome the opportunity to participate in the development of a scientific humanism that emancipates both practitioner and patient from the often debilitating excesses of a "technical fix."

Much of the ambiguity surrounding the terms *caring* and *curing* have roots firmly planted in antiquity.[17] Here, the term *cura* ("care") presented two distinct and somewhat contradictory meanings. As Reich observes, the term "meant worries, troubles, or anxieties," as when one is "burdened with cares," while it also carried the meaning of "providing for the welfare of another."[17] In this last meaning we see the more compelling notion "of care as attentive conscientiousness of devotion."[17] It is interesting to note that the word "cure" comes from the Latin word "cura," which meant, in particular, "care."[15] Moreover, as Pelligrino and Thomasma note, "For the greatest part of medical history these various senses of curing and caring were essentially one. It is only with the beginnings of truly scientific and therapeutically effective discrete therapies that the possibility of cure without care has existed."[15]

Also derived from antiquity is the sense of caring and compassion firmly grounded in religious teachings. Here religious traditions found in all cultures contain promises to care for the sick and needy. The spiritual dimensions of caring have also found expression in the secular thought of several key humanists. Rollo May, for example, defines caring as a state in which something matters. Care is seen as the antithesis of apathy and distance and is the necessary source of eros. It is "the source of human tenderness."[19] For May and other humanists, care is not to be confused with sentimentality, for this emotion is reflecting on sentiment itself rather than experiencing him or her who is the subject of the caring attention. Care is essentially equated with compassion. But it is important to note that within the humanistic tradition, the concept of care conveys a compassionate state of being and not merely an attitude. Indeed, for the humanists, "being" and the ontological presence of humankind are constituted by that which is cared about.[19]

Within the humanistic psychology of Rogers and Maslow is found the essence of "otherness" in the caring relationship. To care for another person in a meaningful sense is to help with growth and "self-actualization." It is a process, a relationship, we call it the therapeutic relationship, wherein the cared for individual is deeply involved in his or her healing journey. Self-actualization, as a process, engages all those concerned in the healing process. Thus, "client-centered" therapy does, in a secular sense, what theological intervention achieves as it integrates mind, body, and spirit. Disjunctions between the "care giver" and the "cared for" become blurred as the relationship brings two or more individuals together in a partnership (covenant) intent on the resolution of a particular problem.[20,21]

Caring, then, involves a profound respect for the "otherness" of the other. It differs considerably from any paternalistic, authoritarian imposition of will or direction upon the other. Thus, with this in mind, therapeutic compliance is not to be seen as enforcement based on the authority of the practitioner but rather as a consequence of an alliance among *all* those concerned with the resolution of a particular problem. Perhaps the better term for compliance is *adherence*. Caring, as situated within the context of pharmaceutical care, finds its expression in helping the other come to care for himself or herself. It requires a relationship where there is a sense of participation in the other, an awareness of that individual's particular need for growth and control over the thera-

Pharmaceutical care means treating the patient as though he/she is your own grandfather/grandmother.

Pharmaceutical care promotes the patient's participation in the therapeutic process.

peutic process. This is frequently dismissed as practitioners assume that more paternalistic posture of the "expert knows best." Any effective and appropriate therapeutic alliance requires that the "voice" of the patient be heard and heeded. On matters that require empirical knowledge, practitioners have a duty to inform, educate, and engage in listening to the patient's needs and preferences. Dialogue is essential, practitioner monologue is not. Mayerhoff, for example, emphasizes the importance of self-actualization: "Caring, as helping another grow and actualize himself [sic] is a process, a way of relating to someone that involves development in the same way that friendship can only emerge in time through mutual trust and a deepening and qualitative transformation of the relationship."[22]

Gaylin offers a somewhat different viewpoint. His understanding of caring attempts to demonstrate that caring is biologically programmed and must be seen as a fundamental fact of human growth and development. His thesis weds biology to culture and reaches out to humanistic philosophy in an attempt to argue a case for innate goodness.[23]

Perhaps the most substantive discourse on the subject of caring and the essential meaning of therapeutic relationships is to be found in nursing. Indeed, the literature is rich with intellectual argument and passion. Benner's work is of particular importance and goes directly to the heart of the matter: "Caring is a relational word, and it shows up in relational contexts. Caring, if it means anything, always means something in a particular context, a particular relationship. Caring is incompatible with radically free individualism and autonomy. Caring means that others can lay claim on your time, your interests, your resources. It means that you cannot remain atomistic, unrelated, outside a community, or outside of relationships."[24]

Surely this captures the essence of any therapeutic relationship. She continues: "Caring unravels the control paradigm and forms one of the few cultural resistances against the anomie, dominance, and oppression of a technological self-understanding. Caring requires both listening and a form of knowing that goes beyond curiosity and dissection, beyond laying bare the facts. Caring requires a truth theory that is true to the knower and the known. Caring is embodied and embedded in a community or social network. Caring unleashes pleasure in the midst of work; a sense that some things are worth doing and some things are good in themselves—a uniting of means and ends."[24] Moreover: "Care sets up what matters, what counts as stressful, what can count as coping, what being related and situated means, and finally, what counts as giving and receiving help."[24]

Benner, in our view, provides us with one of the clearest, most comprehensive treatments of the caring concept, particularly as it relates to the therapeutic relationship as we envisage it within pharmaceutical care.

In essence, nursing theory literature provides us with important ideas to ponder as we develop pharmacy's caring discourse and practice. Some ideas are more controversial than others (e.g., gender ethics); some are more process-oriented or means-oriented; and many see caring as an end in itself. Scholarly work on the epistemological, ontological, and broader philosophical dimensions of caring now fill volumes, and the pharmaceutical care practitioner is urged to explore this body of literature. Nursing theorists have now turned their attention to such important issues as the meanings attached to care, transcultural themes in caring, values, beliefs concerning care and practice (theory and practice relationships), the esthetics of care, the economics and politics of care, the ethics of care, spiritual and religious dimensions of care, and the educational requirements for a "caring profession." These are but a few of the issues central to any caring practice.[25] Pharmacy will have to find the time and the intellectual *stamina* to deal with these and other topics as it develops itself as a caring profession.

Hepler and Strand have asserted that pharmaceutical care is "provided for the direct benefits of the patient and the pharmacist accepts direct responsibility for the quality of that care."[11] Recall, they emphasize that pharmaceutical care "is based on a covenant between the patient, who promises to grant authority to the provider, and the provider, who promises competence and commitment to the patient."[11] To this we would add that the pharmacist is to be held *accountable* for his or her decisions and interventions.

The key term in the original Hepler and Strand position is *covenant*. They use the term to signify a *bond* between the pharmacist and patient. This is the bond that cements the therapeutic relationship. It is to be seen as a common understanding of roles and responsibilities for both parties actively engaged in such a relationship. Essentially, it is an agreement, for all concerned, to work toward the resolution of all experienced and potential drug therapy problems.

Within the therapeutic relationship and the reciprocity of the covenant, certain responsibilities are recognized, assumed, and accounted for on the part of both practitioner and patient. The practitioner of pharmaceutical care agrees to assess the patient's needs, bring whatever resources are required to successfully address these needs, and follow up to ensure that effective, good interventions have taken place. The patient agrees to at least two important things. First, he or she agrees to provide accurate and complete information (data) to the practitioner so that effective decisions can be made by both individuals. Also, the patient agrees to play an active role in the care provided. This means that the patient agrees to set goals, carry out agreed-upon behaviors, and provide information required for beneficial care.

Cooper believes that "a covenant relationship brings the moral and personal aspects of nursing care together."[26] She notes that "a responsiveness to the presence of the patient and his or her needs, an acknowledgment of the indebtedness by the caregiver to the patient for the benefit of practice and engagement, and a recognition of the mutuality and reciprocity that distinguishes the relationship indicate a willingness by nurses to enter a covenantal relationship."[26]

While the concept of a covenant does have a certain appeal, particularly as it fits well into accepted Judeo-Christian understandings of commitment, it does have some limitation. Bishop and Scudder, for example, contend that "A covenant is an agreement that both includes and excludes. For example, in the Judeo-Christian tradition, the people of the Covenant saw themselves as connected to each other through covenant but separate from those who were not of the Covenant."[27]

The central issue, they continue, is that the covenantal relationship is too restrictive in that it emphasizes the practitioner's responsibilities but does not adequately address the patient's involvement. Thus, while we recognize the essential element of good faith implied in covenant relationships and accept the positive implication for professional responsibility—and ultimately accountability—we also recognize the importance of the dialogue that frames the formation of covenantal relationships or, for that matter, those of a more contractual intent. Cooper expresses this well:

Therapeutic relationships are built on dialogue and commitment.

> Unlike a covenant relationship, a dialogical relationship does not assume a common purpose between both parties. Each person meets the other as they are present to each other as persons. They mutually respond to each other's presence in a relationship which recognizes the legitimate right of the other to be. This relationship has been described by Buber (1923) as an I-Thou relationship, in contrast to a I-It relationship in which the person is treated as a thing to be categorized and used. I-Thou relationships are cultivated and developed through dialogue.[26]

Covenant and dialogue clearly have a place in pharmaceutical care. Once the dialogical preconditions are satisfied, both practitioner and patient can enter into a covenantal relationship that is committed to open, not exclusive, conditions. Moreover, such a relationship must very seriously incorporate the desires, wishes, and needs of the patient. Such an alliance must move from the patient to the practitioner. However, we also recognize the essential dialogical preconditions that must frame the agenda and shape the nature of the relationship. We do not see covenantal and dialogical relationships as necessarily mutually exclusive. Rather, we see both as dimensions of the therapeutic relationship and central to effective pharmaceutical care.

Caring, then, initiated and sustained through dialogue, is fundamental to pharmaceutical care philosophy and practice. The covenantal ethic establishes commitment to and respect for persons. Certainly, close inspection of the dynamics of a covenantal relationship reveals that it is essentially dialogue that makes such a relationship possible and maximizes its inclusive probabilities. Hence, the relationship is not simply a mutual understanding, however it is arrived at. It is first and foremost the process of how such a relationship is formed and sustained. Dialogue shapes expectations, desires, methods, and therapeutic commitment. It identifies needs, fosters well-being, and brings to the relationship ongoing reflection on meaning and purpose. Dialogue explores the sense of trust, respect, truth telling, and authenticity. For some, talk may be "cheap," but in a viable therapeutic relationship, not talking can be costly.

As a way of summarizing, it may be instructive to list the characteristics of caring behavior and the vital components of the therapeutic relationship. These consist of the following:

Mutual respect
Honesty/authenticity
Open communication
Cooperation
Collaboration between patient and practitioner
Empathy
Sensitivity
Promotion of patient independence
Seeing the patient as a person
Exercising patience and understanding
Trust
Competence
Putting the patient first
Offering reassurance
Confidence
Paying attention to the patient's physical and emotional comfort
Supporting the patient
Offering advocacy
Assuming responsibility for interventions
Being willing to be held accountable for all decisions made and recommendations given

This list is by no means exhaustive. However, it does present characteristics that are central to the philosophy and practice of pharmaceutical care. Building upon this list may be seen as essentially broadening our conceptualization of both. Certainly, as therapeutic relationships develop and as we learn more about their structure, function, and value, we will doubtless improve our contribution to care. Our understanding of an ethic of care and responsibility will shape our practices, consolidate our professional identity, and effectively extend our knowledge and technical expertise to those in need. Acting in the best interests of others can only contribute to the good of practitioners and profession, alike.

The therapeutic relationship is an alliance between a practitioner and a patient, formed to meet a patient's health care needs.

We have presented a brief overview of issues that are central to pharmaceutical care philosophy and practice. Moreover, our discussion of caring and the therapeutic relationship serves as an introduction to important philosophical discourse as it affects all aspects of patient care. The reader is urged to pursue these issues, develop them further, and integrate them into his or her practice. The therapeutic relationship links a practitioner's philosophy of practice to the actual lived-in world of the patient care process. In this way it provides an ethic of practice.

In summary, a therapeutic relationship is an alliance between a practitioner and a patient and is formed for the very specific purpose of meeting the patient's health care needs. It is an act of caring for and about a person. In this sense it focuses on the whole person and not simply a biological specimen, organ system, or disease state in any reductionistic sense.

THE PRACTITIONER'S RESPONSIBILITIES

The practice of pharmaceutical care is designed to meet the major social problem of drug-related morbidity and mortality based on a caring, patient-centered process, and clearly defined practitioner responsibilities. In the practice of pharmaceutical care, the practitioner is responsible for ensuring that all drug therapies the patient is taking are appropriately indicated and that all indications for drug therapy are being appropriately treated with medications. The practitioner also accepts the responsibility for ensuring that the patient's drug therapies are as effective as possible and are as safe as possible. This is accomplished by identifying, resolving, and preventing drug therapy problems so the patient can realize the intended goals of therapy. Finally, when providing pharmaceutical care, the practitioner is responsible for ensuring that the patient is able to comply with the medication instructions and care plan instructions in order to produce positive patient outcomes. The practitioner's responsibilities, as well as the patient care process, are described in detail in Chaps. 3 and 4.

PHARMACEUTICAL CARE AS PRACTICE

The previous discussion of the meaning of a philosophy of practice allows us to further develop the practice of pharmaceutical care. All health care professionals bring their knowledge and expertise to patients in the form of a service generally referred to as *practice*. Indeed, in common use, *practice* refers to what those with knowledge actually do or can potentially do. At best there is a tacit understanding that the application of specific forms of knowledge to daily actions constitutes practice. Also, there is the confusing but frequent reference to practice as "place" or context—where the action occurs. In short, practice is a concept that all too frequently appears vague, confusing, and somewhat taken for granted.

Practice is more than simply an inchoate configuration of activities, no matter how important these may be to persons conducting them. Most importantly, "practices are not just agents' activities but also the configuration of the world within which those activities are significant."[28] Within the context of pharmacy, the concept of practice has taken on the oversimplified meaning of *doing*. That is to say, practice is generally taken to mean whatever activities pharmacists engage in at any given time. This view is simply too narrow.

Here, our purpose is to broaden the conceptualization of practice and provide it with a deeper meaning than that found in common use. To this end, we begin with a challenging definition offered by MacIntyre: "By a 'practice' I am going to mean any coherent and complex form of socially established cooperative human activity through which goods internal to that form of activity are realized in the course of trying to achieve those standards of excellence which are appropriate to, and partially definitive of, that form of activity, with the result that human conceptions of the ends and good involved, are systematically extended."[29]

Practices, then, are more than the application of knowledge to some ill-defined end. Practices contain a strong commitment to providing good. Thus, for our present purpose, the practice of pharmaceutical care means the application of knowledge to promote the well-being of others. In this sense, practice clearly contains a strong ethical component that defines purpose and end. Morality is to be seen as inescapably an integral part of all practices. Any practice must have a clear, recognizable understanding of its internal goods, goods shared by all members of the community participating in the practice. There must be a common understanding of and commitment to a moral purpose that sets itself apart from the more general, discursive moral frameworks that define goods external to the practice. For MacIntyre, virtues have a key role to play in sustaining practices. He contends that "Every practice requires a certain kind of relationship between those who participate in it. Now the virtues are those goods by reference to which, whether we like it or not, we define our relationship to those people with whom we share the kind of purposes and standards which inform practices."[30]

When we place this within the context of pharmaceutical care, we contend that its practice requires a shared understanding of and commitment to those values and virtues that promote group solidarity (practitioners), circumscribed by a commonly held philosophy that defines rules, roles, responsibilities, and purpose. Moreover, as MacIntyre makes quite clear, practices consist of whole systems of meanings and are not to be seen as confined to those skills and technical interven-

Pharmaceutical care is applying knowledge to promote the well being of others.

tions that tend to dominate as defining characteristics of this concept. Thus, he avers, "brick-laying is not a practice; architecture is. Planting turnips is not a practice; farming is."[29]

Practices must also be sustained over time. In a real sense, this means that their foundations must be solid and provide ongoing reference points for practitioners. Practices build traditions and become socially visible. They act as the source of practitioner identity and prepare nascent members for future growth and development. Like culture, practices exist before any particular individual and "acculturate" future members into the group. Furthermore, they "are identifiable as patterns of ongoing engagement with the world, but these patterns exist only through their repetition or continuation."[28] These patterns "are sustained only through the establishment and enforcement of 'norms'" and standards.[28] Thus, practices depend not on the autonomous (often idiosyncratic) actions of practitioners but on whether they "understand and respond to one another as capable of acting in accordance with norms."[28] It is important to recognize that central to the very notion of a practice is the idea that "practices are understood by their practitioners *as* enforced."[28] The norms that sustain practice must be held in common by all practitioners. Pharmaceutical care, as a philosophy of practice, embraces norms and expectations of performance that must be accepted by all who claim to practice it. This is not to suggest an authoritarian presence but rather to define standards of practice and thereby provide a rationale for all those electing to commit to the practice itself.

In the light of the above discussion, pharmaceutical care practice is defined by its foundational philosophy, dedicated to a patient care process with all its attendant responsibilities, and through its practice management systems is held accountable for all practitioner interventions. This practice is illustrated with its component parts in Figure 1-2. Pharmaceutical care practice provides a visible, consistent *identity* for its practitioners. The identity of such a practitioner will be clear and meaningful to both patients and other health care providers.

THE LANGUAGE AND VOCABULARY OF PRACTICE

The French philosopher Paul Ricoeur concluded that the most significant factor connecting us to the social world is language. Language constructs our realities and shapes our sense of who we are.[31]

Within the context of our discussion of practice, language takes on particular importance. Here, language mediates the realities of practice and also communicates these to others. Moreover, it is only when we put things into words that they take on any meaning, thereby making communication possible.

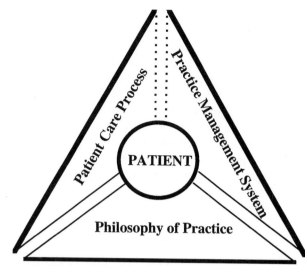

•**Figure 1-2** Pharmaceutical care practice.

All health care professions, over time, have generated a descriptive language for their roles and responsibilities, and they continuously introduce technical vocabularies serving to define and delineate specific tasks and interventions. These frequently function specifically to identify who is carrying out these acts. Thus, we find that physicians customarily establish "diagnoses," nurses conduct "physical assessments," and pharmacists practicing pharmaceutical care, "identify, resolve, and prevent drug therapy problems."

On the surface much of this is self-evident. However, as pharmaceutical care practice develops, the language/vocabulary that describes its unique purpose and function, process, and action(s) taken must also evolve and represent these to others. This cannot be overemphasized, for it is through language/vocabulary that we communicate what we do, for whom, and how we do it. In short, we communicate our identity as practitioners, our responsibilities, and our particular unique knowledge base through our language.

Our language/vocabulary will communicate our practice, its meaning and value, to all other health care professionals, patients, third-party payers, potential clients, university colleagues, and other members of the general public. Furthermore, the language we use is a form of empowerment.[32] It is essential that pharmaceutical care practitioners learn to "speak with authority" on those matters that lie within their area of expertise. To engage in clinical discourse with other health care practitioners requires that pharmacists speak like clinicians and articulate their expert recommendations with a technical clarity that conveys meaning. There is no room for obfuscation in clinical exchange. Lan-

The language of practitioners communicates their identity, responsibilities, and knowledge.

guage is also about legitimacy and recognition. Other practitioners will listen to and respect those who present authoritative knowledge and information in competent, coherent language. This is certainly the case when any unique body of knowledge, sometimes seemingly wrapped in highly technical discipline-bound "jargon," is communicated to "outsiders."

To facilitate a beginning, we have constructed a glossary that provides a point of departure in our attempt to build and communicate the essence of pharmaceutical care practice to other practitioners and to patients. We have included those terms most directly related to pharmaceutical care practice. We encourage readers/practitioners/students/patients to build upon this vocabulary as they focus on the importance of linguistic competency in practice.

PHARMACEUTICAL CARE AS PRIMARY HEALTH CARE

If pharmaceutical care is to flourish as a new professional practice, then it must meet the needs and promote the goals of the evolving health care system. One of the most obvious "movements" to surive the contemporary health care reform era is that of primary care. We will discuss how and why pharmaceutical care is consistent with this agenda after we briefly discuss what exactly primary health care is, since there is much confusion over the meaning of this concept. However, be reminded of the elements of the philosophy of pharmaceutical care practice and it will become obvious as to how pharmaceutical care is completely consistent with the philosophy of primary health care.

The distinguished physician and bioethicist Eric Cassel identifies primary care medicine "as the capstone of twentieth-century medicine," and "the foundation for twenty-first-century doctoring."[33] Primary care is rapidly emerging as the dominant form of medical practice within the context of managed care. Indeed, as Cassell contends, primary care has emerged as a "sophisticated generalism" that is propelled by the mismatch between the high-technology medicine at which we excel and the health care needs of large groups of the population—for example, the poor, chronically ill, aged, and disabled."[33]

Historically, primary health care has been afflicted with ambiguity and has taken on several different meanings. One of the earliest definitions (1920) focused on organizing medical services into primary health centers and teaching hospitals.[34] This organizational framework—"definition by location"—was used to organize medical services until 1978, when an international conference (Alma-Ata) moved the emphasis from medical to health services. This was a significant change, as it broadened the concept and somewhat subverted medical hegemony as the defining force.

This broader, more sociocultural ecological framework also contained explicit acknowledgment of the political nature of all health matters. Indeed, what is essentially an anthropological conceptualization challenged the biomedical model and the professional dominance of the medical profession while at the same time presenting a radical humanistic approach to health that opened all areas of health care to critical scrutiny. At the same time, primary health care was transformed into a more collaborative effort, with numerous health professions participating in the provision of services.

After 1979 discourse on primary care appeared in the form of two distinct views. The first was developed by the World Health Organization (WHO), which focused on operationalizing an "approach" to primary care.[35] This particular approach encompassed a broad range of interests: health education, environmental sanitation, prevention, drugs, nutrition, and traditional medicine. The WHO approach was most commonly accepted in less developed or modernizing countries.

The second view of primary health care was more focused on a constellation of health activities and/or emphasized temporality or a basic "level of service," usually at the point of first contact.[36] These services might include responsive care for episodic illness, continuing care for chronic illness, health screening and monitoring, preventive services, appropriate health education, and integration with care in acute- and long-term-care institutions.[37] This view of primary care was most commonly accepted in developed countries such as the United States.

Practitioners have been differentiated over time as primary, secondary, or tertiary, based on the variety of problems encountered. Primary care practitioners are seen as those encountering greater variety among the most common diagnoses (50 percent of all visits), whereas the secondary and tertiary practitioners see more variety among the rare diagnoses.[34] In addition, a larger percentage of primary health care visits are prevention-related and involve more patients who are continuing in care than are coming into the health care system for the first time.[34]

Regardless of the view taken, either the "approach" of the WHO or the alternatives emphasizing "levels of service," there are common core elements to primary care. These may be summarized thus:

Services that are comprehensive, continuous, coordinated, accessible, and acceptable

Strategies for serving the vulnerable

First-contact care (gatekeeping function)

"De facto" care for most people's problems, most of the time

Care provided by multiple practitioners

Emphasis on health, *not* medicine

Proliferation of generalist practitioners

Pharmaceutical care is a generalist practice that emphasizes health, prevention, and care.

Developed countries such as the United States will have to undergo a significant conceptual shift to move beyond specialized medicine to the concepts of primary health care. Subtle shifts from specialized medicine to a more "generalist" practice of primary care are reflected in the change of focus from illness to health and from cure to prevention and care. Also, important shifts in content must occur. We should expect to see movement from an emphasis on specific problems to one on comprehensive care, from episodic care to continuous care, and from treatment to health promotion. We can also expect the increased emergence of teams whose members are drawn from a number of professions. Solo practice is already a thing of the past.

Primary health care is "based on the centrality of the patient rather than on an organ system or a disease, as is the case with specialism." Moreover, "It is addressed to both the sick and the well. It understands functional impairment and disease to be processes that enter into the patient's life story, so that its interventions are chosen with the development of that story in mind. Because of this, it is as well suited to prevention as to treatment, to children as to adults, and especially to the care of the chronically ill, who make up the largest number of sick in our society."[33]

Cassell concludes: "Primary care medicine can best be provided by generalists who are specifically trained to meet the broad, as well as the intellectually and technically exacting, demands implied in the definition of the term."[33]

Hibbard and Nutting also offer a valuable description of primary care that serves to "situate" pharmaceutical care in this context:

> . . . primary care is distinguished by being "front-line" or "first contact" care, person-centered (rather than disease or organ system-centered), and comprehensive in scope, rather than being limited to illness episodes or by the organ systems or disease process involved. Primary care is distinguished from other levels of care by the scope, character, and integration of the services provided. Primary care practitioners deal with ambulatory patients at the initial interface of the individual with the health care system. Patients present with a variety of illnesses, ailments, and concerns that represent early stages of disease that are not easily classified by organ system or diagnostic label. Often patients have multiple problems, and a rational approach to one problem may make another worse. Primary care thus provides an integrating function, balancing the multiple requirements of the patients problem(s), using information developed from many sources, and developing a strategy to help each individual achieve the highest level of function possible.[38]

This definitional framework leads us to conclude that in all conceptualizations of primary health care, the patient's needs dictate the services required. Therefore, primary care is not the same as specialized services such as disease management, pharmacokinetic services, or drug utilization review. In addition, we can conclude that practitioner-selected services, or those specified by health care plans—such as formulary control, Adverse Drug Reaction (ADR) reporting, and generic/therapeutic substitution—are not necessarily a subset of primary health care, since to be a subset of a patient's care plan the *whole* must exist.

Pharmaceutical care, in theory and practice, is primary health care. Indeed, the basic foci of primary health care and pharmaceutical care are the same. These include:

Patient-centeredness

Addressing both acute and chronic conditions

Emphasizing prevention

Implementing documentation systems that continuously record patient
    need and care provided

Being accessible to front-line first contact

Offering continuous and systematic care

Ensuring integration of care

Being accountable

Placing emphasis on ambulatory patients

Including educational/health promotional intervention

It is clear by now that pharmaceutical care is a generalist practice. This means that the practitioner takes responsibility to identify and resolve all of a patient's drug-related needs. In practice, the pharmacist would seek assistance from a specialist practitioner only when the drug therapy problem reaches a level of complexity that surpasses his/her knowledge, skills, and/or experience.

The reconciliation of the two concepts lies in the fact that primary health care includes *all* of a patient's health care needs, and pharmaceutical care involves only the patient's drug-related needs—but *all* of the patient's drug-related needs.

Pharmaceutical care practice has an important role to play in the alleviation of pain and suffering. Pharmacy, as profession, is heavily populated with well-qualified "drug experts" who can be put to much more valuable use than the dispensing, distributing, and other duties they are asked to perform. Their underutilization must be corrected, and the more demanding roles associated with direct patient care embraced. This chapter has outlined the ideas of a new pharmacy practice. It is an invitation to all pharmacists regardless of degree held, years of experience in the "other paradigm," or practice setting. To practice pharmaceutical care does require responsiveness and a sensitivity to the misfortunes of others as well as a fundamental commitment to an ethic of care. As we will demonstrate, the practice of pharmaceutical care can make a difference in the lives of individuals experiencing drug-related illness. The problems are enormous, the challenges great, the opportunities exciting. Think about it—and create a vision of the possibilities.

Pharmaceutical care is a form of primary health care.

Pharmaceutical care requires responsiveness, sensitivity, and commitment to others.

REFERENCES

1. Dougherty, C.J. *Back to Reform: Values, Markets, and the Health Care System.* Oxford, England: Oxford University Press; 1996.

2. Johnson, J.A., Bootman, J.L. Drug-related morbidity and mortality. *Arch Intern Med* 1995; 155:1949–1956.

3. Johnson, J.A., Bootman, J.L. Drug-related morbidity and mortality and the economic impact of pharmaceutical care. *Am J Health Syst Pharm* 1997; 54: 554–558.

4. Hepler, C.D. Strand, L.M. Oportunitities and responsibilities in pharmaceutical care. *Am J Hosp Pharm* 1990; 47:533–543.

5. Eraker, S.A. Understanding and improving patient compliance. *Ann Intern Med* 1984; 100:258.

6. Strand, L.M. Re-visioning the professions. *J Am Pharm Assoc* 1997; NS 37, (4):474–78.

7. Manasse H., Jr. Medication use in an imperfect world: Drug misadventuring as an issue of public policy. *Am J Hosp Pharm* 1989; 46:924–944; 1141–1152.

8. Mikeal, R.L., Brown, T.P., Lazarus, H.L, Vinson, M.C. Quality of pharmaceutical care in hospitals. *Am J Hosp Pharm* 1975; 32:567–574.

9. Brodie, D.C., Parish, P.A., Poston, J.W. Societal needs for drugs and drug-related services. *Am J Pharm Ed* 1980; 44:276–278.

10. Hepler, C.D. The third wave in pharmaceutical education and the clinical movement. *Am J Pharm Ed* 1987; 51:369–385.

11. Hepler, C.D., Strand, L.M. Opportunities and responsibilities in pharmaceutical care. *Am J Pharm Ed* 1990; 53(winter suppl):75–155.

12. Posey, L.M. Pharmaceutical care: Will pharmacy incorporate its philosophy of practice? *J Am Pharm Assoc* 1997; NS37(2):145–148.

13. Strand, L.M., Cipolle, R.J., Morley, P.C. Documenting the clinical pharmacist's activities: Back to basics. *Drug Intell Clin Pharm* 1988; 22:63–67.

14. Strand, L.M., Morley, P.C., Cipolle, R.J., et al. Drug-related problems: Their structure and function. *DICP Ann Pharmother* 1990; 24:1093–1097.

15. Pellegrino, E.D., Thomasma, D.C. *Helping and Healing.* Washington, D.C.: Georgetown University Press; 1997.

16. Kuhse, H. *Caring: Nurses, Women and Ethics.* Oxford, England: Blackwell; 1997.

17. Reich, W.T., Historical dimensions of an ethic of care in health care, in Reich, W.T., ed. *Encyclopedia of Bioethics.* New York: Macmillan; 1995, p.331.

18. Cipolle, R.J. Drugs don't have doses . . . People have doses. *Drug Intell Clin Pharm* 1986; 20:881–882.

19. May, R., ed. *Existential Psychology.* New York: Random House; 1960.

20. Rogers, C. *On Becoming a Person.* Boston: Houghton Mifflin; 1961.

21. Maslow, A.H. *Toward a Psychology of Being.* Princeton, NJ: Van Nostrand; 1962.

22. Mayerhoff, M. *On Caring.* New York: Perennial Library; 1971.

23. Gaylin, W. *Caring.* New York: Avon Books; 1976.

24. Benner, P. The moral dimensions of caring, in Stevenson, J., Tripp-Reimer, T., eds. *Knowledge about Care and Caring.* Kansas City, MO: American Academy of Nursing; 1990.

25. Leininger, M. Historic and epistemologic dimensions of care and caring with future directions, in Stevenson, J., Tripp-Reimer, T., eds. *Knowledge about Care and Caring.* Kansas City, MO: American Academy of Nursing, 1990.

26. Cooper, C.C. Covenant relationships: Grounding for the nursing ethic. *Advances in Nursing Science* 1988, cited in Bishop, A.H. Scudder, J.R. Jr., in Chinn, P., ed. *Anthology of Caring.* New York, NY: National League of Nursing, 1988.

27. Bishop, A.H. Scudder, J.R. Jr. Dialogical care and nursing practice, in Chinn, P., ed. *Anthology of Caring.* New York, NY: National League of Nursing; 1988.

28. Rouse, J. *Engaging Science: How to Understand its Practices Philosophically.* Ithaca, NY: Cornell University Press; 1996.

29. MacIntyre, A. *After Virtue,* 2d ed. Notre Dame, IN: University of Notre Dame Press; 1984.

30. MacIntyre, A. *Three Rival Versions of Moral Inquiry.* London: Duckworth; 1990.

31. Ricoeur, P. *The Conflict of Interpretations: Essays in Hermeneutics*. Evanston, IL: Northwestern University Press; 1974.

32. Bourdieu, P. *Language and Symbolic Power*, 4th ed. Cambridge, MA: Harvard University Press; 1995.

33. Cassell, E.J. *Doctoring: The Nature of Primary Care Medicine*. Oxford, England: Oxford University Press, 1997.

34. Starfield, B. *Primary Care: Concept, Evaluation, and Policy*. New York: Oxford University Press, 1992.

35. WHO. Division of Strengthening of Health Services, paper number 7, 1978 (cited in Ref. 34).

36. Woodward, K. '76 Primary health care model, in Miller, R.S., ed. *Primary Health Care: More Than Medicine*. Englewood Cliffs, NJ: Prentice Hall; 1983.

37. Lloyd, W. '76 Neighborhood health center. *Bull NY Acad Med* 1977;53:55

38. Hibbard, H. Nutting, P. Research in Primary Care: A National Priority. *AHCPR Conference Proceedings*. Washington D.C.: U.S. Department of Health and Human Services; 1991.

RECOMMENDED READINGS

Argyris, C., Schön, D. *Theory in Practice: Increasing Professional Effectiveness*. San Francisco: Jossey-Bass; 1974.

Bowden, P. *Caring: Gender-Sensitive Ethics*, London: Routledge; 1997.

Bryan, L. *A Design for the Future of Health Care*. Toronto: Key Porter Books; 1996.

Chaiklin, S., and Lave J., eds. *Understanding Practice: Perspectives on Actvity and Context*. Cambridge, England: Cambridge University Press; 1996.

Gerteis, M., Edgman-Levitan, S., Daley, J., Delbanco, T. L., eds. *Through the Patient's Eyes: Understanding and Promoting Patient-Centered Care*. San Francisco: Jossey-Bass; 1993.

Gordon, S., Benner, P., Noddings, N., eds. *Caregiving: Readings in Knowledge, Practice, Ethics, and Politics*. Philadelphia: University of Pennsylvania Press; 1996.

Knowlton, C., Penna, R., eds. *Pharmaceutical Care*. New York: Chapman and Hall; 1996.

Pellegrino, E., Thomasma, D. *A Philosophical Basis of Medical Practice: Toward a Philosophy and Ethic of the Healing Profession*. New York: Oxford University Press; 1981.

Rantucci, M.J., *Pharmacists Talking with Patients: A Guide to Patient Counseling*, Baltimore: Williams and Wilkins; 1997.

Seedhouse, D. *Reforming Health Care: The Philosophy and Practice of International Health Reform*, Chichester, England: Wiley; 1995.

Singer More, E., Milligan, M.A., eds., *The Empathic Practitioner, Empathy, Gender, and Medicine*. New Brunswick, NJ: Rutgers University Press; 1994.

Stewart, M., Brown, J.B., Weston, W.W., et al. *Patient-Centered Medicine*. Thousand Oaks CA: Sage Publications; 1995.

Turner, S. *The Social Theory of Practices: Tradition, Tacit Knowledge, and Presuppositions*, Chicago: University of Chicago Press; 1994.

CHAPTER 2 TWO

DRUG-RELATED MORBIDITY AND MORTALITY: THE CHALLENGE FOR PHARMACEUTICAL CARE

A HISTORICAL OVERVIEW OF DRUG THERAPY

The medical use of pharmaceuticals in the United States is a gargantuan enterprise that, by the twenty-first century, will undoubtedly undergo further growth in volume, diversity, and biotechnological complexity. In 1961, for example, approximately 656 drugs were in use in the United States, whereas today we can identify around 8000 pharmaceutical agents that are available for widespread clinical use.[1]

Clinicians of any stripe confront an exponential growth curve of complex pharmaceutical knowledge requiring much more than a general awareness of a few select variables culled from the *Physician's Desk Reference* (PDR) or derived from highly ritualistic "detailing" encounters that impart limited, oversimplified information to key decision makers in pharmacotherapy.

Pharmacotherapy involves risks and benefits. Indeed, pharmaceuticals are potentially dangerous substances, but danger and risk are essentially found in their use and not simply in their chemical composition. It is far too simplistic—and notably far too common—to claim that *the* problem with the drug-use process is the drug itself. Doubtless, there have been pharmaceutical substances that are of little use to human or beast, but these, if left unused on a shelf, rarely harm anyone, although over time they may decay and discharge into the biosphere, thus becoming harmful. The same may be said for all pharmaceuticals, even those with unquestionable therapeutic value. Here, the central problem is that

Danger and risk are found in how drugs are used, not simply in their chemical composition.

of negligence, bad judgment, or, more generally, human error. For our present purposes we consider drug-related problems, however defined, to be firmly grounded in a complex web of human reason with all its uncertainty. Competent performance is an essential focus if, in short, we are to avoid the objectification of pharmaceutical agents.

The history of humankind is replete with examples of pharmaceutical lore drawn upon to alleviate pain and suffering. Indeed, the health of human populations has derived considerable benefit from folklore, folk medicines, and more recently from the prodigious accomplishments of researchers in synthetic organic chemistry.[2] Twentieth-century developments in medicinal chemistry, pharmacology, and numerous other pharmaceutically related disciplines have continued to spur innovation and research focused on combating disease.

Just how successful medicine has been in fighting disease and illness has become a somewhat controversial issue. One view, considered extreme by some, is that of Illich.[3] In brief, his argument is that medical effectiveness "is an illusion." He acknowledges that pharmaceuticals have "played a significant role in the control of pneumonia, gonorrhea and syphilis, yaws and many cases of malaria and typhoid." Also, he concedes, the "reappearance of malaria is due to the development of pesticide-resistant mosquitos and not to any lack of new antimalarial drugs."[3] Moreover, he lauds the impact of immunization on poliomyelitis, and vaccines for their success against whooping cough and measles: "But for most other infections medicine can show no comparable results. Drug treatment has helped to reduce mortality from tuberculosis, tetanus, diphtheria, and scarlet fever, but in the total decline of mortality or morbidity from these diseases, chemotherapy played a minor and possibly insignificant role."[3]

Illich presents an argument that eschews technological intervention. His polemical prose emerges as an extreme denunciation of medicine because it is not perfect and it fails to realize the absolute goals and certainty found within Illich's idealistic brand of virtue. To use a well-worn cliche, he would have us "throw the baby out with the bathwater."

Illich is not the only protagonist in the debate on medicine's contribution to the fall in the death rate. In 1953 Habakkuk, an economic historian, attributed the modern rise in population to an increase in the birth rate which in itself was a consequence of improved social, economic, and industrial conditions during the eighteenth century.[4] Dubos,[5] Griffith,[6] and McKeown[7] offered similar arguments, each claiming, albeit with different emphasis, that human longevity is largely due to environmental, social, and economic factors rather than the intervention of pharmaceutical agents.[8]

McKinlay and McKinlay[8] continue the debate and conclude:

> In general, medical measures (both chemotherapeutic and prophylactic) appear to have contributed little to the overall decline in mortality in the United States since about 1900—having in many instances been intro-

duced several decades after a marked decline had already set in and having no detectable influence in most instances. More specifically, with reference to those five conditions (influenza, pneumonia, diphtheria, whooping cough, and poliomyelitis) for which the decline in mortality appears substantial after the point of intervention—and on the unlikely assumption that all of this decline is attributable to the intervention—it is estimated that at most 3.5 percent of the total decline in mortality since 1900 could be ascribed to medical measures introduced for the diseases considered here.[8]

McKeown offers a similar conclusion: "The main influences on the decline in mortality were improved nutrition on airborne infections, reduced exposure (from better hygiene) on water and food-borne diseases and, less certainly, immunization and therapy on the large number of conditions included in the miscellaneous group. Since these three classes were responsible respectively for nearly half, one-sixth, and one-tenth of the fall in the death rate, it is probable that the advancement in nutrition was the major influence."[9]

While critics presenting the "limits to medicine" viewpoint are correct to emphasize sociocultural, economic, and environmental factors as major influences in promoting health or producing disease, their reliance on mortality and morbidity statistics past and present does much to weaken their argument. Eighteenth-century data are particularly unreliable. Moreover, little attention is given to the considerable wealth of pharmacological input offered by practitioners of folk medicine and their impact on the quality of life of rural peasants and the rapidly growing urban proletariat.[2] In sum, the history of pharmacological development and the practice of therapeutics is largely ignored by the critics and, to the extent that they touch on it, is trivialized and viewed as a product of industrialization.[2]

Pharmaceuticals, in one form or other, have been used since the dawn of humankind. Possibly the oldest pharmaceutical records in existence are those of the Emperor Shen Nung (c. 2735 B.C.), a Chinese scholar whose writings on herbs formed a formidable pharmacopoeia.[10] He was the first known recorder of the stimulating effect of Ma Huang, now known as *Ephedra sinica*, a plant containing a number of important alkaloids (the most important being ephedrine) isolated in 1887 by the Japanese chemist Nagai.[10]

Ackerknecht's scholarly *Therapeutics: From the Primitive to the Twentieth Century*[11] and Sigrest's *Primitive and Archaic Medicine*[12] document the tremendous wealth of botanicals used by the Egyptians, Babylonians, Greeks, and Romans. Sumerian tablets appearing around 2100 B.C. and assorted papyri reveal "a great amount of sound empirical knowledge and practice."[10] Prescriptions containing such natural products as opium and colchicine were commonplace. Adams observes that "The placebo effect of the more than 800 prescriptions mentioned in Eber's papyrus—augmented by incantation and sorcery—probably produced more cures than their physiological effects, but to the extent that they reduced symptoms and restored well-being, their value to the sick patient was unquestioned. The empiric use of this rather substantial number of drugs preceded, by many centuries, any systematic study of anatomy and physiology or the cause of disease."[10]

What is aptly termed a reversal of the search for botanical drugs occurred in Greece in the fourth century B.C., when Hippocrates (460–377 B.C.) focused attention on inorganic salts as medicine.[10] It was his studies and teaching that laid the foundation for diagnosis and systematic treatment.[10] His medicinal authority lasted throughout the middle ages and may be particularly noted in the materia medica of Basilius Valentis in the middle of the fifteenth century A.D. and of Philipus Aureolus Paraceleus (1493–1541).[10]

Also of great importance in the history of pharmaceuticals is the Greek physician Claudius Galenus (Galen), who lived from A.D. 131 to 200. Galen's influence lasted for over a thousand years. In passing, it is worth noting that it was Galen who "insisted on carefully identifying the kind and age of botanical material and thus foreshadowed the value of controlling the purity of drugs."[10] In his lifetime Galen produced 500 volumes of medical writing, "including a vast materia medica, that dominated medical thinking and practice until the time of the Renaissance."[13]

Paracelsus wrote that "the purpose of chemistry is not to make gold but to study the fundamental sciences and turn them against disease."[13] With this admonition, Paraceleus set the stage for modern medicine and science.

> He did indeed emphasize observation and he recommended reading the book of nature rather than the writing of Galen. With his empiricism he mingled philosophic speculation that far transcended any experience. He emphasized chemical principles in the study of medicine, but to his chemical insight he occasionally added the antics of a mountebank. He combined mystical and poetical intuition with concrete medical observations. And while he brought new and refreshing currents into medicine, he retained a surprising amount of the Galenic and Aristotelian thought he affected to despise.[14]

Paracelsus played a highly significant part in shaping the scientific method that came to dominate eighteenth century medicine and the emergence of what we now know as pharmacology. It was he who "sought the *arcanum*, the healing essence within all effective pharmaceutical preparations, be they animal, vegetable or mineral."[15]

While Paraceleus inspired many with his rejection of herbs and the call for the development of clinical medicine from minerals, herbal medicine did not vanish. Indeed, "it reached its zenith in the seventeenth century."[15] As Sneader observes:

> Its subsequent decline was due to the emergence of physicians who rejected authoritarianism in favor of the experimental method. Opposing

the magic and superstition that had dominated medical thinking, these pioneers demanded evidence for the effectiveness of medicinal preparations, be these the traditional galenicals or merely samples gathered from the hedgerow as domestic remedies for those who could not afford the expensive services of a physician. Gradually, other physicians came to share their views, with the result that towards the end of the eighteenth century, a mood of therapeutic nihilism developed among leading practitioners.[15]

Moreover:, "Wise physicians came to the conclusion that, apart from cinchona bark for malaria and ipecacuanha for dysentery, both remedies having been introduced from the New World during the preceding century, opium and belladonna (the use of which had just been revived) were the only traditional drugs with any real value."[15]

In the early nineteenth century, pharmacology made considerable progress as a respected science, with its attempts to isolate the active principles of drugs used by physicians. Quinine was isolated from cinchona bark, morphine from opium, and numerous other pharmaceuticals of benefit to humankind were discovered through increasingly sophisticated pharmacological research. For example, it was during this period "that the first organic chemical was synthesized from an inorganic source."[15] Additionally, "for the first time it was possible to create, in the laboratory, physiologically active chemicals that were not derived from natural sources."[15]

One of the first pharmacological revolutions was the synthesis of active drug products in the laboratory.

It was the twentieth century that witnessed the greatest pharmaceutical achievements. Research indicates that 195 of the 200 most prescribed drugs (in about 1982) were unknown prior to the twentieth century.[15] Moreover, 150 of the 195 have been available in the health "marketplace" only since 1950[15]: All but a small fraction of the important drug discoveries since the dawn of history have probably occurred in the past 50 years. Over the same 50 years, and more than coincidently, the average life span of Americans has increased by 10 years, accompanied by a vast improvement in the quality of life.[15]

195 of the top 200 prescribed drugs in the early 1980's were unknown prior to the twentieth century.

Adams, in his brief but instructive overview of the societal impact of pharmaceuticals, identifies two pharmacological revolutions. The first was ushered in by the passage of the Biologics Control Act of 1902 and the second by the passage of the Pure Food and Drug Act of 1906. The former set in place mechanisms for the assurance of the safety of all biologics sold in the United States. The latter placed the pharmaceutical industry under the control of the federal government.[13]

In the 1930s the new hybrid discipline of biochemistry appeared and began to make major contributions to drug development. At the same time sulfanilamide and other sulfa drugs emerged as potent antibacterial agents. These were soon to be followed by the successful introduction of penicillin into therapeutics.[16] The impact of antibiotics has been considerable and their contribution to the quality of life immeasurable. Infections such as mastoiditis and osteomyelitis are rarely found in present industrial societies.[13]

New classes of drugs that were highly effective in combating diseases which had failed to respond to earlier treatment were developed in the years following World War II.[13] Nitrogen mustards, formerly used as weapons of war, were known to produce changes in lymphoid tissue and bone marrow, and this generated research interest in their potential chemotherapeutic use. In 1942, research laboratories began to examine the potential of nitrogen mustards as therapeutic agents to treat lymphosarcoma and other malignancies. Work on cytotoxic pharmaceuticals led eventually to the discovery of alkylating agents and antimetabolites. Androgens and estrogens were found to be useful in treating prostate and breast cancer. Cortisone and other corticosteroids appeared in the 1950s and proved highly successful in the treatment of lymphosarcoma, leukemia, and Hodgkin's disease.[13]

Research with cortisone and its derivatives proved useful in the treatment of numerous collagen diseases, dermatological disorders, allergies, ophthalmic conditions, gastrointestinal disorders and respiratory diseases.[13] In the words of Adams, "[no] single group of drugs has ever been approved for such a wide spectrum of diseases."[13]

Vaccines represent another major category of pharmaceutical intervention. The impact of vaccines on poliomyelitis, mumps, rubella, whooping cough, measles, bubonic plague, typhoid, and typhus is well documented. Other major drug classes include analgesics, which, while replete with addictive potential, have vastly improved the quality of life for millions whose alternative is suffering intractable pain. Antipyretic and antirheumatic drugs, drugs affecting nervous transmission, neuromuscular blocking agents, cardiovascular drugs, antihistamines, antiprotozoal drugs, and psychopharmacological agents have all made a major contribution to human health. These and many other pharmaceuticals are but a few examples of therapeutic agents produced during what Adams refers to as "the first pharmacological revolution," which was a consequence of "the elucidation and practical application of the relationship between chemical structure and biological activity."[13] Knowledge accumulated during this first revolutionary stage in the development of pharmaceuticals, based in organic chemistry, shed light on important drug actions at the molecular level. Also, it rapidly became apparent that "the success of future drug research would depend on increased knowledge and better understanding of cellular biochemistry and physiology."[13]

The beginning of the second pharmacological revolution witnessed a significant shift "from the synthesis and testing of large numbers of compounds in the chemical laboratory to the isolation and characterization of biochemical compounds synthesized in the "laboratory" of the living cell."[13] Thus, molecular pharmacy emerged as the paradigm of contemporary pharmacology.

The study of molecular structure and function has produced redesigned molecules that pioneer the reconceptualization of drug development:

The second pharmacological revolution was the isolation and characterization of compounds in the living cell.

Researchers at the Upjohn Company have designed and made modified molecules of vasopressin, a hormone that consists of a short chain of amino acids. Vasopressin increases the work done by the heart and decreases the rate at which the kidneys produce urine; this increases blood pressure. The researchers designed modified vasopressin molecules that affected receptor molecules in the kidney more than those in the heart, giving them more specific and controllable medical effects. More recently, they designed a modified vasopressin molecule that binds to the kidney's receptor molecules without direct effect, thus blocking and *inhibiting* the action of natural vasopressin.[17]

As it is now possible to move DNA from one organism to another, recipient organisms can be made to produce a protein through technical manipulation:

> This is the key concept of biotechnology as it is now applied to the production of health care related products. The first step in this process is to isolate the desirable protein. Very often, it can only be obtained in small quantities, that is, it is a rare protein. After purifying the protein and documenting its physiological activity, its amino acid composition is determined. The amino acid composition provides the information necessary to find the gene for the protein, the piece of DNA which tells the cell how to make that particular protein. The gene is then isolated and spliced into a vector, another piece of DNA which permits the insertion of the gene into a host organism. The metabolic machinery of the host organism, which is often a bacterium, can then be harnessed to produce the protein. In the end, then, the protein can be produced in large quantities, sufficient to use in the clinic or on the farm.[18]

Biotechnology's impact on the pharmaceutical industry is to set in motion processes "by which useful quantities of important proteins can be produced in pure form relatively cheaply."[18] According to Manasse, Gerald J. Mossinghoff, president of the Pharmaceutical Manufacturers Association (PMA), has stated that "only nine biotechnology products have been approved by the FDA to date," but "81 compounds are 'coming around the bend.' Of the 81 compounds 67 are in human clinical trials and 14 are awaiting FDA approval."[1] Biotechnological products already on the marketplace include human insulin, human growth hormone, human alpha interferon, human tissue plasminogen activator, OKT-3 monoclonal antibody, blood factor VIII:C, and erythropoietin.[18]

Future developments include the following: immunomodulators (as noted above, alpha interferon is already approved by the FDA) such as interleukins; growth factors targeting bone, epidermal, and nerve cells; alpha-l-antitrypsin, and other highly specific enzyme inhibitors; recombinant vaccines; biotechnology-derived diagnostics, and other, perhaps more utopian, pharmaceutical agents such as Isoprin-osine and a drug with the potential to extend the life span.[18]

Not only are highly complex, important advances being made in the structure and function of drugs but we may also expect to see highly sophisticated delivery systems developed in the near future.[19] Halperin lists some of these systems, and they are summarized by Manasse thus: controlled release technologies (incremental drug release), magnetic systems (site-specific release of drugs with magnetized particles), monoclonal antibodies (targeting highly toxic drugs to specific antigens on cell membranes), respiratory delivery (delivering large molecules through the respiratory system), liposomes (taking a drug to a specific cell using drugs that are trapped in oil and water emulsions), neurotransmitters (natural peptides that will deliver drugs directly to the brain), and erodible polymer implants (delivering drugs that will require pulsed dosage delivery).[19]

The true value or risk of any pharmacological agent lies in how it is used. This challenge has never been greater than it is today with the new generation of pharmaceuticals which is about to expand the horizons of pharmacological knowledge and place highly complex demands on the safe, efficacious application of "high-tech pharmaceuticals."[20] Given such a set of tasks and responsibilities, it is essential to fully understand the potential harm, that is to say, drug-related problems, associated with their inappropriate use. Understanding the potential harm will allow clinicians to establish the therapeutic monitoring plans necessary to carry out their clinical duties in a highly competent manner. We now turn our attention to the important issue of the nature, type, and magnitude of drug-related problems as identified in the literature. It is this evidence which establishes the need for a practitioner to assume responsibility for the appropriate, effective, safe, and convenient use of drug therapy.

The new biotechnology generation will expand the limits of pharmacology and place new demands on the use of these complex drug therapies.

A HISTORICAL LOOK AT DRUG-RELATED MORBIDITY AND MORTALITY

THE NATURE OF THE PROBLEM

Awareness of the potential and actual harm inflicted by medicine is an ancient part of medical consciousness. Side effects of drugs were studied by the Arabs and recorded by AlRazi as early as A.D. 900. Avicenna (A.D. 980–1037) reported the effects of mercury on the nervous system and warned of its dangers.[21] In short, the potential for medically induced harm is not a recent discovery but rather extends back to antiquity and is as old as medicine itself.[21]

In essence, the issue of drug toxicity is central to the subject of iatrogenesis.[22] All drugs are toxic in some measure. Their toxicity, however, is inextricably linked to their use, and this follows specific judgments made by individuals of variable levels of qualification and competence. More will be said regarding this seemingly obvious but often overlooked relationship.

First, it is necessary to address the issue of terminological ambiguity associated with the negative effects of pharmaceutical agents.[1] Manasse notes that the term *iatrogenic disease* was first used by Pepper in relation to negative drug effects in 1956. This was defined as "a disease that is independent of underlying disease and results from either drug administration, medical or surgical acts for prophylaxis, diagnosis or other therapy."[1]

D'Arcy and Griffin, also cited by Manasse, offer a broad definition of what they term "iatrogenic hazards." These "embrace all the risks for which a doctor may be held responsible in whole or in part. The hazard may lie in something the doctor has done, whether this be a drug prescribed, an investigation requested, a hospital admission arranged, an operation performed, or even a conversation held. It may also lie in something he has not done, whether by accident, design, or indolence."[1]

Both of the above definitions of iatrogenesis provide a general foundation or conceptual framework to use as a starting point. However, in search of greater specificity, researchers have coined numerous other terms to refer to the negative effects of pharmacotherapy. Synoptically, these consist of adverse reactions, complications, drug-induced illness or disease, iatrogenic illness, negative therapeutics, drug intolerance, adverse events, erroneous use and accidents, prescribing errors, adverse drug reactions, excessive therapeutic effects, unwanted pharmacological effects, pathological reaction, superinfection, drug-induced injury, and drug interactions.[1]

Doubtless there are others to be found in the literature, but to a large extent all of these are variations on a theme or points of emphasis, which differ from researcher to researcher. Manasse's work is particularly valuable in offering a distillation of precepts derived from a thorough analysis of the literature characterizing the linguistic idiosyncrasy and terminological confusion of the negative effects of drug use. Following is Manasse's summary of how negative consequences from drugs are characterized in the literature:

> The diverse terminology used to describe drug-related events is not standardized and therefore of minimal use to practitioners.

1. There is an inherent risk to the patient whenever a medical procedure is implemented and, in the case of drugs, when these are administered as a part of the medical-care treatment plan.

2. Causality or attribution is independent of the disease or pathological condition; however, there are known pathological conditions that exacerbate drug effect (increase or decrease).

3. A variety of individuals, structures, and systems may be responsible or accountable.

4. The patient is harmed in some fashion ranging from mildly distraught to death.

5. Problems are likely to be created when multiple chronic illnesses are treated with multiple drug therapies; such problems are especially prevalent in the elderly patient.

6. Negative consequences may occur with one drug prescribed for one condition as well as with multiple drugs prescribed and administered for a single pathological condition.

7. The impact is noxious, undesirable, and unintended at doses that on their face or in the judgment of the prescriber seem appropriate.

8. Any serious failure of expected pharmacological action, including inappropriateness of the prescribed drug(s) for the illness or misdiagnosis (a contingency table of right-wrong drug/right-wrong diagnosis) may be included.

9. Such effects can or will create complications or pathological conditions or manifestations directly attributable to prescribed drug therapy.

10. Culpability or preventability may be remote under some circumstances.

11. Causality may be based on a known or unknown immune response to a drug or drug combination.

12. The event is unexpected and thus unacceptable to either patient or prescriber, and thus is an adverse experience for both.

13. The experience may not be causally related to the drug itself, but rather to erroneous use or errors or accidents in prescribing, preparation, dispensing, or labelling of the drug.[1]

Drug misadventuring describes the risk and negative effects of the use of drugs as a part of a medical-care treatment plan.

Manasse suggests that the term *drug misadventuring* captures the essence of the above precepts. His conceptualization of drug misadventuring may be thought of as an iatrogenic hazard or incident. Manasse's distillation of the issue is one of the simplest, and thereby, perhaps one of the most useful ways to think about the negative effects drug therapy are able to have. Drug misadventuring is that which is

1. an inherent risk when drug therapy is indicated;

2. created through either omission or commission by the administration of a drug or drugs during which a patient is harmed, with effects ranging from mild discomfort to fatality;

3. able to generate an outcome may or may not be independent of the pre-existing pathology or disease process;

4. possibly attributable to error (human or system or both) immunological response or idiosyncratic response;

5. always unexpected and thus unacceptable to patient and prescriber.[64]

In 1955 D. P. Barr, a New York physician published a paper entitled "Hazards of Modern Diagnosis and Therapy—The Price We Pay." This paper, presented to the Section on Internal Medicine of the American Medical Association (Frank Billings Memorial Lecture) urged members to reflect on the ancient admonition *Primum non nocere.* He exclaimed that "We can shudder now when we remember outdoor treatment of pneumonia, cold tub baths for typhoid, starving of fevers, and withdrawal of water in cholera. We hesitate to think of the harm unwittingly done by the use of aminopyrine, cinchophen, and dinitrophenol. Their wrongful use and many other errors plague our recent past and make us insecure in our present judgments."[23] He goes on to state:

> Although incalculable benefits have come to mankind with the introduc-
> tion of these newer diagnostic and therapeutic procedures, hazards of
> medical management have at the same time enormously increased. Not
> one of the occasionally indispensable diagnostic tests may be undertaken
> without risk. The simplest as well as the most complicated possesses
> inherent danger. Infection may be introduced by a needle; sudden death
> may follow the intravenous administration of such a relatively inert sub-
> stance as dehydrocholic acid (Decholin). Furthermore, no agent that can
> modify the internal environment or organic integrity of the body can be
> used without hazard. As yet no drug has been found with a single action,
> and no human body with a single reaction. Risks accompany the use even
> of those remedies that are regarded as safest.[23]

With the introduction of new diagnostic and therapeutic procedures comes increased hazards associated with medication management.

Barr's message was a consequence of his growing concern for the safety of his patients, particularly in the light of increasingly more complex pharmaceuticals entering the marketplace. He arbitrarily selects seven major areas where he concludes that "accidents and misfortunes may result on occasion even with enlightened thoughtful use of diagnostic and therapeutic measures by conscientious and well-informed physicians earnestly trying to help their patients."[23] His list of "possible dangers" includes the following:

1. Accidental drug intoxication (e.g., digitalis, scopolamine, curare, and bishydroxycoumarin)
2. Modification of internal environment, particularly through the use of parenterally given fluids
3. Introduction of infection
4. Allergic reactions
5. Special instances of intoxication (e.g. antibiotics, cortisone, hydrocortisone and corticotropin antihistaminics, phenylbutazone, and chlorpromazine)
6. Hidden and general dangers (e.g., hydralazine hydrochloride)
7. Dangers from multiple procedures

Barr's observations, based on the research of the day and clinical experience, focused attention on what he saw as an increasingly complex part of therapeutics—clinical judgment.

One year later, in 1956, Moser, a resident in cardiovascular disease, published his paper "Diseases of Medical Progress."[24] Here, he reviews the literature with a view to documenting diseases produced by medical progress as those "that would not have occurred if sound therapeutic procedures had not been employed."[24] He admits that this is a somewhat "oblique" approach.

Moser's review focuses on "classes" of diseases of medical progress. The first is that of collagen and collagen-like diseases such as periarteritis nodosa, which he links to the rising use of sulfonamides (since

1936). However, there are numerous reports of periarteritis nodosa in patients who had not taken sulfonamides.[25] Thus, the relationship is not "isomorphic" in any real sense. Other diseases in this class are hydralazine syndrome "occurring in patients successfully treated with the antihypertensive agent hydralazine hydrochloride (Apresoline)."[25] Intestinal pulmonary fibrosis (resembling Hamman-Rich disease, nickel carbonyl poisoning, or pulmonary scleroderma) "is believed to result from prolonged administration of the antihypertensive agent hexamethonium."[25]

Neurological diseases such as epilepsy and parkinsonism follow the use of reserpine. Other examples include psychosis from steroids and reserpine, hepatic coma through the injudicious selection of ammonium chloride as a diuretic to mobilize ascitic fluid, antibiotic-induced eighth-nerve damage, and peripheral neuritis as a toxic side effect of numerous therapeutic agents.

Hepatic diseases such as jaundice from intrahepatic obstruction implicate such drugs as chlorpromazine, arsphenamine, thiouracil, methimazole, methyl testosterone, and atophan-cinchophen. In the case of chlorpromazine, for example, jaundice had a reported incidence of 3 in 71 and 1 in 506 cases in addition to 14 cases from the Mayo Clinic (from a series of unknown size).[25] Toxic hepatitis has been associated with "old" drugs such as male fern, trinitrophenol (picric acid), gold compounds, and sulfonamides. More recent drugs include phenylacetyl urea, phenylbutazone and isonicotinic hydrazide. All of these are well known as agents that incite toxic hepatitis.[74]

Hematological diseases caused by drug therapy are numerous. Moser identifies antigranulocytic, antierythrocyte, antiplatelet, and total bone marrow reactions.

There are also many metabolic diseases, such as secondary gout and uric acid calculi (due to anti–folic acid compounds), retrolental fibroplasia, low-sodium syndromes, digitalis-induced gynecomastia, adrenal exhaustion syndrome, steroid-withdrawal syndrome, hyperchloremic acidosis, and goiter induced by phenylbutazone and cobalt.

Steroid-induced diseases, particularly when steroid therapy is long-term, have been known for a long time. The treatment of rheumatoid arthritis, lupus erythematosus, and asthma has given rise to states similar to Cushing's disease. This is because "the effectiveness of the drug often does not become manifest until dosage is pushed to a point where signs of toxicity resembling Cushing's disease may appear quite insidiously."[25]

Hypertension; mental torpor; hyperglycemia with glycosuria, sodium retention, and potassium loss; acne; buffalo hump; hirsutism and negative nitrogen balance with accompanying muscle wasting; and osteoporosis are also linked to steroid use.[25] Adrenal exhaustion syndrome (as little as 100 mg of a steriod given over a 5-day period has been suspected of causing adrenocortical suppression), steroid withdrawal syndrome, peptic ulcer, and perforation in regional enteritis and ulcerative colitis have also been clinically identified as effects of steroid therapy.[25]

Among the cardiac diseases identified by Moser are digitalis-induced arrhythmias, ranging from paroxysmal atrial tachycardia with block to ventricular tachycardia. He cautions that these arrhythmias "may be attributed erroneously to the underlying heart disease."[25] Other drugs linked with these conditions are quinidine, procainamide (Pronestyl), and rauwolfia (premature ventricular contractions).[25] In addition to the aforementioned arrhythmias, Moser mentions hemorrhagic pericardial effusion thought to be due to diapedesis of red cells from the capillaries of the subepicardial infarcted myocardium resulting from the use of bishydroxycoumarin and related anticoagulants in the treatment of acute myocardial infarction.[25] Fuadin, tartar emetic, and sulfadiazine have been implicated in many cases of nonspecific myocarditis.[25]

The last class of "diseases of medical progress" discussed by Moser is the renal diseases. Here he identifies acute renal shutdown (acute tubular necrosis, lower-nephron nephrosis), drug-induced nephrosis, acute urinary retention, and dermatitis as major drug-related problems.

Moser and Barr provide "landmark" papers. Both brought to the attention of health professionals significant drug-related problems requiring systematic, rigorous, and sustained research. Moser terms his work "a brief review," and Barr by no means considers his contribution to be an exhaustive account of complex clinical issues. But their work clearly documents the essential range and scope of necessary clinical research. We now turn our attention to the work of those who accepted the challenge and attempted to document the magnitude of the problem.

THE MAGNITUDE OF THE PROBLEM

In 1957[26] the Committee on Research, Council on Drugs of the American Medical Association (AMA) produced a report on blood dyscrasias associated with promazine hydrochloride therapy, and in 1960 this same body produced a report on blood dyscrasias associated with chloramphenicol therapy.[27] Following this, in 1962, Erslev and Wintrobe published an important paper on the detection and prevention of drug-induced blood dyscrasias.[28]

Also, in 1962, the Mary Fletcher Hospital, a reporting member of the FDA's Adverse-Drug-Reaction Reporting Program, reported 98 drug reactions (approximately 1 percent of admitted patients). Antibiotics, hypnotics, and tranquilizers were the major classes of drugs implicated.[29]

A major epidemiological study of adverse drug reactions (ADRs) was published in 1965. In this study, carried out at the Johns Hopkins Hospital, Seidl et al. report on data collected on drug usage within the hospital since July 1963.[30] Their methods of surveillance were discussed in detail in a 1964 publication[31] and will receive more detailed attention further on in the present work.

For 3 years a report-of-drug-reaction card system was in use at Johns Hopkins Hospital but proved unreliable in indicating drug-reaction incidents. This called for different methods. In the methicillin pilot study, "all patients in the hospital for whom methicillin was ordered from the pharmacy were followed daily from the time the drug was begun until they left the hospital."[30] The researchers found that the average number of drugs the patients received was 14. Moreover, they "also previously or concurrently had received an average of four other antibiotics."[30] They note that "one desperately ill patient received thirty-two medications including ten other antibiotics."[90] Only two reactions ($n = 37$) "probably caused" by methicillin were found, but 18 patients experienced ADRs to one or more of the other drugs received.

The researchers also reviewed the records of all patients receiving warfarin (over a 3-month period) looking for evidence of adverse effects, particularly bleeding. Some 15 percent of these patients "receiving warfarin under 'routine' conditions had overt adverse reactions probably related to it, and another 21 percent had at least one prothrombin determination below 10 percent, an arbitrarily chosen hazardous range."[30]

5% of admissions to public medical services are caused by drug reactions.

In the Medical Service Study, Seidl et al. visited each of the six wards over a 3-month period and questioned staff about the occurrence of any untoward reactions. Any patient experiencing such a reaction was followed throughout his or her hospitalization. The investigators state that while their analysis is incomplete, "it appears that about 5 percent of all admissions to the public medical service were directly caused by drug reactions, including digitalis excess, sulfadiazine crystalluria, bromism, erythema multiforme caused by phenolphthalein, penicillin 'serum sickness,' thrombocytopenic purpura attributed to sulfisoxazole, glutethimide-induced coma, and hypokalemic dehydration caused by chlorothiazide."[30] Additionally, 15 percent of all patients admitted acquired an ADR while hospitalized.[30] When compared with the population of all patients, those who experienced ADRs were found to be more common in the 41- to 70-year age range. Also, there seemed to be "no racial predilection for developing drug reactions."[30] But women, who made up 45 percent of the population accounted for approximately 62 percent of the ADRs detected.

At least 15% of hospitalized patients experience an adverse drug reaction while being treated.

A West German paper by Lenz in 1966 reviewed malformation caused by drugs in pregnancy. He identified numerous "causal relationships" that require attention. Malformations have been associated with aminopterin, busulfan, androgens and progestogens, cortisone, quinine, insulin, and tolbutamide.[32] Specific teratogenic drugs discussed are thalidomide and cyclophosphamide—an alkylating agent "which caused aplasia of big toes, hernias, and minor facial and digital abnormalities in one infant."[32] Hoddinott et al. carried out a study in an investigative and treatment ward of 31 beds in a Canadian hospital over a 59-day period in 1966. Their purpose was to survey the risks of drug administration on a general medical ward.[33] Their definition of a "drug adverse reaction" is "any noxious or unintended consequence of drugs, normally used clinically for the diagnosis, prophylaxis, or therapy of disease, or for the modification of physiological function."[33] A total of 26 patients were investigated for 29 identified reactions. Of these, 17 were classified as "probable." In effect, 15 percent of the 104 patients had *probable* ADRs.[33] Additionally, in 20 patients, 23 errors were detected, 11 of which followed a change in physicians' orders.

Ogilvie and Ruedy, in another Canadian study conducted in 1967, surveyed all patients admitted to the Montreal General Hospital over a 12-month period. They define an ADR as "any undesired consequence of drug therapy."[34] Failure to achieve an expected therapeutic goal was not defined as an ADR. Of 731 patients, 132 (18 percent) suffered 193 adverse reactions to drugs during the year of the study.[34] Most ADRs were the result of overdose (44.6 percent), side effect (27.0 percent), or cytotoxic effect (9.4 percent). Digitalis, antibiotics, insulin, and diuretics caused 60 percent of the reactions. On the other hand, analgesics, sedative-hypnotics, antidepressants, antihypertensives, hormonal agents (other than insulin), radiographic dyes, anticoagulants, and bronchodilating agents each caused less than 4 percent of the ADRs.[34] Patients who experienced ADRs during hospitalization stayed an average of 20.5 days. Those who did not experience ADRs averaged 11.6 days in the hospital. A breakdown of the data reveals that of the 193 ADRs, 52 were considered minor, 74 were of moderate severity, and 67 were major.[34] The authors note that it "is remarkable that 38% of all adverse reactions in our patients were due to three agents which have been used in medical practice for over 20 years—digoxin, quinidine and insulin."[34] Findings such as these may very well suggest that pharmacotherapeutic monitoring is far from an exact science or, more probably, not executed routinely within hospital settings. One other set of observations is worth noting at length: "If reactions to other acetylsalicylic acid drugs such as phenobarbital, paraldehyde, adrenalin, heparin, thyroid extract and purgatives are added, the percentage of reactions by these 'old' drugs was over 50%. The majority of remaining reactions was due to drugs which have been in use for more than 10 years. It cannot be said that the high incidence of reactions was due to new drugs with which the medical profession has had little experience."[34] The authors conclude by stating that present "methods of predicting drug reactions are unsatisfactory."[34]

In 1963 the Greater Philadelphia Committee for Medical Pharmaceutical Sciences met with the College of Physicians of Philadelphia. During this meeting, a subcommittee on Adverse Drug Reactions met "to plan and develop a registry of such reactions."[35] The subcommittee designed a reporting technique for ADRs and carried out a 2-year study at five medical school hospitals. A total of 809 ADRs were reported to the registry. A total of 772 occurred while the patients were hospitalized. Dermatological conditions and allergic reactions were the most common effects and represent 65 percent of all cases. Penicillin was thought to be implicated in 101 cases, phenobarbital and digitalis preparations in 21, and aspirin in 20. They conclude that the "overall incidence of adverse reactions was 0.49% of all hospitalized patients for the first year of study and 0.41% for the second year."[35]

Batsakis et al. report on the iatrogenic aberrations of serum enzyme activity.[36] They present three forms of iatrogenic alterations in serum enzyme activity "as they relate to the diagnosis of acute myocardial infarct in the pre- or postoperative patient."[36] These are opiate-induced hypertransaminasemia, sensitized creatine phosphokinase (CPK) assay systems (e.g., injections of drugs such as aqueous penicillin are capable of producing a rise in CPK activity up to five times normal levels), and post–cardiac surgery aberrations.

All reports describing adverse reactions emphasize the problem of under-reporting.

Borda et al. in 1968 carried out a comprehensive drug surveillance of 830 patients in the medical wards at Lemuel Shattuck Hospital.[37] Over an 11-month period, the total number of ADRs was 405 and the total number of drug exposures 7078. The "incidence of *alleged* adverse reactions per drug exposure was 5.7%."[37] Approximately 35 percent of the patients experienced at least one ADR. A clinical pharmacologist investigated 73 percent of the adverse reactions and submitted 293 investigated reports. In all, 69 percent of the ADRs were considered to be either "definitely" or "probably" due to the drug identified earlier. In 20 percent of the cases it was concluded that the drug was not responsible for the reaction, and in 11 percent no decision could be reached. It was also found that 26 percent of the reactions were life-threatening and 12 percent did in fact lead to increased hospitalization. The authors note that the reported incidence of ADRs (in the literature) in patients ranges from 5 to 20 percent. However, in the Lemuel Shattuck study, the considerably higher figure of 35 percent was found.

In 1969 Rodney Sweetnam contributed an editorial on corticosteroid arthropathy and tendon rupture to the *Journal of Bone and Joint Surgery*.[38] In this he notes that "the frequent development of severe vertebral osteoporosis in patients receiving prolonged treatment with corticosteroids has awakened orthopaedic surgeons to at least one serious complication of such treatment."[38] He concludes his comments with the assertion that "[we] now have evidence, both clinical and experimental, that apart from the well recognized hazard of infection, intraarticular injections of corticosteroids, certainly if repeated, may be harmful." Moreover, "corticosteroid injection around painful tendons in athletes should be discouraged because of the risk of rupture, particularly if the tendon is to be subjected to continued strain."[38] This practice was considered a common intervention on the part of orthopedic surgeons and the editorial is to be considered an "alert" based on research and clinical experience.

In 1969 Hurwitz published two papers in the *British Medical Journal*. Both report important findings regarding (1) predisposing factors in ADRs and (2) admissions to hospitals due to drugs.

In her first paper, Hurwitz reports the findings of a prospective study which, in part, obtained information on predisposing factors in 118 patients who developed ADRs in the hospital.[39] In this paper, Hurwitz finds that significantly more patients over 60 years old and more women than men developed ADRs. Polypharmacy was implicated in that more patients taking several drugs at the same time (median of total number of drugs was nine) experienced ADRs. Patients who did not experience such effects had a median of four drugs in their therapeutic regimen. Moreover, it was found that a previous ADR "and history of allergic disease were significant factors, while a history of jaundice or the presence of diabetes mellitus and renal disease was not."[39]

In her study "Admissions to Hospital due to Drugs," Hurwitz studied ADRs in the wards of two Belfast hospitals for 52 weeks. She found that 2.9 percent of 1268 patients were admitted to the hospital because of ADRs due to therapy, and 2.1 percent were admitted due to self-poisoning.[40] Patients in the former category were older than those admitted through self-poisoning, and they stayed in the hospital longer. Drugs identified as causing ADRs were digitalis preparations, antibiotics, corticosteroids, anticoagulants, analgesics, and tranquilizers. Hypersensitivity and side effects were the major types of reactions.[40] These findings are consistent with those of other studies.

Shapiro et al., in 1971, published the results of a study focusing on fatal drug reactions.[41] In this study, 6199 deaths were consecutively monitored. Death due to "drugs administered in hospitals" was recorded in 27 cases (0.44 percent). Again we find that most of the deaths were attributed "to commonly used drugs," which may well add to the argument for more rigorous, systematic pharmacotherapeutic monitoring. Potassium supplements and parenterally administered fluid therapy were implicated as contributing to hyperkalemia and pulmonary edema. The researchers list other drug-attributed mechanisms causing death in the patients monitored. These include depression of the central nervous system, superinfection, hemorrhage, cardiorespiratory complications, dehydration and electrolyte depletion, hypoglycemia, anaphylaxis, liver failure, perforated duodenal ulcer, and hypercalcemia.[41]

Caranasos et al.,[42] following completion of a 3-year study, found that "drug-induced illness, excluding suicide attempts and drug abuse, accounted for 2.9 percent of admission to a medical service."[42] They also found (as did Hurwitz, see above) that proportionally more patients over 61 years of age were admitted. Also, considerably "more white women than black women or men were affected." More than 6 percent of these patients died.[42] Eight drugs produced one-third of the illnesses. These were: aspirin, digoxin, warfarin, sodium, hydrochlorothiazide, prednisone, vincristine sulfate, norethindrone, and furosemide. Other findings were that hemorrhagic effects were frequent; the cardiovascular, gastrointestinal, and hemopoietic systems were most often involved. Also, drug allergy was the negative mechanism of the ADR in 17.6 percent of identified illness. Others were "due to pharmacological mechanisms."[42]

Since 1966 the Boston Collaborative Drug Surveillance Program (BCDSP) has carried out intensive monitoring of patients in four countries. An overview of their work provides some useful insights into drug-related problems. Jick et al., in 1968 reported on 97 consecutive patients who received heparin. Adverse drug reactions occurred in 18 of 56 women (32 percent) and 6 out of 41 men (15 percent). The average age of patients experiencing ADRs was over 60. All but one of the ADRs were due to hemorrhage, and one death was due to heparin (intrapulmonary hemorrhage). The investigators concluded that there was a higher risk of hemorrhage in women patients over the age of 60 who receive heparin.[43]

Shapiro et al. studied 2098 consecutive patients in a comprehensive surveillance program where all drugs were monitored.[44] The results with digoxin prescribed for 441 consecutive patients indicate that this treatment was effective in 91.7 percent of the patients and poor in 2.8 percent of all patients monitored, while ADRs were found in 18.4 percent. Following pharmacological analysis, this was confirmed in 82.8 percent of those cases. Prochlorperazine, used to treat nausea and vomiting, was found to be associated with toxicity in these patients.

A study by Jick et al. focused on the clinical effects of hypnotics.[45] This was a controlled clinical trial that compared three hypnotic drugs: chloralbetaine, 750 mg; diphenhydramine hydrochloride, 50 mg; pentobarbital, 100 mg; and a placebo. These drugs: were "introduced into a comprehensive drug surveillance program." This study found that there was some evidence of a higher frequency of side effects among patients receiving hypnotics. The placebo had a greater effect on women than on men, but the hypnotics had an equal effect on both male and female patients. The study concluded that physicians' judgments of drug efficacy and side effects are valid in that they discriminate between hypnotic drugs and placebo when placed under the constraints of a randomized double-blind trial. In a somewhat oblique sense, this study was an exercise in clinical problem solving.

A second paper by Shapiro et al. used an epidemiological approach to study the clinical effects of four of the most commonly prescribed hypnotic drugs: chloral hydrate, diphenhydramine hydrochloride, seco-barbital, and pentobarbital. This study was also carried out in the context of a comprehensive drug surveillance program. The researchers studied 4177 patients and found that, at the time of writing, 2045 (49 percent) individuals were given one or more of the four drugs surveyed to treat insomnia. Treatment with each of these drugs was judged effective in 60 percent to 80 percent of patients. The frequencies of ADRs varied between 1.8 percent and 5.1 percent.[46]

Sloan et al. examined the probable relationship between ethacrynic acid administered intravenously and gastrointestinal bleeding.[47] During routine computer monitoring, such an association ($p<.0001$) was noticed. A detailed study followed, and even when diagnosis, age, sex, blood urea nitrogen (BUN) levels, the presence or absence of heparin sodium therapy, and the severity of specific illness were controlled, it was found that patients receiving ethacrynic acid continued to exhibit a higher frequency of gastrointestinal bleeding than did patients receiving furosemide, meralluride sodium, and/or hydrochlorothiazide and/or chorothiazide orally or in patients who did not receive any of these diuretics ($p<.02$).

Also in 1969 Shapiro et al. reported on drug rash associated with ampicillin and other penicillins.[48] After monitoring 3985 consecutive medical inpatients, they found rash associated with any drug in 9.5 percent of 422 patients treated with ampicillin and in 4.5 percent of 622 patients receiving other penicillins. It was found that the frequency of rash in 2941 patients not receiving these drugs was 1.8 percent. Their research suggests that antigenic impurities may be found in ampicillin and are responsible for dermatological conditions such as rash.

Lewis et al., in 1971, surveyed the side effects of prednisone and serum protein levels.[49] This study revealed a correlation between the frequency of side effects, the mean daily dose, and serum albumin. The investigators found that when serum albumin concentration is less than 2.5 g/100 mL, the frequency of prednisone's side effects is doubled. Hypoalbuminemia can result in increased free prednisone levels in the body.

The BCDSP group produced a study in 1972 that identified adverse reactions to the tricyclic antidepressant drugs.[50] The total ADR rate was 15.4 percent. Major reactions such as psychosis, hallucinations, disorientation, and agitation were found in 4.6 percent of 260 patients.

Also in 1972 this same group conducted a study of tetracycline and drug-attributed increases in blood urea nitrogen.[51] This association was found to be confined to tetracycline recipients who were also on diuretics. The investigators concluded that patients receiving diuretics should not be given tetracycline.

Other studies carried out by the BCDSP group in 1972 include acute adverse reactions to prednisone in relation to dosage,[52] drug-induced concussions,[53] and coffee drinking and acute myocardial infarction.[54]

In 1973 the BCDSP group conducted two studies related to cigarette smoking and ADRs. The first of these looked at clinical depression of the central nervous system (CNS) due to diazepam and chlordiazepoxide in relation to smoking and age.[55] Here, clinical depression of the CNS as indicated by drowsiness attributed to drugs was compared among nonsmokers, light smokers (20 cigarettes per day or less), and heavy smokers receiving diazepam, chlordiazepoxide, or phenobarbital. In the case of the two benzodiazepines, CNS depression was less frequent as fewer cigarettes were used. This was not the case with phenobarbital, where CNS depression with benzodiazepines was more common with increased age.

The second study examined decreased clinical efficacy of propoxyphene in cigarette smokers.[56] Patients receiving propoxyhene hydrochloride for mild or moderate headache pain were monitored. This drug was judged by physicians to be ineffective in the case of 10.1 percent of 334 nonsmokers, 15 percent of 347 individuals who smoked 20 or less cigarettes per day, and 20.3 percent of 153 patients smoking more than 20 cigarettes per day ($p < .01$).

Other studies conducted by the BCDSP group in 1973 focused on (1) drug-induced deafness[57] (drugs implicated: aspirin, 11 per 1000 exposed; aminoglycoside antibiotics, 13 per 1000 exposed; intravenous ethacrynic acid, 7 per 1000 exposed; and quinidine, 3 per 1000 exposed); (2) drug-induced anaphylaxis[58] (1.3 per 1000) following injectable aqueous penicillin and cephalothin sodium; (3) drug-induced extrapyramidal symptoms (found to occur in approximately 1 percent of patients receiving the phenothiazines or tricyclic antidepressants);[59] (4) oral contraceptives and venous thromboembolic diseases, surgically confirmed gallbladder disease, and breast tumors (estimated relative risk for thromboembolism was 11 per 100,000 users; estimated rate attributable to oral contraceptives was 60 per 100,000 per year, and the estimated rate for gallbladder disease was 79 per 100,000 users).[60]

Greenblatt reports on 788 patients (monitored in a drug surveillance program) who received spironolactone during one or more admissions.[61] Adverse drug reactions were attributed to spironolactone in 164 patients (20.8 percent). Hyperkalemia was found in 68 patients (8.6 percent). Hyperkalemia was far more frequent in patients receiving potassium chloride concurrently (15.8 percent) than it was in those not receiving this drug (5.7 percent). Other ADRs included dehydration (3.4 percent), hyponatremia (2.4 percent), gastrointestinal symptoms (2.3 percent), neurological conditions (2.0 percent), and dermatological conditions such as rashes (0.5 percent).

Levy et al. conducted a prospective study of ADRs among 1239 patients in Jerusalem and compared this group with findings from a similar group of 11,891 U.S. patients.[62] The average number of drugs received per patient was 6.3 in Israel and 8.8 in the United States. Adverse drug reactions occurred in 28 percent of the patients and 9 percent of drug exposures in Israel. In the United States these figures were 27 percent and 5 percent respectively. Drug-attributed deaths occurred in 0.44 percent of the total (Israel and United States) population studied.

Levy and the BCDSP also examined the possible relation between long-term regular use of drugs containing aspirin and hospital admissions for gastrointestinal bleeding with no known predisposing factors and newly diagnosed peptic ulcer.[63] There was a statistically significant relationship with aspirin taken regularly for 4 or more days per week ($p<.01$) and major bleeding in patients with no evidence of duodenal ulcer. Similar results are reported for patients admitted with newly diagnosed and uncomplicated duodenal ulcer.

In another BCDSP group study (as reported by Miller), hospital admissions due to ADRs were surveyed among 7017 patients.[64] It was found that in 260 (3.7 percent) of the patients, an ADR either "caused or strongly influenced" admission to the hospital. Five drugs were most often implicated as causes of hospitalization. These were digoxin (42 patients), aspirin (24), prednisone (15), warfarin sodium (9), and guanethidine sulfate (5). The most common adverse events diagnosed were digitalis intoxication (46), gastrointestinal bleeding (24), hypoglycemia (13), rash (13), and gastritis (12). The report also states an important reminder: "Since a major segment of the outpatient population that is served by the wards monitored in this study consume large amounts of many drugs, adverse reactions requiring hospitalization for any one drug are uncommon."[64]

Ballinger and Ramsay, in 1975, surveyed 351 accidents (i.e., ADRs) occurring over a 2-year period in a psychiatric hospital.[65] Their retrospective survey revealed that 77 percent of the accidents involved females and 48 percent involved patients with organic psychoses. In 277 cases, adequate controls were available, and it was found that 75 percent of the patients having accidents had received a psychotropic drug on the day of the accident. This compares to 61 percent of the controls, who received no drug. The authors suggest that their conclusions be treated with caution, since some patients were excluded because of inadequate controls and the well-known defects of retrospective matching. The investigators' interpretation of data are somewhat speculative, but they pose the logical possibility that psychotropic drugs may predispose a patient to accidents.[65]

In 1976 another significant paper was published by McKenney and Harrison.[66] A survey was carried out in a 100-bed general medical ward of a large teaching hospital. All patients admitted to this ward over a 2-month period were interviewed by a pharmacist to identify the following:

1. Prescription and nonprescription drugs regularly administered by the patient
2. Method of administration

3. Patient's compliance with the therapeutic regimen

4. Signs and symptoms of any ADR[66]

During the 2-month study, 59 (27.3 percent) of 216 patients were found to have experienced an ADR leading to hospital admission. Adverse drug reactions and noncompliance with therapeutic regimen "appeared to be the principal drug-related factor [sic] *associated* with hospital admissions."[66] Of the 216 patients monitored, 24 (11.1 percent) experienced an ADR "to at least one drug associated with their hospital admission." However, further analysis revealed that only 17 (7.9 percent) of the 216 patients were hospitalized due to the ADR in any *causal* sense. In the case of noncompliance, 23 (10.5 percent) of the patients were admitted to the hospital due to problems derived from their behavior. Examples of noncompliance and subsequent hospitalization are anticonvulsant therapy and increased seizures as well as antidiabetic drugs and hyperglycemia or diabetic ketoacidosis. These were implicated in almost 50 percent of hospital admissions. Particular importance is assigned to the role of noncompliant behavior in ADRs and hospital admissions. This dimension of the problem has not received the attention it deserves and most certainly requires further research.

In 1976 Caranasos et al. studied drug-associated deaths.[67] A survey of 7423 inpatients revealed that 15 (0.22 percent) died of drug-related causes. During the 3-½ years of the study, a total of 1318 ADRs were identified in 928 of the patients. Thus, 12.5 percent of all patients had at least one ADR. Antineoplastic drugs, azathioprine, prednisone, and heparin sodium were the most frequently implicated drugs. Recall that Shapiro[41] found that among 6199 consecutive inpatients studied, the deaths of 27 (0.44 percent) were attributed to drugs. Caranasos et al. conclude by stating that "Drug associated deaths are relatively uncommon and usually occur in the cases of severely or terminally ill patients with potentially high toxic drugs."[67]

Armstrong et al. report on a study that focused on fatal drug reactions in patients admitted to surgical services.[68] They begin with the observation that while the frequency of fatal drug reactions in medical inpatients has received detailed attention, "little is known about their frequency in surgical patients."[68] Their report presents an estimate of the frequency of drug-related deaths in "a defined population of surgical inpatients."[68] Twenty-two hospitals were studied. In toto, 3748 men (average age, 46.9 years) and 6533 women (average age, 44.4 years) admitted to the surgical services of these hospitals were surveyed. Twenty-nine patients who died in hospitals were evaluated. Following extensive review of the case summaries, the researchers concluded that ADRs may have contributed to 19 of the deaths. Their conclusion is important enough to warrant direct quotation: "The frequency estimated from this study is 0.19 deaths/1,000 inpatients (95 percent confidence limits), 0.02 to 0.71 deaths/1,000." In sum, their data tend to support their conclusion that "drug-related death appeared to have been a rare event."[68]

Drawing on data derived from the vast experience of the BCDSP research program, Porter and Jick found that among 26,462 medical inpatients, 24, or 0.9 percent per 1000, were "considered to have died as a result of a drug or group of drugs."[69] They too found the number of deaths to be "very small relative to the number of patients exposed to individual drugs."[69] Moreover, "Among the 24 drug-induced deaths, six were attributed to anticancer drugs, five each to intravenously administered fluid therapy and digoxin, two to CNS depressant drugs, two to heparin and one each to streptokinase-streptodornase, potassium chloride, allopurinol, and cosyntropin (Synacthen)."[69]

Two French studies made a significant contribution to the literature in 1979. Auzepy et al. reported the results of severe drug complications (prevalence) among patients admitted to adult intensive care units.[70] This retrospective study covered nine teaching hospitals and 63,717 patients admitted to mixed intensive wards over a 10-year period. In this population there were 1132 drug complications (1.8 percent). Mortality was high (252 patients, or 22.2 percent), particularly among older patients. The most common ADR was anaphylactic shock and anticoagulant-induced hemorrhage.

Jaeger et al. report a single case of a 25-year-old patient who "during discontinuous treatment with a venotropic agent containing catechines suffered from intravascular hemolysis, thrombocytopaenia and acute renal failure, the course of which was favorable with treatment by haemodialysis."[71]

In another study of an international nature, Levy et al. conducted a comparative study of ADRs leading to hospitalization in Jerusalem, and Berlin.[72] This study focused on 2499 medical admissions in Jerusalem, and 2933 in Berlin. In the former population, 103 (4.1 percent), and in the latter, 167 (5.7 percent) admissions were considered to be due to ADRs. The most frequent ADRs found in Berlin were digitalis intoxication and in Jerusalem reactions to antibiotics. In the case of side effects, the most common major problems were arrhythmias, allergic reactions, bleeding, and hypoglycemia.

In 1980, Ghose carried out a survey at Cumberland Infirmary, Carlisle, United Kingdom, to ascertain the number of patients admitted for ADRs and subsequent duration of inpatient treatment in one of the "general medical units."[73] Ninety-three percent of the patients were admitted as emergencies. The most common cause of admission was ischemic heart disease (21.6 percent), acute self-poisoning (9.9 percent), and—more specific to our present interest—drug-related problems (8.8 percent). Prior to hospitalization, 18.7 percent of patients admitted to one unit experienced drug-related problems (including self-poisoning). Within the British context, it seems that, as Ghose puts it, "drug-related problems (even excluding self-poisoning) appear to be a major cause of hospitalization, comparable with bronchopulmonary diseases or complications of diabetes mellitus."[73] His conclusion finds support in the research of George and Kingscombe (Southampton, 17.2 percent)[74] and Wood et al.[75] (London, 17 percent), but, as the author notes, these figures are considerably higher than, for example, those of Miller[76] (Boston, 6 percent).

Another study, emphasizing the effects of ADRs on length of hospitalization, is that of Spino et al.,[77] who studied the effects of ADRs on the duration of hospitalization of 204 patients receiving furosemide. The mean length of stay for patients with no identified ADRs was 13.5 days; in patients experiencing one or more ADRs, it was 27.2 days. Of course, one of the methodological problems with reporting results in this manner is that it does not distinguish "whether ADRs prolonged hospital stay or whether patients had more ADRs because they were in the hospital longer."[77] The researchers identified the dependent variable by keeping the drug exposure periods constant. It is argued that when ADRs did prolong hospital stay, "there were additional factors which had a greater influence on the duration of stay than ADRs." Moreover, the authors conclude that "Intuitively, the severity of illness would appear to be the single most important determinant of hospitalization."[77] In sum, the authors find that "Since many factors influence the duration of hospitalization, including severity and nature of primary disease, presence of concomitant diseases, patients age, number of drugs, types of drugs, nature of institution, cost of hospitalization and availability of care outside of hospital, it is not surprising that ADRs had little or no effect on prolongation of stay."[77] These findings support the contention that there is a need for cautious interpretation of previous drug surveillance literature.[77]

In 1986 Lakshmanan et al. published a paper on hospital admissions "caused by iatrogenic disease." Their study focused on 834 admissions [729 patients were admitted 45 times (5.4 percent) for iatrogenic reasons]. There was a total of 47 iatrogenic occurrences, and two of the patients died (both were severely ill) as a direct result of the iatrogenic problem.[78] In toto it was found that there were 35 drug-related illnesses (4.2 percent). Of these, the drugs implicated were as follows: antihypertensives (8 cases), physiological modulators (7), cancer therapy (6), diabetes therapy (5), anticonvulsants (4), cardiac medications (2), antibiotics (2), miscellaneous (1).[78] Of these, 19 (54 percent) were classified as side effects, 8 (23 percent) were therapeutic overdoses, 7 (20 percent) were immunological, and one was a drug-disease interaction. The study found no drug-drug interactions or idiosyncratic reactions. Finally, 29 of the ADRs were "definite" and six were considered as "probable."[78]

Ives et al., in 1987, produced another important study on drug-related hospitalization. This study, carried out over a 1-year period (293 admissions), identified 45 (15.4 percent) drug-related illnesses. In 29 admissions (9.9 percent), a drug-related problem was identified as "the primary cause of hospitalization."[79] The most common types of drug-related admissions were ADRs (17 of 45, or 37.8 percent) and drug abuse 14 of 45, or 31.1 percent). Adverse drug reactions were most often found in patients over age 70.

An Italian study carried out in 1987 by the Italian Group on Intensive Care Evaluation (IGICE) monitored "clinically relevant" events possibly attributable to drug exposure.[78] The study was conducted in 27 general intensive care units for a period of 6 months. A total of 54 events identified as drug-related were found in 51 patients during hospitalization. There was an overall incidence of 1.35 percent. Furthermore, 24 of the 4537 monitored admissions were a result of "life-threatening emergencies linked to the administration of drugs."[80]

In an earlier study, Trunet et al. (1980) had reported preventable drug-related transfers from acute to intensive care.[81] They showed that 4.3 percent of 325 admissions were due to preventable ADRs or therapeutic error. In 1986 their study reported on 1651 hospitalizations and showed that 2.6 percent were preventable and drug-related. There were 97 (5.88 percent) admitted due to drug-induced illness.[82]

Triazolam, the most recent benzodiazepine used in the treatment of insomnia, received considerable attention during the 1980s. For example, in 1982, Einarson and Yoder present a single case report on a 56-year-old white female suffering "an acute exacerbation of depressive symptomatology."[83] The patient experienced tactile hallucinations and anterograde amnesia, a known effect of the benzodiazepines. The authors suggest that a triazolam syndrome does exist and idiosyncrasy "seems to be the determining factor."[83]

Carskadon et al., at Stanford University School of Medicine Sleep Research Center, conducted a study where they evaluated 13 elderly (ages 64 to 79) insomniacs receiving triazolam (0.25 mg) or flurazepam (15 mg).[84] Vigilance was impaired by flurazepam and unchanged with triazolam. It was found that both drugs improve nocturnal sleep in elderly insomniacs, but there is "a significant residual sedation" in the case of flurazepam; if daytime alertness is necessary, this drug is not recommended.

Britton and Walker report on a 49-year-old black female patient treated with cimetidine 300 mg for more than 18 months for Zollinger-Ellison syndrome.[85] This woman "experienced lethargy, dizziness, ataxia, and auditory and visual hallucinations after receiving triazolam 0.375 mg for sleep."[85] Cimetidine has been observed to decrease the "apparent" oral clearance of triazolam, "resulting in increased triazolam plasma concentrations with the potential for exaggerated pharmacologic effects."[85] It is concluded that cimetidine may be responsible "for the unusually large elimination half-life in this patient."[85] The researchers urge caution when using the combination of triazolam and cimetidine.

Psychiatric inpatients receiving triazolam for a 2-week period experienced "greatly intensified psychopathology."[86] The drug-induced behavioral changes occurred in all patients ($n = 5$) and consisted of anxiety, memory impairment, confusion, paranoid ideation, and hallucinations. The authors, recognizing the limited sample in their own research, urge more clinical studies using larger patient samples to further elucidate what they consider to be a serious clinical problem associated with these two drugs used in combination.

A major study conducted by Dubois and Brooks presents an important conclusion to this brief survey of drug-related problems.[87] In a nonrandom sample of deaths in 12 hospitals, a majority of medical reviewers classified 17 of 70 deaths in patients with pneumonia as preventable; half of those were due to inadequate fluid management or improper antibiotics. Nine of 50 deaths in inpatients with cerebrovascular accidents were preventable, and 24 percent were attributed to inadequate fluid management or inadequate management of sepsis. There were 23 preventable deaths in patients with myocardial infarction. Of these, 16 percent were judged due to inadequate control of arrhythmias and 5 percent were due to inadequate management of sepsis. Of great importance here is the conclusion that a considerable number of drug-related deaths are preventable.

The results of a highly significant 1995 study provide detailed data concerning the incidence of adverse drug events (ADEs) at two large tertiary-care hospitals, one containing 726 beds, the other having 846 beds.[88] The study population consisted of patients admitted to any of 11 units over a 6-month period. Two surgical intensive care units were studied for 3 months to provide information concerning surgical ICUs in addition to medical units. During the 6-month period there were 214,486 patient days in the two hospitals (combined adult, nonobstetric) and a total of 21,412 patient days on the study units. This meant that "10% of all patient days fell within the study sample." The authors state that:

> These 21,412 patient days included 4,031 admissions to study units. We found 247 ADE's of which 70 (28%) were preventable, and 194 potential ADE's, of which 83 (43%) were intercepted before the drug was given. . . Thus, the crude rates of ADE's were 11.5 per 1000 patient days and 6.1 per 100 admissions. When these figures were extrapolated to determine hospital-wide rates, the results were approximately 3800 ADE's between the hospitals, or an average of 1900 ADE's per hospital per year. The adjusted rates per 100 admissions were 6.5 for ADE's and 5.5 for potential ADE's. Also, in every 100 admissions there were 7.3 preventable occurrences (preventable ADE's and potential ADE's combined).[88]

Generally, this study found that ADEs were common and almost one-third were preventable. Additionally, they found that "for each preventable ADE, there were nearly three times as many potential ADEs or near misses." Errors were most often made at the prescribing level, but a large number occurred at the administrative stage. Other studies report similar findings, and all point to a serious problem found within hospital settings.[88]

Leape et al., studying the same hospitals and patient population reported in the Bates study[88] found that dosing errors were the "most common type of error, occurring more than three times as frequently as the next most numerous error type and accounting for 28 percent of all errors."[89] By far most of the wrong-dose errors (50 of 95) were found in the physician prescribing stage. Of these, 70 percent were intercepted, and only 6 percent of the 34 wrong-dose errors were intercepted at the nursing administration stage. Moreover: "Of the common errors, wrong choices and wrong doses were most likely to have actually caused an injury (42% of all ADE's), while errors in frequency or timing seldom caused an ADE."[89]

Lack of pharmacological knowledge was found to be the most common "proximal cause" of error, accounting for 72 (22 percent) of some 334 errors: "At the physician ordering stage, these included such things as lack of awareness of drug interactions (such as warfarin and trimethoprim-sulfamethoxazole) and use of inappropriately large doses of haloperidol in the elderly. At the nurse administration stage, examples were overdose of antiemetics, mixing drugs in incompatible solutions and overly rapid infusions of intravenous (IV) drugs."[89]

In sum, at the physician stage it was found that lack of knowledge of the drug, and the patient, accounted for 60 percent of all proximal causes of error. At the nursing stage, lack of pharmacological knowledge was the most common proximal cause of error, accounting for 15 percent of the problems associated with drug administration. Other nursing-related errors consisted of misuse of infusion pumps and other systems (13 percent), memory lapses (12 percent), inaccurate drug identity checking (10 percent), and faulty dose checking (10 percent).

At the pharmacy dispensing stage, failure to check drug identity (29 percent), and stocking or delivery problems (29 percent) combined to form the leading proximal cause of error. The authors conclude that, in essence, their data reveal more than individual practitioner error, for whatever reason, and indicate systems failures on a grand scale.[89] Sixteen major systems failures are identified: drug knowledge dissemination (98 errors), dose and identity checking (40 errors), patient information availability (37 errors), order transcription (29 errors), allergy defense (24 errors), medication order tracking (18 errors), interservice communication (17 errors), device use (12 errors), standardization of doses and frequencies (12 errors), standardization of drug distribution within unit (11 errors), standardization of procedures (10 errors), preparation of intravenous medications by nurses (6 errors), transfer/transition problems (physical transition of patient, 4 errors), conflict-resolution issues between different practitioners and authority figures (4 errors), staffing and excessive workloads/assignments, availability of nurses, feedback about ADEs lacking (figure missing).[89]

System failures—fragmented organizational culture—contribute to individual error. Indeed, this is the actual cultural context where decisions are made, for no one individual has *all* the responsibility for clini-

Much of the drug-related morbidity and mortality problem is the result of system failures.

cal decisions as they unfold and engage others functioning in any set of interconnected systems that make up hospital culture.

LIMITS OF THE EVIDENCE

There are important problems with most of the studies reviewed here. In 1968 Weston asked the question: "How can one reconcile the variation in incidence of less than 0.5% to 17%?"[90] She concludes that studies employ different definitions of the problem studied and are either prospective or retrospective, but rarely are they systematically rigorous or methodologically sound in their approach. Moreover, she states that *quantitative* data are lacking to provide accurate numerators and denominators "and/or accurate comparative incidence ratios."[90] She continues, "One cannot help but wonder again whether this whole question of adverse experience to drugs may not be completely out of relation to reality. One also wonders if we may have inadvertently slipped into encouraging a new period of therapeutic nihilism entirely unwarranted by the potency, effectiveness, and relative safety of many of the drugs available today."[90]

Weston's faith in the physician's clinical judgment is affirmed in her final paragraph: "Bleak though the total outlook may be, there is enough solid data not available to permit the physician who thinks for himself and who utilizes the responsible sources of drug information to make reasonable, *qualitative* judgments until such time as clearer and more unequivocal, *quantitative* data become available. But in this area, as in almost every other area of medicine, what is new about that?"[90]

Weston's paper was published more than twenty years ago and perhaps there was an argument to be made in support of her position at the time. But, what of subsequent research? Is there in fact any greater availability of reliable quantitative data to more accurately provide "numerators" and "denominators," or accurate comparative incidence ratios?

In 1974 Talley and Laventurier published a letter in *JAMA* asserting that there were indeed reliable data providing estimates of the number of deaths in the United States due to ADRs.[91] They argued that "If you assume that 0.1% of all hospital admissions will result in ADR mortality, and there were 32 million inpatient admissions in the United States in 1971 . . . it is possible to make a conservative estimate that deaths due to ADRs were approximately 30,000 in 1971."[91]

The authors then state that they believe their initial figures to be "too conservative." They cite the 1971 report of the BCDSP, which reported a mortality of 0.44 percent due to ADRs in hospitalized patients: "Extrapolating these findings to the total number of acute general hospital admissions in the United States, one can make a gross estimate that the incidence of lethal ADRs ranges from a low of 60,000 (0.18% incidence) to a high of 140,000 (0.44% incidence) for hospitalized patients. . . . We can conjecture the range of 60,000 to 140,000 ADR deaths to be probably extremely conservative since we have no data measuring drug-induced deaths in the ambulatory and extended care populations."[91]

As Talley and Laventurier observed, their paper touched off a storm of controversy and became a "cause celebre." C. Joseph Stetler of the Pharmaceutical Manufacturers Association replied to their letter and took issue with the origins of the 30,000 ADR death estimate.[92] In short, Stetler argues that Talley and Laventurier have confused the issue through their inattention to the specifics of the studies they cite as evidence of the magnitude of the ADR problem. Stetler's argument is persuasive given the convoluted history of the debates, and the reader is urged to read the letters in question. Suffice it to say the argument is essentially one of the reliability and validity of epidemiological data. But, one does need to emphasize that it is also an argument concerning the *interpretation* of data—an issue that pervades all studies reviewed here. Stetler suggests a qualified estimate of 2000 to 3000 deaths "associated with drug reactions in patients suffering from apparently nonlethal diseases."[92]

This debate serves to illustrate the controversial nature of drug-induced illness. Clearly the issues are methodological and, to some extent, ideological. As Jick has correctly observed, "[t]he problem of adverse drug reactions is of broad scientific, political, economic and moral concern."[93] Jick, in 1974, asserted that data derived from the BCDSP can be used "to determine with considerable accuracy how often drugs are used and how toxic they are."[93] Moreover, "Although these data do not provide direct quantitation of the proportion of drug toxicity that is either "unnecessary" or due to "promotional excesses" of the drug industry, they generally confirm the notion that the overall problem of drug toxicity is of substantial magnitude."[93]

The methods used by the BCDSP to obtain information on short-term drug toxicity are twofold. First, all attending physicians' judgments that an ADR had taken place were recorded by nurse-monitors. The circumstances are investigated "and a tentative judgment is made regarding the likelihood that the drug implicated has actually caused the event reported."[93] Second, the means used to quantify acute drug toxicity "involves analysis of the entire body of data, relating drug exposures to a series of adverse events that have been recorded, regardless of any judgment about drug cause."[93]

In the case of clinical judgments made by physicians, causality is usually based on "the time relation between the administration of the drug and the appearance and disappearance of an event, together with the knowledge of the pharmacologic properties of the drug implicated."[204] Moreover, "In many cases clinical events can be attributed to a drug with certainty. For example, if an intravenous infusion is begun and phlebitis develops at the site of infusion, a causal connection is certain. If chills and fever develop shortly after the start of a blood transfusion or if acute anaphylaxis or deafness develops while a drug infusion is being given or if hypoglycemia develops after insulin therapy a causal connection is again virtually certain."[93]

The longitudinal, comprehensive nature of the BCDSP involves quantitative analysis of specific drugs, with particular attention to gross rates of efficacy and toxicity in addition to consideration of the influence of dosage, route of administration, patient characteristics, and assessment of interaction between drugs.[94]

Karch and Lasagna, in 1975, fault ADR studies for their lack of terminological uniformity, criteria for evaluation, confusion between the event in question and the patient's underlying illness, complications from polypharmacy (i.e., confounding inferences and interpretation), subjectivity of symptomatic complaints, lack of proper controls, and, in the extreme, imagined symptoms often taken as "real."[95] "Also, the problem of establishing a clear cause and effect relationship between the drug and the reaction; This is often difficult or impossible. The interpretation involves complex clinical judgments, usually based on limited data and without the benefit of standardized mechanisms for identifying adverse drug reactions."[95]

Karch and Lasagna correctly note that we must develop greater consistency and clarity in the definition of the "firmness" of the link between drug and effect. As we have seen in the literature review section, terms like _possible, probable, conditional, doubtful,_ and _definite_ abound. But upon close scrutiny, it is clear that these terms are used quite vaguely, often with the assumption that their meaning is generally understood. The authors also argue that almost all surveys on the incidence of ADRs have focused on hospitalized patients on acute medical wards. In our review we have noted exceptions to this criticism. Also criticized by Karch and Lasagna is the weight placed on the clinical judgment of the physician. It is reasonably well known that clinical judgment is not, by any means, too reliable and must be questioned as a major source of valid data.[96] This is particularly true for judgments a propos of pharmaceutical agents. Karch and Lasagna draw a number of conclusions from their review of the literature (up to 1975). It is instructive to reflect upon them in some detail. Their analysis suggests that

1. Estimates of the magnitude of the problem of adverse drug reactions are characterized by a data base that is incomplete, arbitrary, unrepresentative and uncontrolled and by cost estimates whose accuracy is questionable.

2. Most reported drug reactions whether minor or serious, seem to be due to older, standard, and relatively unpromoted drugs.

3. It is not clear how much of the problem results from inept prescribing by physicians and how much is preventable by decreasing such prescribing, or by educating doctors and patients about drug-drug interactions, drug-disease interactions, and scrupulous adherence to directions.

4. Most drug reactions are difficult to categorize unequivocally as to cause, except in the case of gross overdosage, accidental or intentional.[96]

They conclude their discussion by stating that we need an in-depth analysis of the following:

1. The operational identification of drug reactions.

2. A method for assigning a reaction causally to a specific drug. No one has described a logical system for assigning blame to a drug for an untoward event. What is needed is a systematic approach—perhaps an algorithm that would analyze each reproducible agreement on drug reaction.

3. The problems involved in evaluating the causes of drug reactions.

4. The extent to which adverse reactions are a reflection of inherently imperfect drugs rather than of improper use.

5. The need for data on control groups for estimates of the 'background noise' that should be subtracted from the observed incidence.

6. Stratification of populations, since the nature of drugs, the risks-benefit situations etc., will differ greatly (e.g., a cancer hospital is obviously different from an obstetrical hospital).

7. Quantification of the benefit derived from drugs and the costs of under-prescribing drugs."[96]

Following this critique of ADR research, Karch et al. published a second paper extending their argument with some research of their own.[97] Their purpose was to demonstrate the accuracy or inaccuracy of clinical judgments in the identification of ADRs. To address this problem, they had three clinical pharmacologists independently evaluate 60 selected cases to determine if medication, alcohol, or "recreational drugs" had caused hospitalization.

In effect, the results are somewhat surprising. The three clinical pharmacologists agreed on only 30 cases (50 percent), and 27 of these were considered to be unrelated to medications. In 19 of the 20 cases where disagreement existed, the clinical pharmacologists "disagreed on whether or not a medication or alcohol-related event had occurred at all."[97] Moreover, the clinical pharmacologists "disagreed with the physicians treating the patient in 22% to 37% of the cases, but because of the differences among the pharmacologists, the treating physicians agreed with at least one of them in 95% of the cases. Complete agreement between the clinical pharmacologists and the treating physicians occurred in 47% of the cases."[97] The authors conclude that the evaluation of ADRs is "subjective and unprecise. The accurate identification of ADRs awaits the development of an objective technique for recognizing ADRs."[97]

> The rate of adverse drug reactions mandates that each practitioner make rational decisions on a patient-by-patient basis.

In 1982 four researchers in the Medical Department, Drug Monitoring, Ciba-Geigy carried out a comprehensive study of "the quality and completeness of articles on adverse drug reactions."[98] In this study 5737 articles from 80 countries published between 1972 and 1979 were evaluated. The researchers specifically examined articles that related to Ciba-Geigy products that they claim "are used in all branches of medicine all over the world [and] articles relating to them are likely to be representative of all articles on adverse drug reactions."[98]

Only 61 percent of the articles reviewed contained information on the number of patients treated and the number experiencing ADRs. These data are essential for calculating the incidence of ADRs. Additionally, in only 55 percent of the papers could the researchers calculate the incidence of a particular ADR. They conclude:

> Our results show that many articles on large numbers of patients treated with a particular drug and containing information on adverse drug reactions lack important data. We think that most researchers would have basic information on the number of patients treated, the number who have adverse drug reactions, the number of adverse reactions, the age of the patients, the dose of the drug, the duration of treatment, and the galenic form of the drug, yet only 19% of the articles contained all this information. Nor could we find any evidence that things are improving. Our results show that this is a problem in all countries where large numbers of studies are undertaken and in most international journals.[98]

There can be no doubt that drug-related morbidity is a highly significant problem. Studies examined in this chapter attest to both the magnitude and severity of the problem. Thus, while there is some controversy over the precise amount of drug-related morbidity and mortality, there is general agreement that the problem is significant enough to warrant very serious attention by all those engaged in pharmacotherapy of any kind.

Human costs associated with the quality of life, health, and general well-being are clearly of utmost importance to any health care system professing to be humane and caring. Drug-related morbidity and mortality are clearly not in anyone's best interest, and all health care practitioners should strive to reduce the harmful effects of "drug misadventuring."

Pharmaceutical care practice makes an individual responsible for the drug-related needs of patients in such a way a that drug therapy can be monitored in enough detail, and with a rational, systematic approach, that all drug therapy problems, actual and potential, can be identified, their causes determined, and solutions for their resolution offered. But, even more important, pharmaceutical care practice requires the practitioner to *prevent* drug therapy problems, like those reported here, from developing in the first place.

REFERENCES

1. Manasse, H.R. Jr. Medication use in an imperfect world: Drug misadventuring as an issue of public policy: Part I. *Am J Hosp Pharm* 1989; 46:930.

2. Scarborough, J., ed. *Folklore and Folkmedicines.* Madison, WI American Institute of the History of Pharmacy, 1987; Sneader, W. *Drug Development: From Laboratory to Clinic.* New York: Wiley; 1986; Sneader, W. *Drug Discovery: The Evolution of Modern Medicines.* Chichester, England: John Wiley & Sons, 1985.

3. Illich, I. *Limits to Medicine.* London: Marion Boyars; 1976.

4. Habakkuk, H.J. English population in the eighteenth century. *Econ Hist Rev* 1953; 6:117–133.

5. Dubos, R. *Mirage of Health.* New York: Doubleday; 1959. See also his *Man Adapting.* New Haven, CT: Yale University Press; 1965; and *Man Medicine and Environment.* London: Pall Mall Press; 1968.

6. Griffith, T. *Population Problems in the Age of Malthus.* London: Frank Cass; 1967.

7. McKeown, T. *The Modern Rise of Population.* London: Edward Arnold; 1976. See also his *The Role of Medicine: Dream. Mirage or Nemesis.* London: Nuffield Provincial Hospitals Trust; 1976.

8. McKinlay, J.B., McKinlay, S.B. Medical measures and the decline of mortality, in Conrad, P., Kern, R., eds. *The Sociology of Health and Illness,* 2d ed. New York: St. Martin's Press; 1986.

9. McKeown, T., Brown R.G., Record, R.G., and Turner R.D. et al. An interpretation of the decline of mortality in England and Wales during the twentieth century. *Population Studies,* 1975, 29:391–422. Cited in McKinlay and McKinlay, Ref. 12, p. 12.

10. Burger, A. *Drugs and People: Medications, Their History and Origins and the Way They Act.* Charlottesville, VA: University of Virginia Press; 1986.

11. Ackerknecht, E.H. *Therapeutics: From the Primitive to the Twentieth Century.* New York: Hafner; 1973.

12. Sigerist, H.E. *Primitive and Archaic Medicine.* New York: Oxford University Press; 1967.

13. Adams, J.G. *The Societal Impact of Pharmaceuticals: An Overview, Cost-Effectiveness of Pharmaceuticals.* Report Series. Washington, DC: Pharmaceutical Manufacturers Association; 1984.

14. King, L.S., ed. *A History of Medicine.* Harmondsworth, England: Penguin Books; 1971.

15. Sneader, W. *Drug Discovery: The Evolution of Modern Medicines.* Chichester, England: Wiley; 1985. For a comprehensive account of this accomplishment and its problems, see Sneader, W. *Drug Development,* Ref. 2.

16. Parascandola, J., ed. *The History of Antibiotics: A Symposium.* Madison, WI: American Institute of the History of Pharmacy; 1980.

17. Drexler, K.E. *Engines of Creation: The Coming Era of Nanotechnology.* New York: Anchor Books; 1986.

18. Montague, M.J. The Impact of Biotechnology on the Practice of Pharmacy in the Year 2000. Paper presented at the *Pharmacy in the 21st Century Conference.* Williamsburg, VA: October 11–14, 1989.

19. Halperin, J.A. Challenge, opportunity, promise and risk: The pharmaceutical industry moving toward the 21st century. *Drug Int J* 1988; Vol 22:25–32. Cited in Ref. 1.

20. Check, W.A. New drugs and drug delivery systems in the year 2000, in Bezold, C., et al., eds. *Pharmacy in the 21st Century.* Bethesda, MD: Institute for Alternative Futures, 1985.

21. Ackerknecht, E.H. Zur Geschichte der Iatrogenen Erkrankungen der Nerven systems. *Rev Ther* 1970; 27(6):345–346. See also his Zur Geschichte der Iatrogenen Krankheiten. *Gesnerus* 1970; 27:57–63.

22. For detailed discussion of the historical dimension of clinical iatrogenesis, see the following works: D'Arcy, P.F., Griffin, J.P. *Iatrogesic Diseases.* New York: Oxford University Press; 1972; Moser, R.H. *The Disease of Medical Progress: A Study of Iatrogenic Disease.* Springfield, IL: Thomas; 1969. Duchesnay, G. *Le Risque Therapeutique.* Paris: Doin; 1954. Heintz, R. *Erkrankungen durch Arzneimittel: Diagnostik, Klinik, Pathogenese, Therapie.* Stuttgart: Thieme; 1978.

23. Barr, D.P. Hazards of modern diagnosis and therapy—The price we pay. *JAMA* 1955; p 1452.

24. Moser, R.H. Disease of medical progress. *N Engl J Med* 1956; pp 606–614.

25. Blankenhorn, M.A., Knowles, H.C. Periarteritis nodosa: Recognition and clinical symptoms. *Ann Intern Med* 1954; 41:887–892.

26. Report of the Subcommittee on Blood Dyscrasias of Committee on Research, Council on Drugs. Blood dyscrasias associated with promazine hydrochloride therapy. *JAMA* 1957; 165:685–686.

27. Report of the Subcommittee on Blood Dyscrasias of Committee on Research, Council on Drugs. Blood dyscrasias associated with chloramphenicol therapy. *JAMA* 1960; 172:2044–2045.

28. Ersler, A.J., Wintrobe, M.W. Detection and prevention of drug-induced blood dyscrasias. *JAMA* 1963; 181:114–119.

29. MacDonald, M.G., MacKay, B.R. Adverse drug reactions: Experience of Mary Fletcher Hospital during 1962. *JAMA* 1964; l90:1071–1074.

30. Seidl, L.G., Cluff, L.E., Thornton, G., et al. Epidemiological studies of adverse drug reactions. *Am J Public Health* 1965; 55:1170–1175.

31. Cluff, L.E., Thoburn, R., Johnson, J.E., et al. Studies on the epidemiology of adverse drug reactions: Methods of surveillance. *JAMA* 1964; 144–151.

32. Lenz, W. Malformations caused by drugs in pregnancy. *Am J Dis Child* 1966; 112:99–106.

33. Hoddinott, B.C., Gowdey, C.W., Coulter, W.K., et al. Drug reactions and errors in administration on a medical ward. *Can Med Assoc J* 1967; 97:1001–1006.

34. Ogilvie, R.I., Ruedy, J. Adverse drug reactions during hospitalization. *Can Med Assoc J* 1967; 97:1450–1457.

35. Registry of Adverse Drug Reactions. Report of the Drug Reaction Registry Subcommittee of the Greater Philadelphia Committee for Medical-Pharmaceutical Sciences. *JAMA* 1968; 203:85–88.

36. Batsakis J.G., Preston J.A., Briere, R.O., et al. Iatrogenic aberrations of serum enzyme activity. *Clin Biochem* 1968; 125–133.

37. Borda, I.T., Slone, D., Jick, H. Assessment of adverse reactions within a drug surveillance program. *JAMA* 1968; 205:645–647.

38. Sweetnam, R. Corticosteroid arthropathy and tendon rupture. *J Bone Joint Surg* 1969; 51:397–398.

39. Hurwitz, N. Predisposing factors in adverse reactions to drugs. *Br Med J* 1969; 536–539.

40. Hurwitz, N. Admissions to hospital due to drugs. *Br Med J* 1969; 539–540.

41. Shapiro, S., Slone, D., Lewis, G.P., et al. Fatal drug reactions among medical inpatients. *JAMA* 1971; 216:467–472.

42. Caranasos, G.J., Stewart R.B., Cluff, L.E., et al. Drug-induced illness leading to hospitalization. *JAMA* 1974; 228:713–717.

43. Jick, H., Slone, D., Borda, I.T., et al. Efficacy and toxicity of heparin in relation to age and sex. *N Engl J Med* 1968; 279–284.

44. Shapiro, S., Slone, D., Lewis, G.P., et al. The epidemiology of digoxin: A study in three Boston hospitals. *J Chronic Dis* 1969; 22:361.

45. Jick, H., Slone, D., Shapiro, S., et al. Clinical effects of hypnotics. I. A controlled clinical trial. *JAMA* 1969; 209:2013.

46. Shapiro, S., Slone, D., Lewis, G.P., et al. Clinical effects of hypnotics. II. An epidemiological study. *JAMA* 1969; 209:2016.

47. Slone, D. Intravenously given ethacrynic acid and gastrointestinal bleeding. *JAMA* 1969; 209:1668.

48. Shapiro, S. Drug rash with ampicillin and other penicillins. *Lancet* 1969; 2:969.

49. Lewis, G.P., Jusko, W.J., Graves, L., et al. Prednisone side-effects and serum protein levels. A collaborative study. *Lancet* 1971; 2:778–780.

50. Boston Collaborative Drug Surveillance Program. Adverse reactions to the tricyclic-antidepressant drugs. *Lancet* 1972; 1:529.

51. Boston Collaborative Drug Surveillance Program. Tetracycline and drug-attributed rises in blood urea nitrogen. *JAMA* 1972; 220:377.

52. Boston Collaborative Drug Surveillance Program. Acute reactions to prednisone in relation to dosage. *Clin Pharmacol Ther* 1972; 13:694.

53. Boston Collaborative Drug Surveillance Program. Drug induced convulsions. *Lancet* 1972; 2:677.

54. Boston Collaborative Drug Surveillance Program. Coffee drinking and acute myocardial infarction. *Lancet* 1972; 2:1278.

55. Boston Collaborative Drug Surveillance Program. Clinical depression of the central nervous system due to diazepam and chlordiazepoxide in relation to cigarette smoking and age. *N Engl J Med* 1973; 288:277.

56. Boston Collaborative Drug Surveillance Program. Decreased clinical efficacy of propoxyphene in cigarette smokers. *Clin Pharmacol Ther* 1973; 14:259.

57. Boston Collaborative Drug Surveillance Program. Drug induced deafness. *JAMA* 1973; 224:515.

58. Boston Collaborative Drug Surveillance Program. Drug induced anaphylaxis. *JAMA* 1973; 224:613.

59. Boston Collaborative Drug Surveillance Program. Drug-induced extrapyramidal symptoms. *JAMA* 1973; 224:889.

60. Boston Collaborative Drug Surveillance Program. Oral contraceptives and venous thromboembolic diseases, surgically confirmed gallbladder disease and breast tumors. *Lancet* 1973; 1:1399.

61. Greenblatt, D.J., Koch-Weser, J. Adverse reactions to spironolactone. A report from the Boston Collaborative Drug Surveillance Program. *JAMA* 1973; 225:40.

62. Levy, M., Nir, I., Birnbaum, D., et al. Adverse reactions to drugs in hospitalized medical patients: A comparative study. *Isr J Med Sci* 1973; 9:617.

63. Levy, M., Boston Collaborative Drug Surveillance Program. Aspirin use in patients with major upper gastrointestinal bleeding and peptic ulcer. *N Engl J Med* 1974; 290:1158–1162.

64. Miller, R., Boston Collaborative Drug Surveillance Program. Hospital admissions due to adverse drug reactions. *Arch Intern Med* 1974; 134:219–233.

65. Ballinger, B., Ramsay, A. Accidents and drug treatment in a psychiatric hospital. *Br J Psychiatry* 1975; 126:462–463.

66. McKenney, J.M., Harrison, W.L. Drug-related hospital admissions. *Am J Hosp Pharm* 1976; 33:792–795.

67. Caranasos, G., May, F.E., Stewart, R.B., et al. Drug-associated deaths of medical inpatients. *Arch Intern Med* 1976; 136:872–875.

68. Armstrong, B., Dinan, B., Jick, H., et al. Fatal drug reactions in patients admitted to surgical services. *Am J Surg* 1976; 132:643–645.

69. Porter, J., Jick, H. Drug-related deaths among medical inpatients. *JAMA* 1977; 237(9):879–881.

70. Auzepy, P.H., Durocher, A., Gay, R., et al. Accidents medicamenteux graves chez l'adulte: Incidence actuelle dans le recrutement des unites de reanimation. *Nouvelle Presse Med* 1979; 8(16):1315–1318.

71. Jaeger, A., Rodier, L., Tempe, J.D., et al. Hemolyse aigue immunoallergique, thrombopenie et insuffi-

sance renale aigue dues a un traitment par les catechines. *Nouvelle Presse Med* 1979; 8:3741–3743.

72. Levy, M., Kewitz, H., Altwein, W., et al. Hospital admissions due to adverse drug reactions: A comparative study from Jerusalem and Berlin. *Eur J Clin Pharmacol* 1980; 17:25–31.

73. Ghose, K. Hospital bed occupancy due to drug-related problems. *J R Soc Med* 1980; 73:853–856.

74. George, C.F., Kingscombe, P.M. Can adverse drug reactions be prevented? *Drug and Therapeutics Bulletin*. 1980; 18(Suppl 3):288–290.

75. Wood, S.M., Turner, P., Vere, D. Clinical Pharmacology and general patient care in two teaching hospitals. *J R Soc Med* 1980; 73(5):355–358.

76. Miller, R. and Boston Drug Surveillance Program. Hospital admissions due to adverse drug reactions. *Arch Intern Med* 1974; 134:219–233.

77. Spino, M. Effect of adverse drug reactions on the length of hospitalization. *Am J Hosp Pharm* 1978; 35:1060–1064.

78. Lakshmanan, M.C., Hershey, C.O., Breslau, D. Hospital admissions caused by iatrogenic disease. *Arch Intern Med* 1986; 146:1931–1934.

79. Ives, T.J., Bentz, E.J., Gwyther, R.E. Drug-related admissions to a family medicine inpatient service. *Arch Intern Med* 1987; 147:1117–1120.

80. Italian Group on Intensive Care Evaluation (IGICE). Epidemiology of adverse drug reactions in intensive care units: A multicentre prospective survey. *Eur J Clin Pharmacol* 1987; 31:507–512.

81. Trunet, P., LeGall, J.R., Lhoste, F., et al. The role of iatrogenic disease in admission to intensive care. *JAMA* 1980; 244:2617–2620.

82. Trunet, P., Borda, I.T., Rouget, A.V., et al. The role of drug-induced illness in admission to an intensive care unit. *Intens Care Med* 1986; 12:43–46.

83. Einarson, T.R., Yoder, E.S. Triazolam psychosis— A syndrome? *Drug Intell Clin Pharm* 1982; 16:330.

84. Carskadon, M.A., Seidel, W.F., Greenblatt, D.J., et al. Daytime carryover of triazolam and flurazepam in elderly insomniacs. *Sleep* 1982; 5:361–371.

85. Britton, M.L., Waller, E.S. Central nervous system toxicity associated with concurrent use of triazolam and cimetidine. *Drug Intell Clin Pharm* 1985; 19: 666–668.

86. Soldatos, C., Sakkas, P.N., Bergiannaki, J.D., et al. Behavioral side effects of triazolam in psychiatric inpatients: Report of five cases. *Drug Intell Clin Pharm* 1986; 20:294–297.

87. Dubois, R.W., Brook, R.H. Preventable deaths: Who, how often, and why? *Ann Intern Med* 1988; 109:582–589.

88. Jick, H., Versey, M.P. Case-control studies in the evaluation of drug-induced illness. *Am J Epidemiol* 1978; 107:1–7.

89. In reference to the problems of interpretation, it may very well be useful to critically examine the philo-sophical issues raised by the contemporary study of hermeneutics. See for example: Ricoeur, P. *Herme-neutics and the Human Sciences*, edited and translated by Thompson, J.B. Cambridge, England: Cam-bridge University Press; 1981. Bernstein, R.J. *Beyond Objectivism and Relativism: Science, Hermeneutics, and Praxis*. Philadelphia: University of Pennsylvania Press; 1983.

90. Weston, J.K. The present status of adverse drug reaction reporting. *JAMA* 1968; 203:89–91.

91. Talley, R.B., Laventurier, M.F. Drug induced ill-ness. (letter). *JAMA* 1974; 229:1043. [The authors refer to their paper "Drug utilization and peer review in San Joaquin," read before the American Associa-tion of Foundations for Medical Care, Sea Island, GA., Aug. 28, 1972.

92. Stetler, C.J. Letter to editor. *JAMA* 1974; 229: 1043–1044.

93. Jick, H. Drugs—remarkably nontoxic. *N Engl J Med* 1974; 824–827.

94. Jick, H., Miettinen, O.S., Shapiro, S., et al. Com-prehensive drug surveillance. *JAMA* 1970; 213: 1455–1460.

95. Karch, F.E., Lasagna, L. Adverse drug reactions. *JAMA* 1975; 234:1236–1241.

96. See, for example, Schwartz, S., Griffin, T. *Medical Thinking: The Psychology of Medical Judgment and Decision-Making*. New York: Springer Verlag; 1986. Dowie, J., Elstein, A., eds. *Professional Judgment: A Reader in Clinical Decision Making*, Cambridge, England: Cambridge University Press, 1988. Cebul, R.D., Beck, L.H., eds. *Teaching Clinical Decision Making*. New York: Praeger; 1985. Gale, J., Mars-den, P. *Medical Diagnosis: From Student to Clinician*. Oxford, England: Oxford University Press; 1983.

97. Karch, F.E., Smith, C.L., Kerzner, B., et al. Adverse drug reactions—a matter of opinion. *Clin Pharmacol Ther* 1976; 19:489–492.

98. Venulet, J., Blattner, R., von-Bulow, J., et al. How good are articles on adverse drug reactions? *Br Med J*, 1982, 284:252–254.

RECOMMENDED READINGS

Hartzema, A.G., Porta, M.S., Tilson H.H., eds., *Pharma-coepidemiology: An Introduction*, 2d ed. Cincinnati, OH: Harvey Whitney Books; 1990.

Stewart, R.B. *Tragedies from Drug Therapy*. Springfield, IL: Charles C. Thomas; 1985.

Strom, B., ed. *Pharmoepidemiology*. New York: Churchill Livingstone; 1990.

CHAPTER THREE

IDENTIFYING, RESOLVING, AND PREVENTING DRUG THERAPY PROBLEMS: THE PHARMACIST'S RESPONSIBILITY

INTRODUCTION TO DRUG THERAPY PROBLEMS

Chapter 2 reviewed and summarized our present understanding of the enormous negative impact that drug-related morbidity and mortality have on the health and welfare of our society. Clearly, there is a substantial social need to address this insidious problem directly. However, there are several aspects of our health care systems and industry that have inhibited any effective methods aimed at addressing the widespread harm and financial impact of drug-related morbidity and mortality. These include the following:

1. The causes of drug-related morbidity and mortality are multi-faceted.
2. There is little agreement among various practitioners as to the causes of drug-related morbidity and mortality.
3. Patients suffer from drug-related morbidity and mortality because of system failures in the use of pharmaceuticals.
4. Most patient care practitioners function in an interconnected health care system.
5. No single health care practitioner has accepted primary responsibility for drug-related morbidity and mortality.

On a population level, drug-related morbidity and mortality is made up of many drug therapy problems that occur at the individual patient level. Only by addressing drug therapy problems on an individual patient-by-patient basis can we hope to impact the present social

Pharmaceutical care is a unique approach to the complex problem of drug-related morbidity and mortality.

The practice philosophy is the connection between theory and practice.

problem of drug-related morbidity and mortality. Drug-related morbidity and mortality represents a set of multifaceted, unique, systemic, pharmacological, scientific, social, ethical, economical, cultural, ethnic, and communicative problems. Any solution designed to address problems of this nature must surely represent such a multifaceted approach. Pharmaceutical provides the means by which the practitioner is able to address problems of this broad scope.

To this point, the philosophy of pharmaceutical care includes rather general precepts of meeting a social need, taking a patient-centered approach, and caring for a patient's drug-related needs. It is now time to focus on the last precept in the philosophy which is quite precise and establishes *specific* practitioner responsibilities. The practitioner has three different responsibilities:

1. To make sure the patient's drug therapy is appropriately indicated, the most effective available, the safest possible, and able to be taken as intended.
2. To identify, resolve, and prevent any drug therapy problems that might interfere with the first set of responsibilities.
3. To make sure the patient's goals of therapy are met and optimal outcomes are realized.

We have described the principles that define the philosophy of pharmaceutical care practice. This philosophy remains at a level of abstraction until the practitioner *acts* in a manner consistent with this philosophy and thereby makes the essential connection between theory and practice. This is accomplished by first understanding the relationship between the three responsibilities described above which are explained in this chapter and by becoming proficient at the patient care process described in Chap. 4. With these tools the practitioner can begin to provide pharmaceutical care to a patient.

The first responsibility, to ensure that all of a patient's drug therapy is appropriately indicated, the most effective available, the safest possible, and that it can be taken as intended, is a significant responsibility. To accomplish this, the practitioner must be able to take into account numerous patient characteristics which can impact outcomes. The number of medical conditions which require consideration can be enormous, and the categories of drug therapies available keep expanding exponentially. None of this occurs in a vacuum. The practitioner who assumes this responsibility must be aware that it requires cooperation and participation of not only the patient, but many other health care providers, the support of information systems, and much, much more.

But perhaps, most importantly, assuming this responsibility requires the practitioner be prepared and qualified to make decisions which can lead to dramatically positive and/or negative consequences. Therefore the practitioner needs a decision-making process which promotes consistent, systematic, comprehensive, and well-reasoned results.

The most effective decision-making process we have found that allows the practitioner to assume this responsibility is the clinical process that is already utilized by nurses and physicians to assume their patient care responsibilities. This problem-solving process is described as the Pharmacist's Workup of Drug Therapy and is the organizing force for the patient care process in pharmaceutical care. However, for this process to have meaning, it is necessary to explain the centrality of drug therapy problems.

A problem-solving process is relatively useless until a unique set of problems, in this case, health care problems generally, and drug therapy problems specifically, are defined as the focus of this activity. This is why we have devoted an entire chapter to understanding drug therapy problems. The next responsibility is to identify, resolve, and most importantly, prevent drug therapy problems from interfering with positive patient outcomes.

The last of the three responsibilities, to make sure the patient's goals of therapy are met and optimal outcomes are realized, are again, a by-product of the problem-solving process described above. These responsibilities will be met if, and when, the practitioner is able to identify, resolve, and prevent all actual and potential drug therapy problems from occurring. Drug therapy problems become the framework in which the practitioner works to organize and apply the very sophisticated and extensive knowledge, skills and experience necessary to accomplish this objective.

A DRUG THERAPY PROBLEM DEFINED

We will begin by explaining exactly what a drug therapy problem is. A drug therapy problem is any undesirable event experienced by the patient that involves or is suspected to involve drug therapy and that actually or potentially interferes with a desired patient outcome.[1]

In this context, pharmacists providing pharmaceutical care use the term *problem* to denote a drug-related event amenable to detection, treatment, or prevention. A drug therapy problem always has two primary components:

> Drug therapy problems interfere with desired patient outcomes.

1. An undesirable event or risk of an event experienced by the patient. This event can take the form of a medical complaint, symptom, diagnosis, disease, impairment, disability, or syndrome. The event can be the result of psychological, physiological, sociocultural, or economic conditions.[1]
2. Some relationship must exist (or be suspected to exist) between the undesirable patient event and drug therapy. This relationship can be (a) the consequence of drug therapy, suggesting an association or even a cause and effect relationship, or (b) an event that requires drug therapy for its resolution or prevention.[1]

All drug therapy problems can be classified into one of seven categories of drug therapy problems.

Pharmacists frequently perceive that an infinite number of different types of drug therapy problems exist. This might seem logical due to the fact that, during 1995, there were 1.58 billion prescriptions dispensed from community pharmacies throughout the United States.[2] However, although many thousands of different drug products are available, we have been able to identify only seven major categories of drug therapy problems. The categories we have created are based on a description of the patient's problem and not the drug's problem or the practitioner's problem. The traditional criteria for categorizing drug therapy problems include the right dose, route, frequency, and duration of drug therapy, making the drug product and not the patient the focus of the pharmacist's problem-solving efforts. Instead, we think it is very important that both the empirical problem as well as the patient's perception of the problem become the focus of all the deductive energies of the pharmacist. Pharmacists providing pharmaceutical care should have the skills, knowledge, and support systems to identify, prevent, and resolve the seven types of drug therapy problems that can occur in their patients.

The key to the pharmacist's ability to identify drug therapy problems and to create a plan to appropriately respond to the drug-related needs of individual patients is to begin with the patient. Patients have a number of different health care needs that they present to the pharmacist, and it is important for the pharmacist to differentiate the needs he or she can address from those for which another practitioner is more appropriately responsible. Therefore, the pharmacist must be able to differentiate drug-related needs from other, more general health care needs. To accomplish this the pharmacist needs very specific and complete information from the patient. We should not forget that this information belongs to the patient. A therapeutic relationship is necessary for the patient and the pharmacist to work together to establish and achieve desired therapeutic goals. For a moment, let us assume such a relationship has been developed and that the necessary information can be elicited from the patient. Just how does the pharmacist identify the patient's drug-related needs and then translate those into a problem solving format so that action can be taken to resolve the drug therapy problem, prevent future problems, or meet desired drug therapy goals?

A therapeutic relationship is required to determine a patient's understanding, expectations, and concerns about drug therapy.

TRANSLATING DRUG-RELATED NEEDS INTO DRUG THERAPY PROBLEMS

Drug therapy problems are the "heart and soul" of the practice of pharmaceutical care.

Drug-related needs include any concerns, expectations, or lack of understanding identified by the patient or practitioner and related to a drug substance. A drug substance can be any product obtained via a prescription or purchased as a nonprescription drug item. A drug product can include food supplements, vitamins, and other products taken internally, products applied topically, and even naturally occurring products. Any drug-related need expressed by a patient can become a drug therapy problem if that need is not appropriately addressed. Therefore it is most important for a pharmacist to identify a patient's drug-related need early and to meet that need. As meeting a patient's drug-related needs is the most basic responsibility of a pharmacist providing pharmaceutical care, we will examine drug-related needs in detail.

It is important to effectively and efficiently identify these needs. This is why establishing therapeutic relationships with patients is the cornerstone of the pharmaceutical care encounter. The major objective of the initial discussion with patients is to determine what they understand about drug therapy, what expectations they have about therapy, and what concerns they may have. This information allows the pharmacist to determine if any drug therapy needs exist. For the pharmacist to perform his or her responsibilities, it is necessary to translate the patient's drug-related needs into a problem-solving format. This allows the pharmacist to address the patient's needs using the knowledge, skills, and experience he or she has to determine if any drug therapy problems exist and to prevent future problems from developing. During this translation step, the pharmacist must assess whether the patient understands why he or she is taking the medication (the *indication* for the drug), if patient expectations are consistent with the stated *effectiveness* of the medication, and if the concerns the patient might have about taking the drug are consistent with the *safety* profile of the medication. All of this patient-specific information will then help the pharmacist to determine if the patient can adhere to the drug regimen as designed. This organized, structured translation step from patient-specific information gathering to professional problem-solving responsibilities describes the organized, structured, rational approach to drug therapy that is central to pharmaceutical care practice. This translation step is summarized in Table 3-1, beginning at the left and moving to the right.

All patients require drug therapy to be (1) appropriately indicated, (2) effective, (3) safe, and (4) convenient.

TABLE 3-1 TRANSLATING DRUG-RELATED NEEDS INTO DRUG THERAPY PROBLEMS

PATIENT'S EXPRESSION	DRUG-RELATED NEEDS	DRUG THERAPY PROBLEMS
Understanding	Indication	1. Additional drug therapy
		2. Unnecessary drug therapy
Expectations	Effectiveness	3. Wrong drug
		4. Dosage too low
Concerns	Safety	5. Adverse drug reaction
		6. Dosage too high
Behavior	Compliance	7. Compliance

The pharmacist depends, in large part, on the patient to provide the information needed to make a comprehensive assessment of the patient's drug-related needs and determine if the patient has a drug therapy problem. This is why the therapeutic relationship between the patient and the pharmacist is so important. Without the proper information, inappropriate decisions will be made and the wrong action taken. The process whereby the pharmacist elicits the appropriate information to assess the patient's drug-related needs is the patient care process. Before this process is examined in detail, it is necessary to have a very clear understanding of the purpose for it—namely, to identify, resolve, and prevent drug therapy problems and to make certain that the goals of drug therapy are met for the patient.

A TAXONOMY FOR DRUG THERAPY PROBLEMS

To organize the cognitive processes required to identify drug therapy problems in individual patients and to ensure that a comprehensive assessment of all potential drug therapy problems can be conducted, we have divided drug therapy problems into seven major categories. Knowing that all of the drug therapy problems one will ever see in practice are from one of only seven categories is a very empowering concept. Each pharmacist needs to become intimately familiar with these categories and their common causes. Only then can the pharmacist identify, resolve, and prevent them with confidence and success. The seven categories of drug therapy problems are listed in Table 3-2.

TABLE 3-2 CATEGORIES OF DRUG THERAPY PROBLEMS

1. The patient has a medical condition that requires the initiation of new or additional drug therapy.
2. The patient is taking drug therapy that is unnecessary given his or her present condition.
3. The patient has a medical condition for which the wrong drug is being taken.
4. The patient has a medical condition for which too little of the correct drug is being taken.
5. The patient has a medical condition resulting from an adverse drug reaction.
6. The patient has a medical condition for which too much of the correct drug is being taken.
7. The patient has a medical condition resulting from not taking the drug appropriately.

These categories are not specific to pharmacological class, area of practice specialty, medical service, or level of pharmacist education and training. Nor are they specific to a unique patient group based on age, disease state, or health care plan. All pharmacists who deliver pharmaceutical care must be able to identify, prevent, and solve each of the seven types of drug therapy problems for each patient. When the pharmacist identifies that a patient has a drug therapy problem, the practitioner is obligated to resolve that problem. This will occur through the patient care process described in Chap. 4.

> Pharmaceutical care meets a patient's drug therapy needs by identifying, resolving, and preventing drug therapy problems.

Each of the seven types of drug therapy problems can also be stated as a potential drug therapy problem that requires care, interventions, and monitoring to ensure that the problem is prevented. Many of the most cost-effective forms of pharmacotherapy focus on the prevention of illness. Therefore, the prevention of drug therapy problems should be a major focus of the practitioner's activities. Each of the seven types of drug therapy problems can also be stated as a potential drug therapy problem that requires care, intervention, and monitoring to ensure that a problem is prevented. Examples include vaccinations in infants and/or high-risk elderly patients, prophylactic antibiotics for patients undergoing surgical procedures where bowel contamination is a risk, prophylactic heparin therapy for patients at high risk to develop deep venous thrombosis, low-dose aspirin prophylaxis in patients at high risk to develop a myocardial infarction or stroke, prenatal vitamin supplementation for expectant mothers, and immunosuppression for transplant patients to prevent the immune system from rejecting the transplanted organ. The seven categories of drug therapy problems are stated as potential problems in Table 3-3.

TABLE 3-3 POTENTIAL DRUG THERAPY PROBLEMS

1. The patient is at a high-risk to develop a new medical condition for which additional drug therapy is indicated.
2. The patient is at risk to develop a new medical condition that is the result of taking an unnecessary drug for which there is no valid medical indication.
3. The patient is at risk to develop a new medical condition because the wrong drug is being taken.
4. The patient is at risk to develop a new medical condition because too little of the correct drug is being taken.
5. The patient is at risk to develop a medical condition from an adverse drug reaction.
6. The patient is at risk to develop a new medical condition because too much of the correct drug is being taken.
7. The patient is at risk to develop a medical condition that is the result of not complying with the prescribed or recommended drug therapy.

The prevention of drug therapy problems and providing care require the practice of pharmaceutical care to be proactive.

The delivery of a comprehensive level of pharmaceutical care requires that the practitioner provide proactive care rather than simply being prepared to react to prescriptions, changes in drug therapies, or questions from patients or other care providers. This patient-specific method to identify drug therapy problems helps to provide preventive care in which the patient remains the focus of all inquiries and investigations. This patient-centered focus must be established and maintained if one is to adequately identify potential problems, especially those for which no drug has yet been prescribed or recommended. If one's efforts are limited simply to reviewing a list of medications that have already been prescribed for or consumed by the patient, then there is little chance that all the potential problems that the patient might develop will be identified; certainly they will not be prevented. The level of risk that determines if the potential drug therapy problem requires an intervention will, of course, vary from patient to patient and will depend on the patient's condition and/or risk factors, the risk of the proposed preventive pharmacotherapy, and the patient's perception of those risks.[3] The foregoing combined with the clinical competence and judgment of the practitioner allow for each patient to be cared for on an individual basis.

Drug therapy problems can be resolved or prevented only when the cause of the problem is clearly understood. Therefore, it is necessary to identify and categorize not only the drug therapy problem but also its cause. Only then can the pharmacist move on with confidence to its resolution or its prevention. The common causes of drug therapy problems are summarized in Table 3-4 (pages 82–83). These should become second nature (a tacit understanding) to the practitioner. By identifying the cause, the practitioner and patient can rationally construct a care plan that resolves the drug therapy problems, thereby making it possible for the patient to realize the maximal potential benefit of drug therapy. A description of the drug therapy problems, their major causes, and common examples of each type of drug therapy problem will be presented further on in this chapter.

DRUG THERAPY PROBLEMS IN PRACTICE

The following sections describe each of the seven categories of drug therapy problems and provide common and uncomplicated examples to demonstrate the nature of such problems as they occur in practice. How each practitioner might design a care plan to resolve each of these drug therapy problems will obviously vary depending on specific patient, disease, and drug information.

APPROPRIATE INDICATIONS FOR DRUG THERAPY

It is the responsibility of the pharmacist to ensure that there is an appropriate indication for every drug the patient is taking.

It is the responsibility of the pharmacist to ensure that all of the medications that are appropriately indicated for the patient are available to the patient.

There are two categories of drug therapy problems that must be addressed to make certain each patient's medications are all appropriately indicated. If a patient needs additional drug therapy for a new or changing medical condition, the pharmacist must create a plan to respond to this unmet drug-related need. Similarly, if the patient is receiving drug therapy for which there is no longer a valid indication, the pharmacist must create a plan to respond to this drug-related need. First, let us examine drug therapy problems in which the patient requires additional or new drug therapy.

Drug Therapy Problem Category 1: Patient Needs Additional Drug Therapy

A most common unmet drug-related need and, therefore, drug therapy problem is the circumstance when a patient is suffering from an illness or develops a new or worsening condition and is in need of pharmacotherapy. Such situations include a patient who requires new drug therapy to treat a new illness or a patient who requires the addition of a second or third drug to treat a condition optimally. A patient who is at risk to develop a new illness or disease and the addition of a form of drug therapy designed to prevent that illness or disease would also be described as constituting an indication for additional drug therapy that is yet unmet.

Data from the Minnesota Pharmaceutical Care Project indicate that almost one out of five drug therapy problems involve patients who require additional or new drug therapy in order to fully meet their drug-related needs. The major causes for requiring new or additional drug therapy are as follows:

- To treat a previously untreated condition
- To add synergistic or potentiating drug therapy
- To fill the need for prophylactic or preventive drug therapy

Many patient encounters involving this type of drug therapy problem are very straightforward, as, for example, the patient who is suffering from seasonal allergic rhinitis who requires antihistamine therapy, such as diphenhydramine or chlorpheniramine, for the relief of bother-

TABLE 3-4 CAUSES OF DRUG THERAPY PROBLEMS

DRUG THERAPY PROBLEM	POSSIBLE CAUSES OF DRUG THERAPY PROBLEMS
Need for additional drug therapy	The patient has a new medical condition requiring initiation of new drug therapy.
	The patient has a chronic disorder requiring continuation of drug therapy.
	The patient has a medical condition that requires combination pharmacotherapy to attain synergism/potentiation of effects.
	The patient is at risk to develop a new medical condition preventable by the use of prophylactic drug therapy and/or premedication
Unnecessary drug therapy	The patient is taking a medication for which there is no valid medical indication at this time.
	The patient accidentally or intentionally ingested a toxic amount of a drug or chemical, resulting in the present illness or condition.
	The patient's medical problem(s) are associated with drug abuse, alcohol use, or smoking.
	The patient's medical condition is better treated with nondrug therapy.
	The patient is taking multiple drugs for a condition for which only single-drug therapy is indicated.
	The patient is taking drug therapy to treat an avoidable adverse reaction associated with another medication.
Wrong drug	The patient has a medical problem for which this drug is not effective.
	Patient is allergic to this medication.
	Patient is receiving a drug that is not the most effective for the indication being treated.
	The patient has risk factors that contraindicate the use of this drug.
	The patient is receiving a drug that is effective but not the least costly.
	The patient is receiving a drug that is effective but not the most safe.
	The patient has an infection involving organisms that are resistant to this drug.
	The patient has become refractory to the present drug therapy.
	The patient is receiving an unnecessary combination product when a single drug would be appropriate.
Dosage too low	The dosage used is too low to produce the desired response for this patient.
	The patient's serum drug concentrations are below the desired therapeutic range.
	Timing of prophylaxis (presurgical antibiotic given too early) was inadequate for this patient.
	Drug, dose, route, or formulation conversions were inadequate for this patient.
	Dose and interval flexibility (insulin sliding scales, "as needed" analgesics) were inadequate for this patient.
	Drug therapy was altered prior to adequate therapeutic trial for this patient.
Adverse drug reaction	The drug was administered too rapidly for this patient.
	The patient is having an allergic reaction to this medication.
	The patient has identified risk factors that make this drug too dangerous to be used.
	The patient has experienced an idiosyncratic reaction to this drug.
	The bioavailability of the drug is altered due to an interaction with another drug or food the patient is taking.

DRUG THERAPY PROBLEM	POSSIBLE CAUSES OF DRUG THERAPY PROBLEMS
	The effect of the drug has been altered due to enzyme inhibition/induction from another drug the patient is taking.
	The effect of the drug has been altered due to a substance in the food the patient has been eating.
	The effect of the drug has been altered due to displacement from binding sites by another drug the patient is taking.
	The patient's laboratory test result has been altered due to interference from a drug the patient is taking.
Dose too high	Dosage is too high for this patient.
	The patient's serum drug concentrations are above the desired therapeutic range.
	The patient's drug dose was escalated too rapidly.
	The patient has accumulated drug from chronic administration.
	Drug, dose, route, formulation conversions were inappropriate for this patient.
	Dose and interval flexibility (insulin sliding scales, "as needed" analgesics) were inappropriate for this patient.
Compliance	The patient did not receive the appropriate drug regimen because a medication error (prescribing, dispensing, administration, monitoring) was made.
	The patient did not comply (adherence) with the recommended directions for using the medication.
	The patient did not take the drug as directed owing to the high cost of the product.
	The patient did not take the drug(s) as directed because of lack of understanding of the directions.
	The patient did not take the drug(s) as directed because it would not be consistent with the patient's health beliefs.

TABLE 3-4 CAUSES OF DRUG THERAPY PROBLEMS (CONTINUED)

some nasal congestion, and who would certainly be considered to have a drug therapy problem of this type. With the advent of numerous effective medications that are available without a prescription—such as nonsteriodal anti-inflammatory drugs (NSAIDs), peptic ulcer agents, antifungal agents, and antihistamines—pharmacists will increasingly care for patients who present with a condition or illness for which a nonprescription drug is indicated and likely to be effective.

Continuity in drug therapy is very often important. This is frequently the case in chronic diseases and disorders that require prolonged therapy for relief of discomforting signs and symptoms, such as pain in a patient with rheumatoid arthritis or weight loss and steatorrhea in a patient with chronic pancreatitis. Continuous and long-term use of antiinflammatory/analgesics such as naprosyn and chronic continuous use of pancreatic enzyme replacements such as pancreatin might be indicated in these two different patients. A drug therapy problem might occur if these patients were transferred from one hospital or one health plan to another, from one physician's care to another, or from one pharmacy to another and their therapies were not continued. In these situations, the continuity of drug therapy might be interrupted, resulting in a drug therapy problem.

Other examples of patients who might experience the first type of drug therapy problem (an indication for a drug) are patients requiring combination drug therapy, such as an individual with stage III Hodgkin's disease requiring combination chemotherapy to effect a greater cell kill than could be achieved with monotherapy. Similarly, at least two antimicrobial agents are often necessary to eradicate active tuberculosis because of the risk of emergence of resistance and continued infection associated with single-drug therapy. Therefore, solutions used in current practice for this type of drug therapy problem (tuberculosis requiring chemotherapy) include combinations of agents with different mechanisms, like isoniazid and rifampin designed to rapidly eliminate extracellular organisms from sputum, thus rapidly decreasing the patient's infection (isoniazid) and also eradicating the slowly dividing organisms within granulomas and macrophages (rifampin).

A common drug therapy problem is the underutilization of effective medications.

In summary, this first type of drug therapy problem, that of a new indication for drug therapy not yet being treated, is very common and requires the pharmacist to be proactive and take responsibility for the care of patients who may not yet be receiving any medications and therefore have no patient profile to review.

Examples:

An untreated condition:

A 55-year-old business executive who has been experiencing "upset stomach" after dinner and in the evening just before bedtime.

Synergistic or potentiating therapy:

A 55-year-old business executive who has been treated for a gastric ulcer with ranitidine (Zantac) 150 mg orally twice daily for the past 6 weeks and is still experiencing "upset stomach" after dinner and in the evening just before bedtime. This is the third treatment course he has had over the past year.

Prophylactic or preventive therapy:

A 66-year-old retired executive who has stable coronary disease and should be taking aspirin to reduce his risk of developing a myocardial infarction and cardiovascular mortality.

Drug Therapy Problem Category 2: Patient Is Taking Unnecessary Drug Therapy

This category of drug therapy problems frequently tends to be overlooked. It is the pharmacist's responsibility to see that people are not exposed to potent drugs for which there is no valid medical indication. Patients who are exposed to unnecessary drug therapies can only realize the toxic potential of that drug and have little or no chance of realizing any positive outcome associated with such unnecessary treatment. The cost of unnecessary drug therapy should also be considered. Drug therapy is considered unnecessary for the patient if there was not or there is no longer a valid medical indication for a particular drug. However, it is important to keep in mind that we use medications for several reasons, not only to treat diseases and relieve pain and suffering but also for prophylaxis and prevention and to aid in the diagnostic process.

If a patient is receiving combination therapy when a single drug would be expected to be equally effective, then the patient would be experiencing a drug therapy problem that must be resolved. This type of drug therapy problem associated with combination drug therapies commonly occurs in patients who receive their care in long-term-care facilities. In fact, the guidelines for those who assess patient and staff drug use in these facilities are specifically directed to identify patients who receive more than one analgesic, or more that one antidiarrheal, or more than two laxatives for the same indication. Clearly, the pharmacists who are retained by long-term-care facilities to conduct drug regimen reviews are responsible to see that patients do not experience this type of drug therapy problem.

Data from the Minnesota Pharmaceutical Care Project indicate that 7 percent of the drug therapy problems identified and resolved by pharmacists arose when patients took medications that were not necessary. These problem situations expose patients to unnecessary toxicities or side effects and force upon both patients and payers the direct expenses associated with the consumption of unnecessary drug therapies.

Unnecessary drug therapy can arise from several common causes, including the following:

- No medical indication
- Addictive/recreational drug use
- Nondrug therapy more appropriate
- Duplicate therapy
- Treating an avoidable adverse drug reaction

Usually, when we conceptualize pharmaceutical care, we focus our attention on legal drugs, obtained by prescription or over the counter from a legitimate source. Of course this does not mean that pharmacy, as a profession, has ignored illicit drugs and individuals who abuse them. When we set aside the heavy rhetoric, political ideology, moral posturing, and the criminal justice system's aggressive prosecution of drug users as first and foremost criminals, we cannot fail to recognize drug abuse as a serious public health issue. However, within the context of pharmaceutical care as defined and developed here, we believe that

Illicit drug use is clearly within the domain of pharmaceutical care.

more can be done. Pharmaceutical care is, after all, about harm reduction across the broadest spectrum of drug use.

Harm reduction, or risk reduction associated with *all* drugs, is the mandate of pharmacists practicing pharmaceutical care. While laws may vary from country to country (or within a particular country), it can be argued that ethical standards of patient care, and the pharmacist's responsibilities in this process, should be held constant. Thus, any patient in need of pharmaceutical care should receive it. Illegal drug-taking activities, while subject to prosecution, do not in themselves exempt a practitioner from providing pharmaceutical care. Certainly, the pharmacist must work within the law but act at a clinical level to reduce harm to anyone at risk regardless of judicial decrees or moral disapproval of an individual's conduct. Here, it is important to know the law and fully understand the ethics of the situation. Frequently, the pharmacist will find himself or herself carrying out a delicate balancing act between patient autonomy (and confidentiality) and acts of mandatory reporting and disclosure. Conflicts between rights and responsibilities are never easily resolved, but they are a common characteristic of interpersonal relationships found in daily practice. Indeed, any therapeutic relationship is certain to generate some degree of such tension. Pharmacists have little choice but to acquire skills that can be applied to conflict situations.

The boundaries of pharmaceutical care are not determined by the legal or political status of a drug.

Drug abuse is not simply the abuse of an illegal substance (e.g., crack cocaine, heroin)—it involves numerous licit drugs as well, both prescription and over-the-counter products. The pharmacological properties are of interest to the pharmacist, for it is these factors that create the type of harm that can be reduced or eliminated by pharmaceutical care interventions. Within the context of an ethic of care, the legal status of a particular drug should, in itself, not determine need or prohibit pharmaceutical care interventions, be they preventive, health promotional/educational, or palliative. The resolution of drug-related morbidity and mortality means that *all* drugs are subject to the pharmacist's clinical intervention.

Drug abuse is a major public health problem. It results in excessive utilization of health care resources by predisposing users at high risk to develop other illnesses, including serious and life-threatening infections, nutritional and immunological deficiencies, and psychiatric disturbances.

The dire consequences of drug and alcohol abuse, along with such popular substances as caffeine and nicotine, need not be told here. Suffice it to say that the pharmacist practicing pharmaceutical care should be well informed about all of these noxious substances and factor them into any conceptualization of drug therapy problems. Future developments in pharmaceutical care should more rigorously move in the direction of drug, alcohol, and tobacco abuse. To do otherwise is to ignore a highly complex set of drug therapy problems, problems that can benefit from the expert intervention of pharmacists committed to a broad-based practice of pharmaceutical care.

Examples:

No medical indication:

A 55-year-old business executive has been successfully treated for his first episode of a duodenal ulcer with ranitidine 150 mg orally twice daily for the past 8 weeks. He presents to the pharmacist requesting a refill of his prescription to continue ranitidine at that dose.

Addictive/recreational drug use:

A 55-year-old business executive has been successfully treated for his first episode of a duodenal ulcer with ranitidine 150 mg orally twice daily for the past 6 weeks and still has stomach discomfort associated with his excessive coffee and nicotine consumption.

Nondrug therapy more appropriate:

A 55-year-old business executive has been successfully treated for his first episode of a duodenal ulcer with ranitidine 150 mg orally twice daily for the past 6 weeks. He asks about methods to reduce the stress that he believes has caused or aggravated his ulcer condition.

Duplicate therapy:

A 55-year-old business executive has been successfully treated for his first episode of a duodenal ulcer with ranitidine 150 mg orally twice daily for the past 4 weeks. He is also using cimetidine (Tagamet HB), which he purchased without a prescription.

Treating avoidable adverse drug reaction:

A 55-year-old business executive has just begun treatment for his first episode of a duodenal ulcer with ranitidine 150 mg orally twice daily for the past 2 weeks. He asks about continuing to use aspirin to treat his recent headaches, which are sometimes severe and seem to be associated with his new ranitidine therapy.

The Most Effective Drug Therapy Available

The pharmacist is responsible to do whatever is necessary to ensure that a patient's drug therapy is effective.

Two categories of drug therapy problems must be addressed to make certain that each patient's drug therapy is as effective as possible. If the medication the patient is taking is the wrong drug for the current illness, then the pharmacist must create a plan to respond to this drug therapy problem so as to ensure that the patient's condition is properly treated. Similarly, if the dosage of medication the patient is taking is too low to produce the desired beneficial outcome, then the pharmacist must create a plan to respond to this drug therapy problem.

Drug Therapy Problem Category 3: The Patient Is Taking the Wrong Drug

Introducing a chemical entity (the drug) into a biological system (the patient) leads to an uncertain response.

If a patient is not experiencing the intended positive outcomes from a certain drug regimen, then the practitioner should consider that the patient may be receiving or taking the wrong drug. Unfortunately, patients are exposed to this type of drug therapy problem far too frequently. Data from the Minnesota Pharmaceutical Care Project indicate that 17 percent of the drug therapy problems identified and resolved by community pharmacists involved patients who were receiving the wrong drug. This situation occurs despite corporate efforts by managed care and pharmacy benefits companies to control the use of drugs. This control is exercised through formularies, disease state management protocols, drug utilization reviews, and countless electronic error messages sent to pharmacy computers, often associated with a refusal to pay for the prescription. It is clear that the most effective place in the health care system to identify patients who are on the wrong drug is at the individual patient-practitioner interface.

When caring for patients, one is always dealing with probabilities. A drug therapy can represent the wrong drug if the patient is not experiencing the intended outcome or if it is likely that the patient will not experience the intended outcomes. If a patient is prescribed a medication and an alternative drug therapy exists, and this alternative has a higher probability of producing the desired outcome, then the patient might be said to be receiving the wrong drug. However, if the patient is actually experiencing the desired outcome from the originally prescribed drug therapy, then one would conclude that the patient is not experiencing a drug therapy problem. Probabilities of the drug therapy being effective and probabilities of the drug therapy producing toxic effects must constantly be balanced when deciding which form of pharmacotherapy will best suit a particular patient's needs. A balance between these two pharmacological probabilities that improves the quality and comfort of a patient's life is what practitioners and patients must continually seek.

Although very few data exist, use of the wrong drug is not as common as one might initially believe. Drug therapy problems are often described as being due to the "wrong drug" when what is actually the case is that another agent might be expected to have a higher probability of producing the intended outcomes. Too often a patient's drug therapy is changed and care can be compromised. Unnecessary changes in drug therapy can result from discontinuing a drug that has a lower expectation of being effective and initiating a drug that has a higher expectation of being effective. A drug therapy regimen that is expected to be effective in 70 percent of all patients (from the literature, clinical trails, and experience) and another that is expected to be effective in 90 percent of all patients can both be right for a specific patient who shows positive results. In other words, a drug that is effective in only three out of ten patients is the wrong drug in seven of the patients but might be the right drug in those three patients. Just as in most fields where decisions are made in areas of uncertainty, drug therapy decisions based on probabilities are seldom 100 percent right, and neither are they often 100 percent wrong.

As with all forms of therapy, the success and effectiveness of drug therapy is contingent upon the identification and eventual diagnosis of the patient's medical problem or problems. All of the components that constitute making drug therapy the correct regimen for a given patient can also contribute to making a particular drug therapy the wrong treatment for that patient. These include the patient's medical condition, the severity of the condition, the infectious process and organism involved, and finally the age and general health status of the patient—including renal, hepatic, cardiovascular, neurological, cognitive, and immune functions. For example, an adult patient with chronic asthma who is being treated for essential hypertension with propranolol therapy might be described as being on the wrong drug for blood pressure control due to the bronchoconstrictive properties of the beta blocker. Certainly one could offer several alternative antihypertensive therapies that do not carry the risk that propranolol might in this patient. Furthermore, this patient might be described as having a drug therapy problem despite apparent adequate control of blood pressure from the beta blocker. Patients who have an allergy to a particular drug or who receive drug therapy when contraindications to it exist might have a drug therapy problem of the "wrong drug" type even though published data support the drug's efficacy. All drug therapy must be patient-specific, not simply disease-specific.

If an effective drug is being used to treat a patient's medical condition but there is an equally effective but less expensive drug available, then it could be argued that the wrong drug is being used. There is an important question here that is often ignored, and that is: "What is the actual evidence that these two agents are equally efficacious?" There is a significant conflict between not being aware of any difference in efficacy of two drugs and having actual data that indicate that two drug therapies are equally effective. Of course, one must also consider the potential toxicity of each agent as well as the patient's thoughts and preferences in any of these types of burdens-to-benefits determinations.

Before changes are made in a patient's drug therapy, practitioners are obligated to ascertain the patient's preferences and wishes. Small differences in price may not be important enough for some patients to agree to change drug therapies from those that they perceive to provide relief from their condition to an "unknown" that costs a bit less. Here the consensual theme of patient involvement is central to the decision-making process. However, a case can certainly be made that practitioners would be obligated to recommend changing from one form of drug

> Decisions concerning a drug's effectiveness are always based on probabilities, not certainties.

> In pharmaceutical care the decision making process accommodates the patient's preferences and wishes.

therapy to another if the second drug therapy was thought to be equally effective and safer for the patient. Practitioner-patient dialogue on such an issue is preferred to the more "authoritative allocation" of pharmacist values presented either paternalistically or in an authoritarian manner. Recall that the essence of a therapeutic relationship is "partnership," and patient input should be sought at all times.

There are, of course, several common causes for patients receiving the wrong drug therapy—instances in which pharmacists will need to institute or recommend changes. Any given drug regimen might be considered wrong for a specific patient at a given time if the dosage form is inappropriate, contraindications are present, the patient's condition is refractory to the drug, the drug is not indicated for the patient's condition, or more effective drug therapy is available.

Examples:

Dosage form inappropriate:

A 53-year-old man who recently began experiencing anginal attacks once or twice a month when engaging in strenuous activities is prescribed nitroglycerin (Nitro-Dur) transdermal patches to be applied daily as needed.

Contraindications present:

A 22-year-old pregnant woman with acne vulgaris presents with a prescription for isotretinoin (Accutane) 20 mg twice daily for 2 weeks.

Condition refractory to drug:

A 2-year-old girl with her third episode of otitis media is prescribed amoxicillin 125 mg three times a day for 10 days. Her last episode, during the previous month, was initially treated with amoxicillin, but after 7 days of no relief, a change to cotrimoxazole was made, which successfully resolved her infection.

Drug not indicated for condition:

A 54-year-old woman borrowed a sample of salmeterol xinafoate (Serevent) from a friend down the street who also has asthma. She has been using it to relieve her own acute asthmatic episodes, which occur about once a week.

More effective medication available:

A 14-year-old girl who sprained her ankle in a basketball game on the previous day has been taking two tablets of acetaminophen (Tylenol) 325 mg every 4 h. She has experienced little pain relief and is still very uncomfortable.

Drug Therapy Problem Category 4:
The Patient Is Taking Too Little of the Correct Drug

Drug therapy problems resulting from patients receiving inadequate doses of potentially effective medications can be a serious and expensive health care problem. The best diagnostic, assessment, and patient care skills can all be nullified if the patient is not receiving an appropriate dosage regimen given his or her unique needs. In general, drug therapy dosage regimens are considered to be too low for a patient if the patient has an appropriate indication for the drug, is not experiencing any therapy-limiting side effects, yet is not realizing the desired benefit from the medication.

Experience from the Minnesota Pharmaceutical Care Project indicates that 14 percent of drug therapy problems occur in patients who are being underdosed on their medications and that adjusting their dose and/or dosage intervals can noticably improve their clinical outcomes. The following exemplify these common causes of drug therapy problems.

Examples:

Wrong dose:

A 2-year-old girl with her first episode of acute otitis media is prescribed amoxicillin suspension 40 mg orally (40 mg/5 mL) three times a day for 10 days.

Frequency inappropriate:

A 2-year-old girl with her first episode of acute otitis media is prescribed amoxicillin 20 mg/kg suspension once daily for 10 days.

Duration inappropriate:

A 5-year-old boy with a respiratory infection is prescribed amoxicillin 250 mg three times daily for 3 days.

Incorrect storage:

A 2-year-old girl with her first episode of acute otitis media is prescribed amoxicillin/clavulanate potassium (Augmentin) 125 mg suspension three times daily for 10 days. Her mother keeps the drug in the cupboard.

Incorrect administration:

A 4-year-old girl with her first episode of acute otitis media is prescribed amoxicillin, suspension (125 mg/5 mL), 1 teaspoonful three times a day for 10 days. At the child's day-care center, the aide uses a plastic baby teaspoon to measure and administer the dose of liquid amoxicillin.

People like to use safe drugs. It is easy to make drugs reasonably safe: simply underdose everyone. If one examines the most frequently prescibed medications on a year-to-year basis, it is noteworthy that the most frequently used drugs have two common characteristics—they are all quite efficacious for their respective indications and they are reasonably safe in general use. Examples of these most commonly used medications that are quite safely used in general practice include amoxicillin, penicillin V, ibuprofen, hydrochlorothiazide, acetaminophen, conjugated estrogens (Premarin), fluoxetine (Prozac), ciprofloxin (Cipro), levothyroxine (Synthroid), and ranitidine (Zantac).

There is a fine line between using a safe drug and making a drug regimen safe for a particular patient. No allopathic practitioner would ever intentionally provide subtherapeutic doses for a patient, but pub-

Safety is the patient's major concern.

lished dosing guidelines are often so conservative that patients are required to suffer through days, weeks, and longer of ineffective drug therapy because they are instructed to take the "recommended" dose. The tools, knowledge, and successful approaches to the dosing of drugs based on patient-specific pharmacokinetic parameters play an important role in the provision of pharmaceutical care. Clinical pharmacists developed many useful and successful guidelines to improve our ability to ensure that each and every patient receives a dosage regimen that is based on personal/individual clinical parameters, in the broadest sense, and therefore can be maximally effective.

There are also many instances in which patients are started on drug therapies using a very low or conservative dosage regimen in order to "see what happens." This logical and often benign approach requires that the practitioner is committed to follow-up at scheduled intervals to evaluate the patient's status and make any necessary dosage adjustments. Without this critical follow-up evaluation step, the patient is destined to suffer unnecessary periods of inadequate treatment and continued illness because the dose received is too low to produce the desired outcomes.

Prescribers—including physicians, dentists, and nurses—are more comfortable prescribing drugs that are safe and do not frequently result in toxic effects. Nurses are often much more comfortable administering or prescribing drugs that are safe and do not cause the patient any noticeable harm. Physicians very often practice "safe" medicine in light of proliferating litigation, cost-consciousness, or managed care "directives." Similarly, pharmacists are more likely to recommend drug regimens that do not result in undesired effects for the patient. However, this propensity to provide safe drug therapy all too often results in the patient receiving too little of the correct drug. Although it may be a fundamental, positive tenet of homeopathic medicine, too little (a suboptimal amount) of the correct drug within the allopathic paradigm is certainly a common type of drug therapy problem. One might consider this the most egregious type of drug therapy problem because the patient's problem has been identified and a potentially useful drug has been selected, but because the dose regimen is not optimized, the patient is not able to realize the full benefit of the drug. To make matters worse, the patient may very well experience an undesired effect from the drug, including economic cost, even though the desired clinical outcome is not realized.

There are several patient parameters which, if not attended to, might result in suboptimal pharmacotherapy. Age and body weight can often be useful parameters to assist in determining the optimal drug dose for a patient. On a per-kilogram basis, a 6-month-old infant might require a higher digoxin dose than a 60-year-old adult. Also "therapeutic ranges" for most drugs are first established in adults and later applied to pediatric patients, often without sufficient verification as to the appropriateness of the adult-derived guidelines. For instance, a therapeutic range for an adult patient requiring chloramphenicol therapy was established to be 10 to 20 μg/mL. However, there is some evidence that a desired chloramphenicol concentration of 50 μg/mL may be more appropriate in some pediatric patients. Children can also vary greatly in body weight even within the same age range. A 10-year-old boy who weighs 90 lb might very well require more acetaminophen to relieve pain from a knee injury suffered in the school's physical education class than a 10-year-old girl, who is in the same fifth grade class but who weighs just 50 lb. Parents instructed to use *weight* dosage recommendations might give the girl a dose of two caplets (320 mg) using acetaminophen (Junior Strength Tylenol), while giving the boy three caplets (480 mg), while a parent who decides to follow the *age* dosage recommendations might give each of these 10-year-old youngsters the recommended dose of 2 1/2 caplets (400 mg), thus underdosing the 90 lb fifth grade boy and not achieving the rapid relief of pain he needs.

A patient who is experiencing an inappropriately prolonged dosing interval might also be considered to be experiencing a drug therapy problem in the category of too little of the correct drug. For example, the Kapseal formulation of phenytoin (Dilantin) is labeled as "extended" and provides support for once-daily dosing. The selection of a more rapidly absorbed preparation of phenytoin for once-daily dosing in a patient with a seizure disorder may lead to widely fluctuating serum concentrations and the potential for loss of seizure control. Similarly, a patient who has a seizure disorder and requires chronic phenytoin administration to prevent the recurrence of a seizure should be taking a dose of phenytoin that has been individualized to maintain serum concentration within a range that is most likely to reduce the risk of seizure activity. This is often between 10 and 20 μg/mL. A patient taking the prescribed dosage regimen but whose phenytoin concentration is consistently well below this range and who is experiencing repeated "breakthrough" seizures might also be receiving too little of the correct drug.

The drug therapy problem of too little of the correct drug can also be a result of the specific medical condition being treated or of using a drug regimen that is not continued long enough to realize full benefits. For example, antimicrobial therapy for two different 25-year-old female patients with urinary tract infections involving *Escherichia coli* might require very different pharmacotherapy if one patient is suffering from an acute, uncomplicated lower urinary tract infection cystitis and the other patient is thought to have acute pyelonephritis. The patient with the acute pyelonephritis might well be underdosed and receive too little of the correct drug if she received the increasingly popular single-dose regimen of two double-strength tablets of cotrimoxazole; however, this dosage regimen would be expected to result in a resolution of the infection in the woman with the acute cystitis. The patient with acute pyelonephritis would likely require at least a full 10 days or 2 weeks of antimicrobial therapy, such as 1 double-strength cotrimoxazole tablet every 12 h.

There is a substantial body of literature[4,5] indicating that patients with a Gram-negative pneumonia should receive enough tobramycin to produce peak serum concentrations in the range of 6 to 10 µg/mL, while patients with intraabdominal or soft-tissue infections can often realize a cure with tobramycin in doses that produce peak concentrations of only 4 to 6 µg/mL. Therefore, a patient with a Gram-negative pneumonia involving a susceptible pathogen whose tobramycin dosing regimen consistently fails to produce peak concentrations of 6 to 10 µg/mL might be described as experiencing a drug therapy problem that is a consequence of treatment failure, or risk of treatment failure, associated with a subtherapeutic tobramycin dosage regimen. This is an example of what several practitioners have recognized: that as a result of our increasing ability to quantitatively individualize drug dosing through the application of new assay technology, pharmacokinetics, and pharmacodynamic principles, a substantial portion of patients require higher doses than previous recommendations suggested. In practice, it is not unusual for a patient to require doses well above the approved manufacturers' published guidelines due to rapid drug clearance secondary to a hypermetabolic state associated with the disease process present. Many practitioners think of measuring serum, or blood-drug concentrations, simply to avoid high concentrations and their associated risk of dose or concentration-dependent toxic effects. However, patients often need their drug dosage regimen individualized based on serum or blood concentration determinations to ensure adequate drug dosing and to avoid the drug therapy problem of too little of the correct drug.

The rapidly advancing field of immunosuppressive pharmacotherapy has added yet another example of the potential danger of too little of the correct drug or drugs. It is becoming increasingly apparent that a patient who has received a kidney transplant requires long-term, probably lifetime, multiple-drug immunosuppressive regimens, but one of the primary risk factors for late rejection is ineffective immunosuppression secondary to subtherapeutic drug dosage regimens. As chronic therapy continues with these potent agents, which can cause troublesome or even dangerous adverse effects, there has been a tendency to reduce doses of the immunosuppressant agents to minimize side effects. However, evidence[6] is now accumulating that too rapid a deescalation of dosage can put the transplant patient at a high risk to reject the transplant kidney and thus experience a treatment failure secondary to too little of the correct drug or drugs.

Some of the most commonly encountered drug-drug interactions are a result of combining the known and expected pharmacology of two agents. These types of drug-drug interactions are usually predictable and can be avoided or quickly corrected through structured assessment of all medications to be taken by a patient. For example, prostaglandin inhibitors—such as ibuprofen, naproxen, and indomethacin—can antagonize the diuretic and hypotensive actions of furosemide and thiazide diuretics through a pharmacodynamic mechanism of water retention and hypertension. In this situation, the expected pharmacology of one agent (naproxen) can counteract the expected pharmacology of another drug (hydrochlorothiazide), resulting in a treatment failure or even a possible worsening of the patient's blood pressure or fluid and electrolyte imbalance.

The possibility of a patient experiencing an adverse event resulting from a physical or chemical interaction between a particular drug and food consumed is always present. For example, milk and other dairy products can inhibit the absorption of iron preparations from the gastrointestinal tract in patients with iron deficiency anemia. In this case, if the patient's microcytic, hypochromic anemia does not respond to the oral iron therapy, the patient could be described as having experienced a drug therapy problem secondary to a drug-food interaction. On the other hand, beverages such as orange juice can improve the absorption of iron from the gastrointestinal tract and might be considered beneficial for some patients.

In summary, each patient's drug therapy must not only be appropriately indicated, but the dosage regimen the patient receives must provide the best possible opportunity for the patient to actually experience the intended desired outcome if the risk of toxicity from drug exposure is to be justified. Drug therapy in which the dose is too low, often places the patient at risk for toxic effects, while robbing the individual of any potential beneficial effects.

There are several common causes for a patient's drug regimen to be considered too low to produce the desired outcomes. These include the following:

- The dose is too low.
- The dosing frequency is inappropriate.
- The duration of therapy is too short.
- The drug has not been appropriately stored and thus has lost its potency.
- The drug is administered inappropriately, thus the actual dosage received by the patient is too low.
- Another drug interferes causing a drug interaction.

The Safest Drug Therapy Possible

The pharmacist is responsible to ensure that all of the drug therapies the patient is undergoing are as safe as possible and cause the patient no harm.

Two types of drug therapy problems related to safety can develop for a patient. First, adverse drug reactions can occur. Second, the dose of a drug can be too high. Each is discussed in the following section.

Drug Therapy Problem Category 5:
The Patient Is Experiencing an Adverse Drug Reaction

Safety must be balanced with effectiveness, because underdosing a patient results in treatment failures.

When one uses the term *drug therapy problem*, many practitioners inappropriately interpret this to be a synonym for *adverse drug reaction*. These two events represent very different concepts within the realm of pharmacotherapy and within the practice of pharmaceutical care. An adverse drug reaction is only one of the seven types of drug therapy problems that can prevent or inhibit a patient from experiencing the full benefits of drug therapy.

Pharmacists, physicians, epidemiologists, and others have defined, described, and quantified adverse drug reactions (ADRs) more extensively than any other category of drug therapy problem. However, the lack of a uniform definition and the collective inability of health care systems to create and support an effective infrastructure to identify, document, resolve, and report ADRs has resulted in an amazingly sparse amount of practical information that practitioners can apply to protect patients from serious and life-threatening experiences. The need for a uniform definition is clearly illustrated in the list of terms used to describe various types of undesired reactions to medications. Table 3-5 lists terms commonly used to describe adverse drug reactions.

Within the practice of pharmaceutical care, the definition of an adverse drug reaction is intended to encompass undesirable negative effects caused by the medication that were not predictable based on the dosage or concentration dependency of the agent or known pharmacology of the drug. This definition excludes normal, expected consequences of the known pharmacology of the drug.

The data from the Minnesota Pharmaceutical Care Project indicate that adverse drug reactions are quite common. In fact, when we examined a group of patients who received continuous pharmaceutical care services for an entire year, adverse drug reactions were the most common type of drug therapy problem identified. Almost one in four

TABLE 3-5 TERMS USED TO DESCRIBE ADVERSE DRUG REACTIONS

Adverse event	Excessive therapeutic effects
Adverse drug reactions	Erroneous use and accidents
Adverse reactions	Iatrogenic disease
Complications	Iatrogenic illness
Drug-induced illness	Negative therapeutics
Drug-induced disease	Pathological reaction
Drug-induced injury	Prescribing errors
Drug intolerance	Side effect
Drug interaction	Superinfection
Drug misadventuring	Unwanted pharmacological effects

(24 percent) of the drug therapy problems identified and resolved were associated with an adverse drug reaction.

There are several common causes for a patient to experience an adverse drug reaction:

- The patient is receiving a drug product considered to be unsafe.
- The patient has an allergic reaction to the drug.
- Incorrect administration of the drug product causes an adverse reaction.
- Interaction with another drug precipitates an adverse drug reaction.
- The dosage is increased or decreased too rapidly and results in an adverse reaction.
- The patient experiences an undesirable effect that was otherwise not predictable.

Examples:

Unsafe drug for patient:

A 45-year-old man with uncontrolled hypertension has been experiencing nasal congestion. He was given a recommendation by a friend to take two tablets of pseudoephedrine HCl three times a day to relieve his symptoms.

Allergic reaction:

A 2-year-old with her first episode of acute otitis media is prescribed amoxicillin 125 mg suspension three times a day for 10 days. Following her second dose, she develops a rash covering her back, chest, and both arms.

Drug interaction:

A 19-year-old woman is prescribed amoxicillin 500 mg three times daily for 10 days for a respiratory infection. She is currently taking norethindrone/mestranol (Ortho-Novum) 1/35 for contraception.

Dosage increased or decreased too fast:

A 32-year-old woman who has been taking prednisone 20 mg every day for the last 6 months for arthritis symptoms due to systemic lupus erythematosus was instructed to take 10 mg for 2 more days then discontinue medication.

Undesirable effect:

A 24-year-old man with his first episode of seasonal allergies has been taking chlorpheniramine 4 mg three times daily to control his runny nose, sneezing, and itchy eyes. He complains of being very fatigued, visual disturbances, dry mouth, and drowsy since beginning to take the antihistamine.

The definition of *adverse drug reaction* as used in the practice of pharmaceutical care makes an important distinction in that it explicitly does not include normal, expected extensions of the known pharmacology of the agent. For example, if a patient who has never been exposed to a sulfonamide develops a rash when given a first dose of cotrimoxazole, it would be classified as an adverse drug reaction. In this case, the offending cotrimoxazole would most likely be discontinued and therapy with another antimicrobial agent from a different chemical class would be initiated. However, if an antihypertensive medication is given to a patient to lower blood pressure but results in hypotension, it might very well be considered an expected extension of the normal, known dose-related pharmacology of the drug, and reducing the dose would likely prevent future hypotensive episodes.

As stated earlier, how a drug therapy problem is described and the subsequent classification of the drug therapy problem directs the practitioner's response, interventions, and construction of a care plan for the patient. Therefore, placing any and all undesired outcomes of drug therapies into a general category of "adverse drug reaction" is not very useful in practice. Not only does clumping all negative drug effects into such a category not help to direct the appropriate practitioner response, but it also tends to render pharmacoepidemiology data about these varying negative drug effects rather meaningless.

It is often difficult to determine if there is a causal relationship between the active ingredient of a drug product, its preservatives, vehicles or metabolites, and the undesired event experienced by a patient. Often the patient's underlying disease, illness, or other drugs can confound the determination of a suspected adverse drug reaction. Criteria used to establish whether a patient is experiencing an adverse reaction to a particular drug product include

- The temporal relationship between the patient being exposed to the suspected agent and the onset of the adverse event
- Whether the patient's condition improves when the drug is discontinued
- In some situations, whether the adverse event recurs when the patient is rechallenged with the suspected agent[7]

Using these criteria, adverse reactions have been classified as follows:[7]

Highly probable: A reaction that follows a reasonable temporal sequence from administration of the drug or in which the drug concentration has been established in body fluids or tissues. The reaction follows a known response pattern to the suspected drug and is confirmed by improvement on discontinuing or reducing the dosage of the drug and reappearance of the reaction following repeated exposure.

Probable: A reaction that follows a reasonable temporal sequence from administration of the drug and follows a known response pattern to the suspected drug, but could have been produced by the patient's clinical state (disease or illness) or other therapies administered to the patient.

Remote: Any reaction that does not meet the criteria above, especially if the event has no reasonable temporal association with use of the drug.

In general, several noxious or unintended responses to drug therapy that occur are not considered or classified as adverse drug reactions. These include:[7]

Any drug product can be very safe, or very toxic. It all depends on how it is used.

- Inadequate doses resulting in continued illness
- Bioavailability problems that result in therapeutic failure
- Drug abuse
- Nonncompliance
- Accidental or intentional poisoning

Each of these undesired events can be classified as one of the other types of drug therapy problems in the systematic approach to the classification of drug therapy problems used in the practice of pharmaceutical care and presented in this text. This verifies the clinical usefulness of categorizing drug therapy problems by a more descriptive method than simply adverse drug reactions and other noxious events.

Several years ago, Rawlins categorized adverse events as type A or type B.[8] Type A reactions are defined as those events that are thought to be normal and expected extensions of the pharmacological actions of the drug. Type A reactions to drugs occur quite commonly. They are frequently dose- or concentration-dependent and therefore are often predictable and potentially avoidable. On the other hand, type B reactions to drugs represent allergic and other idiosyncratic reactions that are independent of drug dose or concentration of the drug.

A strong case can certainly be made that, if a rational approach to drug therapy were applied to every patient's therapy, only type B reactions to drugs would create serious problems and be of great concern to patients and practitioners. One of the assumptions underlying this discussion of pharmaceutical care is that the pharmacist is playing a proactive role in the patient's drug therapy and thus is doing whatever is necessary to protect the patient from preventable type A reactions to drugs. Most type A reactions to drugs are extensions of the known and anticipated pharmacology of the drug and therefore predictable and preventable if all of the essential patient, disease, and drug characteristics have been incorporated into determining the patient's drug-related needs, the care plan, an individualized drug dosage regimen, and an effective follow-up evaluation plan. Upon receiving pharmaceutical care, a patient should expect that the probability of experiencing a type A reaction to a drug will be as low as current knowledge and technology will permit and that the undesired consequences and associated discomfort, should a type A reaction occur, will be minimized.

On an individual patient basis, some type A reactions to drugs are not predictable or at least not entirely preventable. Examples might include some degree of drowsiness associated with various over-the-counter antihistamine dosage forms, dry mouth and other anticholinergic effects associated with many antidepressants agents, and abdominal pain and nausea associated with erythromycin. These reactions should be anticipated, and patient preferences should be considered an essential part of the clinical decision-making process. This is particularly useful when there is some degree of trade-off involved, because the patient

Pharmaceutical care will reduce Type A adverse reactions.

may be faced with the prospect of selecting some discomfort or inconvenience from a range of possible adverse reactions to various drug alternatives.

In practice, of course, not all adverse reactions to drugs are predictable or preventable in a given patient. Individual patient sensitivity to certain drugs makes it challenging to predict who will and who will not experience even a concentration-dependent drug reaction. For instance, what could be more predictable than a patient bleeding secondary to an anticoagulant drug like warfarin or heparin? It is known that higher heparin doses expose patients to a higher risk of experiencing serious bleeding, and several studies have also demonstrated that elderly females are at a very high, about 50 percent, risk of bleeding from heparin therapy. In addition, there is considerable evidence that heparin dosing is better controlled when a patient's dose is determined based on body weight. If one takes into account several individual patient parameters including age, gender, and body weight when determining a patient's heparin dosage regimen, the risk of bleeding can be substantially reduced. However, there is still considerable variation in response, patient sensitivity to heparin, and the risk of bleeding.[9] By replacing traditional unfractionated heparin with the newer low-molecular-weight heparin preparations, the risk of any given patient to experience a bleeding episode can be greatly reduced, although not to zero.

Drug-drug interactions are among the most frequently mentioned potential causes of drug therapy problems, but they also seem to be the least well studied and most seldomly confirmed events. Drug-drug interactions are often no more complicated than the pharmacology of one drug combined with the pharmacology of another drug. Therefore, the practice of pharmaceutical care requires a thorough understanding of the normal, expected pharmacology of the drugs most commonly used in practice.

The literature is full of case reports of drug-drug interactions and small uncontrolled series of patients who experienced similar adverse events while receiving the same multiple drug combination. Drug-drug interactions are not only very difficult to identify, verify, and document, but their resolution is often extremely complex due to the intricate nature of the interaction. Some drug-drug interactions can involve disturbance in drug absorption, distribution, metabolism, and/or clearance.

Drug-drug interactions can occur not only across pharmacological classes but also in patients who require therapy with several drugs within the same therapeutic class. Anticonvulsants are among the agents most commonly associated with drug-drug interactions that can result in considerable patient discomfort, toxicity, and inconvenience. For example, a dose of phenytoin may need to be adjusted upward in a patient whose seizure therapy requires the addition of a second anticonvulsant such as carbamazepine. This dosage adjustment would be required to prevent a drug therapy problem resulting from the drug-drug interaction of carbamazepine inducing the metabolism of phenytoin, thus potentially reducing the serum phenytoin concentrations and placing the patient at risk to experience continued seizure activity.

In addition to one drug altering the metabolism of another agent, some drugs can alter the metabolism of themselves as well as that of other agents. Some patients experience severe drowsiness and lethargy associated with initial carbamazepine therapy for control of seizure disorders. This drug therapy problem most often occurs early in therapy or whenever the dose of carbamazepine is increased. Autoinduction of the hepatic enzyme systems that are responsible for the metabolism of carbamazepine and other anticonvulsants is thought to be the underlying cause of this complex drug interaction.

Patients who require pharmacotherapy with agents that are extensively protein-bound are also at risk to experience a drug therapy problem if a second drug that competes for similar binding sites is added to their regimen. This drug-drug interaction might result in a transient but dangerous elevation in the circulating free concentrations of one or both of these drugs and produce an undesired toxic event. For example, high-dose salicylates can displace some oral hypoglycemic agents from protein binding sites and thus potentiate hypoglycemia in diabetic patients.

In summary, many unwanted events experienced by patients who require drug therapy are attributed to drug interactions, but the vast majority of these events are the consequence of normal expected pharmacology of the two or more agents and therefore are predictable and usually preventable drug therapy problems.

> Most drug interactions are a function of the known pharmacology of the drugs.

Drug Therapy Problem Category 6:
The Dosage Is too High for the Patient

If a little is good, more is better.

When a patient receives too high a dose of an agent and experiences a dose-dependent or more often a concentration-dependent toxic effect, he or she is experiencing a drug therapy problem. This type of drug therapy problem is not to be confused with the adverse-reaction type of drug therapy problem described earlier. Rather, the "too much of the correct drug" category of drug therapy problems is a result of the predictable, pharmacological action of an agent.

Drug therapy problems can result from too high a drug dosage derived from several common causes. These include the following:

- The wrong dose
- An inappropriate dosing frequency
- Inappropriate duration
- A drug interaction

Examples:

Wrong dose:

A 12-month-old girl with her first episode of acute otitis media is prescribed amoxicillin 500 mg suspension three times daily for 10 days.

Frequency inappropriate:

A 75-year-old woman with osteoarthritis was prescribed acetaminophen 500 mg, two tablets every 4 h for pain.

Duration inappropriate:

A 10-year-old girl with her first episode of strep throat was prescribed penicillin V 250 mg three times daily for 3 weeks.

Dose-dependent drug effects can appear in the form of systemic reactions or localized effects. For example, an elderly patient with atrial fibrillation who needs digoxin therapy for control of ventricular rate and whose pulse rate is reduced to less than 55 beats per minute might be experiencing bradycardia secondary to too much of the correct drug (digoxin). The slowing of the heart rate is the desired pharmacological effect. However, owing to too much drug, this has developed into an undesired effect and may place this patient at a high risk to fall and suffer an injury while rising from bed or while getting up from a chair.

An example of a localized undesired effect might be the common problem of nausea associated with oral iron replacement therapy. Individual doses containing high amounts of elemental iron can often be the cause of local gastrointestinal irritation and make the patient feel nauseous following each dose. This patient may benefit from changing to an iron product that has less elemental iron per dose but is administered more frequently throughout the day. In this situation, the patient can receive the same total amount of daily iron but minimize the discomfort of nausea.

Patients who are often at the greatest risk of experiencing this type of drug therapy problem include elderly patients who frequently have reduced renal function, which can make an elderly patient more vulnerable to drugs that are dependent on renal function for their elimination from the body. Some elderly patients also often have reduced cardiac reserve, which can make them especially vulnerable to the hypotensive effects not only of cardiovascular drugs but also of tricyclic antidepressants and some antipsychotic agents, which can also lower blood pressure.

Obviously, patients with renal dysfunction can accumulate drugs or metabolites that are dependent upon the kidneys for elimination and produce toxic complications. For example, patients with compromised renal function will accumulate *N*-acetylprocainamide (NAPA), the active metabolite of procainamide. Therefore, if a patient has the potential to experience or actually experiences adverse effects, the dose and/or dosing interval must be adjusted according to the level of accumulation. The value of measuring serum or blood drug concentrations and pharmacokinetic monitoring with dosage individualization cannot be overemphasized in preventing or correcting this type of drug therapy problem. Over the past two decades, the application of pharmacokinetics to individualized drug dosing has progressed from the research arena to everyday standards of practice and is now included in the recommended dosing guidelines that appear in some approved product literature for commonly used drugs, including phenytoin, gentamicin, digoxin, potassium chloride, flecainide, procainamide, and theophylline.

In an effort to reduce the frequency and severity of dose-dependent toxic complications associated with commonly used psychotropic drugs, the 1990 Omnibus Budget Reconciliation Act (OBRA)[10] requires biannual documentation of efforts made every 6 months to reduce dosage levels of antipsychotic medications for Medicare recipients (and Medicaid when applicable) in long-term-care facilities. Additionally, this legislation has resulted in documents that provide dosage recommendations for patients over the age of 65 who receive psychotropic medications in a long-term-care facility. This represents an attempt on a national basis to prevent or reduce dose-dependent toxic complications in a vulnerable population. Most of the dosage recommendations call for a simple reduction in dose for patients who are over 65 years of age. One will note that the usual maximum daily antipsychotic dosages for patients aged 65 and older are all 50 percent of the usual maximum daily dosage for other patients. This pervasive halving of the dose is questionably helpful in the treatment of individual patients and probably should be reserved for the intended purpose of general, facilitywide retrospective review of antipsychotic drug use in many patients treated by multiple practitioners.

These general drug usage guidelines are not intended to determine what dose or dosage regimen an individual resident in a long-term-care facility might actually require. Rather, these indicators are provided to reviewers who assess whether pharmacists are adequately conducting drug regimen reviews in long-term-care facilities. Therefore, they are to be primarily seen as "administrative" in the bureaucratic rather than the clinical sense of the word. In practice, more quantitative dosage individualization may be possible through pharmacokinetic and pharmacodynamic monitoring of patients receiving these agents.

In recent years, numerous pharmacokinetic and pharmacodynamic models have been proposed and evaluated in various patient populations in attempts to develop and refine tools to assist practitioners to rapidly and effectively determine the appropriate amount of drug for an individual patient with a specific drug therapy problem. Most of these models are based on measurements of drug in serum or blood and estimates of the patient's elimination or clearance to calculate the appropriate replacement dose to maintain a predetermined, desired, serum or blood concentration of the drug. There are often numerous assumptions in these models, including the following:

- The patient is at steady state.
- The patient is compliant with the directions.
- The desired serum or blood concentration will have some relationship to either desired outcomes or undesirable toxic events in this patient.
- The effects that are observed are associated with the compound that is being measured (i.e., metabolites that are not measured have little or no activity).

In practice, all of these assumptions are seldom, if ever, completely true. However, understanding these assumptions and how they might apply to an individual patient permits the practitioner to maximize the information that can be derived from the clinical application of pharmacokinetic and pharmacodynamic tools when providing pharmaceutical care.

The drug therapy problem of too much drug can also be minimized for patients who require anticoagulant therapy. Even though we do not have reliable and accurate drug assays for heparin or warfarin, drug toxicity in the form of bleeding can be minimized by the application of pharmacodynamic models. In the case of patients who require long term anticoagulation with warfarin (Coumadin) therapy, the prothrombin time measurements and the International Normalized Ratio (INR) are useful determinants of whether the patient's dosage regimen is likely to result in excessive antithrombotic activity and precipitate a bleeding episode. Several risk factors are known to place patients at a higher risk of bleeding while receiving warfarin, but the drug dosage and resultant coagulation times are clearly the greatest risk factor for bleeding in warfarinized patients. In fact, recent studies have resulted in a reduction in the recommended desired prothrombin time ratios for some patients requiring warfarin therapy. This reduction is designed to maintain the beneficial antithrombotic activity while reducing the patient's risk of bleeding from receiving too much warfarin. This less intense warfarin therapy calls for individualizing treatment to provide some patients with a prolongation in the prothrombin time ratio of only 1.3 to 1.5, rather than the traditional prolongation of 1.5 to 2 or even 2.5 time baseline or control values. However, the prothrombin time is best reported using the INR to avoid the substantial variation that exists among the sensitivity and procedures used by laboratories when determining a patient's prothrombin time. INRs between 2 and 3 are currently considered optimal for atrial fibrillation patients. So, not only have the desired pharmacotherapeutic end points changed to reduce the risk of bleeding, but the reporting of the test results themselves is being standardized to reduce over dosage and adverse episodes.[11]

As is the case with patients who require long-term anticoagulation with warfarin therapy, patients who require acute, short-term antithrombotic therapy with heparin are also at risk of bleeding as a result of receiving too much drug. Due to the great heterogeneity of heparin preparations, no useful heparin assay is available; therefore practitioners must rely on coagulation tests to determine the appropriate heparin dose for each patient. The most commonly used tests are the activated partial thromboplastin time and the activated clotting time. In both of these cases, pharmacodynamic models are useful to individualize a patient's dose and avoid serious bleeding due to too much drug.[12-15]

In another situation, a patient being treated for stable exertional angina pectoris with nitroglycerin patch therapy may not receive the full benefit of the drug if the slow release patches are applied every day and left in place for the full 24 h. The patient can develop a form of tolerance from continuous nitroglycerin exposure and thereby be unprotected from chest pain. This patient might be considered to have a drug therapy problem as a result of too much exposure to the correct drug. Moreover, this patient may realize more effective antianginal therapy by removing the nitroglycerin patch each evening and reapplying a new patch the following morning, thus providing a 6- to 8-h nitrate-free interval each day, thereby reducing dosage exposure and thus the risk of developing tolerance to chronic nitrate therapy.

COMPLIANT BEHAVIOR

It is the responsibility of the pharmacist to make certain the patient understands and is willing and able to adhere to the drug therapy and care plan instructions.

Drug Therapy Problem Category 7: Patient Is Noncompliant

Compliance represents a behavior. Most would agree that effective pharmacotherapy requires the medication be consumed in a particular dosage, at specified times, and for a specific period of time. Therefore, patients who are noncompliant need to be cared for in the context of altering their behavior. When patients visit their physician and receive a prescription and then go to their pharmacist for their medication, they have every intention of using that medication to improve their health status. For some patients, this positive, well-intentioned behavior is then altered or disrupted.

Patients frequently do not take drugs as prescribed or instructed for a number of reasons. One common reason is that the patient perceives that the drug has caused or will cause some adverse event or at the very least will be an inconvenience to the point that the decision to discontinue taking the drug seems, from the patient's perspective, to be a logical action.

There is a reason for all noncompliance. Find it!

There is always a reason for noncompliance. In the practice of pharmaceutical care, it is the pharmacist's responsibility to identify whether a patient is or is not compliant and the cause or reason for any noncompliance. The cause or reason for the lack of compliance determines the interventions and care that are necessary to alter the patient's behavior and improve compliance.

The patient's understanding and knowledge about his or her illness and medications are clearly important issues in determining the success of any form of pharmacotherapy. Most approaches to address drug therapy problems associated with compliance have focused on "educating" patients as to the appropriate use of prescribed and recommended drugs. Many clinical interventions to date have been based on the premise that much of the reason that patients do not comply with intended drug regimens is a lack of understanding of the instructions, bad memory, and/or inconvenience. Useful aids can result in a dramatic improvements in one's ability to remember to take prescribed medications. Examples of compliance aids include

- Drug-dosing calendars
- Use of large, visible print on prescription labels
- Auxiliary directions to explain appropriate use
- Telephone reminders when refills are needed
- Eliminating nonessential medications
- Using uncomplicated once-a-day schedules

When the pharmacist takes the time to counsel patients and explain the purpose and appropriate use of each medication, patient compliance tends to improve. This improvement may be associated with an increased awareness of the proper directions or is more likely a result of the less obvious but more powerful influence of the extra attention and care the pharmacist has shown the patient combined with a demonstration of genuine concern for the individual's comfort, safety, and well being. In all cases, the pharmacist must work to understand the patient's perception of illness and treatment, so that, when appropriate, behavior can be changed to achieve the desired pharmacotherapeutic outcome. A positive pharmacist-patient relationship has a strong influence on patient behavior and thus on compliance.

All patients have their own health care beliefs, understanding of their illness and medications, expectations, and concerns. They may have had negative experiences, fears, cultural influences, habits, coping mechanisms, or personality traits that play important and even dominating roles in day-to-day decisions to take or not to take medications. Each of these factors interacts with and can be constantly influenced by the therapeutic relationship that develops between the patient and the pharmacist providing pharmaceutical care. It is important to understand that compliance, as well as noncompliance, is to a considerable extent learned behavior and not simply a lack of knowledge about drug therapy. There is strong evidence that simply trying to teach patients about their drug therapy will not significantly alter drug-taking behavior.

Patients may decide to consume a medication in a manner quite different from how it was prescribed, or they may decide not to take the medication at all. Also, they may not actually receive and consume the intended drug therapy for a number of reasons, those within the patient's control and those outside of the patient's sphere of influence. Noncompliance with a prescribed or recommended drug regimen occurs often and for a variety of reasons that fall into both of these categories. Some reports indicate that as many as 20 percent to 71 percent of patients do not comply with prescribed drug regimens.[16]

Noncompliance among patients receiving prescription medications has been studied quite extensively.[17-19] This common drug therapy problem has most often been examined from the point of view of the practitioner rather than the more influential attitude of the patient. Considerable efforts have been expended to identify the social characteristics of patients that might be indicators of who will and who will not comply with a given medication regimen. Most social factors—including age, sex, race, social class, marital status and religion—have proven to not be of particularly high predictive value in identifying compliant and noncompliant patients.

In order to successfully follow any set of directions, one must first understand the instructions. Pharmacists often use language and terminology that is unclear or not understood by the patient. A patient's interpretation of the phrase "two times a day" may differ widely from the practitioner's intended meaning of two doses, taken about 12 h apart, since common activities such as washing hands, telephoning friends, or surfing the internet "two times a day" seldom reflect a 12 h interval. Patients' understanding of certain commonly used terms can greatly influence intended compliance. Imagine the potential confusion with jargon pharmacists have adapted for their own use, like:

Successful communication requires a common vocabulary between patient and practitioner.

"Profile"	Isn't that a picture an artist draws? Or a view from the side?
"Counseling"	Isn't that what psychiatric patients need?
"Over the counter"	Everyone knows that "under the counter" usually means not legal, or secretive.
"On a drug"	Is that like being "on a table" or "on the floor"?
"Progress"	Progress is almost always good unless your illness is "progressing," which means it is getting worse.

Most patients can make rational decisions. Not only are patients capable, but they actually make decisions concerning their own health and well-being throughout the various stages of the diagnostic and therapeutic processes. Each patient decides whether to be concerned about signs, symptoms, or the discomfort present and decides to agree or not to agree with the diagnosis that is presented. Furthermore, patients decide whether they believe that the proposed therapy is likely to achieve their desired outcome. Too often a patient's cognitive abilities and emotional strengths are overlooked by clinicians, who decide a priori that the patient is helpless and vulnerable. Thus, while vulnerability and other signs of dependency may be real issues in many cases, each individual must be assessed to establish his or her unique abilities and strengths.

Just as the pharmacist is responsible for using special knowledge, skills, and experience to assess the appropriateness of the drug's indication—the likelihood of its being effective and the safety—patients consider these same benefits and risks using their own understanding, expectations, and concerns to determine their compliance behavior. Therefore, to maximize the positive impact of patient counseling and important education efforts, those efforts must be individually tailored to address the unique, personal needs of each patient.

> Patients have beliefs and expectations about drug therapy before the prescription is written.

Similarly, people do not begin taking medication without their own preconceived ideas. Nor do they enter a health care system without their own ideas. They have their own health care beliefs, ideas about medications, and, most importantly, ideas about what they want and when they want it. Patients weigh the advantages and disadvantages of drug therapy, the risks and benefits, and they weigh the discomfort they will have to endure in terms of changing their own behavior against the likelihood of a positive outcome that they consider beneficial.

Compliance is a matter of faith. Just as with any person who is asked or expected to follow a set of directions, the patient must determine whether doing what the professional practitioner has recommended is really going to be in his or her best interest. If patients believe that it will be, then they are likely to do their best to comply with the intended drug regimen. On the other hand, all of the patient package inserts and coaching by pharmacists and physicians will be of little value if patients do not perceive that a condition can cause harm or discomfort or if they do not believe that the recommended therapy will reduce the threat or discomfort caused by the ailment. Patients usually have what they consider to be a good reason for not accepting advice and complying with their prescription instructions. Pharmacists must internalize the fact that patients' perceptions and health care belief systems are major driving forces that ultimately influence the decision to seek or not seek care and to follow or not follow advice.[19]

There are several common causes for inappropriate compliance. These include the following:

- The product the patient needs is not available.
- The patient cannot afford to obtain the needed medication.
- The dosage form cannot be swallowed, tolerated, or administered.

- The patient does not understand the instructions.
- The patient prefers not to take the drug for personal reasons.
- The patient forgets to take the medication.

Examples:

Drug product not available:

A 28-year-old man was prescribed azelastine hydrochloride (Astelin), two sprays per nostril twice a day, for his allergic rhinitis. The medication was just released on the market and it has not been added to the approved formulary of the patient's insurance plan.

Patient cannot afford the drug product:

A 2-year-old girl with her first episode of acute otitis media is prescribed amoxicillin/clavulanate potassium (Augmentin-125) suspension given as 5 mL three times daily for 10 days. The family cannot afford the prescription.

Patient cannot swallow, tolerate, or administer the drug:

A 2-year-old girl with her first episode of acute otitis media is prescribed amoxicillin/clavulanate potassium (Augmentin-125) chewable tablets, one tablet three times a day for 10 days. The child cannot chew and swallow these tablets.

Patient does not understand instructions:

A 33-year-old man with a back injury was prescribed naproxen (Naprosyn) 500 mg three times daily for 10 days. After the first 5 days he is still uncomfortable because he has been taking it only when the pain becomes quite unbearable.

Patient prefers not to take the medication:

A 2-year-old girl with her first episode of acute otitis media is prescribed amoxicillin/clavulanate potassium (Augmentin-125) suspension given as 5 mL three times a day for 10 days. The child does not like the banana flavoring and refuses to take her doses.

Patient forgets to take the medication:

A 37-year-old man with asthma is prescribed triamcinolone acetonide (Azmacort), two sprays four times daily. The man works during the day and seldom remembers to carry his inhaler and use it while on the job.

The vast majority of noncompliance problems direct the focus toward the patient's behavior. However, some modern, expensive, sophisticated health care delivery systems can also be the cause of noncompliance drug therapy problems. A drug distribution or administration system that fails the patient can also precipitate an apparent noncompliance type of drug therapy problem. For example:

- If the drug the patient needs is not stocked in the pharmacy.
- If the drug is lost in the mail.
- If the drug product is not on the approved formulary list.

- If the drug product is not approved for reimbursement by the patient's third-party carrier and thereby not available to the patient.
- If the wrong drug is dispensed.
- If the caregiver fails to administer the drug.
- If the drug delivery device or pump is not functioning properly.

Economics obviously plays an important role in drug therapy problems that result in the patient not taking or not being able to take the medication. Poverty often precludes a patient from even obtaining the appropriate medication. In 1996, the average cost of a new prescription in the United States was $27.21.[20] Expense of medications can also play an influential role in formulary decisions and drug distribution systems and thus influence what drugs will and will not be made available. Formulary committees insist on continually battling budgets by trying to limit the availability of expensive medications. These groups are quick to point out that if the patient really needs the expensive medication, their system will see that it is provided. This "pharmacological safety net" sometimes has serious holes in it. These administrative barriers to patients receiving the medications they need are often just enough of an annoyance to influence the patient to give up trying or not to expend the additional energy required to obtain a drug that is in fact clinically indicated but hidden somewhere in "the system."

Programs designed to improve patient compliance can reasonably be expected to have a positive yet transient influence on patient drug-taking behavior. Intuitively, one should expect improved patient compliance to enhance patient outcomes associated with drug therapy. However, practitioners must also allow for the probability of increased toxicity resulting from enhanced compliance. Improving compliance in a patient who was previously missing several doses each week will increase exposure to the drug, might improve effectiveness, but also has the propensity to cause the side effects and toxicity associated with the drug. What could be assured from a rapid nationwide increase in compliance would be increased drug costs and increased toxicity. We would like to believe that increased compliance always has a positive result, but in reality this is not the case.

The level of noncompliance identified in the Minnesota Pharmaceutical Care Project, which is 12 percent of all drug therapy problems identified, is significantly less than that reported in other literature. We believe that one plausible explanation for this is that the practitioner first identified all other drug therapy problems (Categories 1 through 6) and only when the drug therapy for a patient was first determined to be appropriately indicated, the most effective available, and the safest possible, did the practitioner consider compliance to be a potential problem. After all, 24 percent of the drug therapy problems found in this study involved patients taking the wrong drug or unnecessary drug therapy. Certainly, increasing compliance with these medications would not result in positive outcomes. The practice of pharmaceutical care is essential if we want to assure rational decisions about drug therapy in our societies.

STATING DRUG THERAPY PROBLEMS

Categorizing drug therapy problems into the seven categories of patient problems can be an *empowering process* for a number of reasons. First, this process illustrates how adverse drug reactions (drug therapy problem number 5) are but one category of drug therapy problems. Also, it becomes clear that pharmacists must be able to proactively identify, resolve, prevent, quantify, predict, and intervene in drug therapy problems of all types in order to ensure that each patient experiences safe and effective pharmacotherapy. Second, these categories help to clarify and demarcate the professional responsibilities and accountability of the pharmacist in a team-oriented health care delivery system. Few practicing physicians, nurses, health care administrators, or payers need to be convinced that these problems are important, their prevention necessary, and their resolution in need of an expert. As pharmacy practitioners and pharmacy managers develop systems that put into operation this type of proactive professional practice, the practice of pharmaceutical care, justification for pharmacy personnel, and support services should cease to be distasteful or impossible tasks. Third, categorizing the drug therapy problems can serve as the focus for developing a systematic process whereby the pharmacist contributes significantly to the overall positive outcomes of patients. A systematic process will not only aid the pharmacist in achieving successful outcomes on an individual patient basis but also aid in the pharmacoepidemiologist's development of a national or even international database concerning drug therapy problems.[1]

The fourth function of this categorization is to bring to the clinical work of the pharmacist a vocabulary consistent with that used by other health care professionals. By defining the pharmacist's function in terms of identification, resolution, and prevention of drug therapy problems, the function of the pharmacist is placed in a patient-care context consistent with the responsibilities of other health care practitioners. In the practice of pharmaceutical care, the patient and not the drug product is the major focus of the pharmacist's energies, skills, knowledge, decisions, and actions. If we accept these seven categories of drug therapy problems as a model, or representation of clinical reality, then perhaps the disciplined order provided will effectively structure clinical perceptions in a manner consistent with a truly patient-centered professional practice.

The centrality of drug therapy problems to the practice of pharmaceutical care cannot be over-emphasized. As the presence of drug therapy problems prevent patients from experiencing the desired therapeutic goals associated with their medications, it is absolutely essential that pharmacists who intend to provide pharmaceutical care can internalize the understanding, descriptions, and identification of not only the *concept* of drug therapy problems but of each and every type and common *cause* of drug therapy problems. The responsibility to identify, resolve, and prevent drug therapy problems serves not only as the unique contribution that pharmaceutical care practitioners make to a patient's health care but can also serve as a sort of gyroscope that can guide or refocus the pharmacist's activities in cases involving patients with numerous complex and difficult therapeutic dilemmas. Constant referral to the seven categories of drug therapy problems ensures that a consistent, rational, comprehensive, and effective care plan can be established for even the most complicated case.

The way a drug therapy problem is stated determines the content of the care plan.

One must be aware that the way in which a drug therapy problem is stated or described can greatly influence the care of a patient. Simply stating that a patient is experiencing "toxicity" from drug therapy is not very useful. The type of toxicity (i.e., nephrotoxicity, leukopenia, thrombocytopenia, pseudomembranous colitis, diarrhea, bleeding) and the specific drug thought to be associated with this concentration-dependent or non-concentration-dependent toxic reaction should be identified as part of the statement of the patient's drug therapy problem.

The pharmacist must give considerable thought to how the drug therapy problem is stated. Keep in mind that patients or health care practitioners might treat the problem using their own ideas or using recommendations that are very different from the interventions offered by the pharmacist, but the fact remains that the patient is likely to treat the drug therapy problem based on how it was presented or described by the pharmacist. How a drug therapy problem is stated will not only determine the therapy employed but also often dictate other components of the care plan to be considered, including the follow-up evaluation and specific monitoring parameters.

Experienced practitioners are mindful of the benefit of stating drug therapy problems in a format that is most useful and with an appropriate level of specificity for the patient's condition at the time of intervention. The level of specificity can easily direct all subsequent considerations, including:

- Goals of therapy
- Alternative therapeutic approaches
- Drug recommendations chosen
- Monitoring plans
- Evaluation of outcomes

A problem stated as: *"Toxic trough concentrations resulting from too high a dose of theophylline"* might very well be approached differently than a problem stated as: *"Toxic trough concentrations resulting from theophylline being administered too frequently."* In the first case one might reduce the dose and in the second case one might prolong the dosing interval. Similarly, one might intervene with very different recommendations whether the drug therapy problem in a 7-year-old child is presented simply as a compliance problem or as a more specific problem description such as a difficulty taking a medication four times a day, as prescribed, during the school day.

The manner in which the drug therapy problem is defined can directly guide the solution pursued. For example, if the drug therapy problem is defined as "inappropriate drug therapy," the problem statement is not sufficiently comprehensive to be helpful in identifying a successful resolution. Thus, the pharmacist is not sure if he or she should

1. Change the drug
2. Increase the dose
3. Decrease the dose
4. Add a new drug
5. Discontinue all drug therapy
6. Take some other action

If, instead, the drug therapy problem is defined as the patient receiving too little of the correct drug, it is clear that the pharmacist must recommend an increase in the amount of drug the patient is receiving.

The terminology used to describe a drug therapy problem will influence not only how a patient or other health care practitioner perceives the problem but also how the problem in resolved. Terminology that implies cause and effect must be differentiated from terminology that implies a weaker association. Consider the different therapies that might be initiated to resolve drug therapy problems stated in the following fashion:

- Continued breakthrough seizures associated with subtherapeutic phenytoin concentrations
- Noncompliance with phenytoin therapy, resulting in continued breakthrough seizures

- Gastrointestinal bleeding caused by aspirin
- Gastrointestinal bleeding in a patient presently taking low-dose aspirin as prophylaxis to prevent a second myocardial infarction

- Renal dysfunction possibly associated with gentamicin therapy
- Renal dysfunction secondary to gentamicin therapy

- A rash requiring topical corticosteroid therapy
- A rash from cotrimoxazole therapy

PRIORITIZING DRUG THERAPY PROBLEMS

Pharmaceutical care represents a rational thought process for drug therapy decisions.

Once identified, each drug therapy problem can be prioritized as to the urgency with which it needs to be addressed. This prioritization depends on the extent of the potential harm each problem might inflict on the patient, the patient's perception of the potential harm, and the rate at which this harm is likely to occur. Organized intelligence is the best method to solve problems. Unregulated inquiries can make things worse. As René Descartes (1596–1650) said in his *Discourse on Methods and the Meditations*:[21]

Analyze the problem

Clean it of prejudices

Divide it into as many parts as possible

Decide what is relevant

Conduct thought in order

Simplest to complex

Recapitulate the chains of reasoning to be certain that there are no omissions

In patients with multiple drug therapy problems, some drug therapy problems are identified but are considered to be of such a low priority that they are not resolved or the effort to resolve is delayed until drug therapy problems with a higher priority are first resolved. However, it remains essential to document that those drug therapy problems with a lower priority are identified so that they eventually do receive the attention required and are not simply ignored or forgotten. This raises the question of who determines if there is a drug therapy problem.

Obviously, pharmacists hold a great deal of the responsibility for identifying drug therapy problems. Much of this responsibility stems from their special knowledge and experience in the fields of pharmacology, pathophysiology, and toxicology. However, patients often identify their own drug therapy problems. This occurs through self-diagnosis, self-examination, and introspective comparisons with previous states of health or the condition of friends, colleagues and acquaintances.

When a patient has or at least feels that he or she has identified a drug therapy problem, it must receive the full attention of the pharmacist. When a patient identifies a drug therapy problem, the patient-centeredness and caring philosophy of pharmaceutical care dictate that it is to be seen as a drug therapy problem. One might ask, in a patient-centered practice, "Who better to recognize drug therapy problems than the patient?" An example of the potential impact of patients' perception of what is and what is not a drug therapy problem can be found in the evidence that indicates some 65 percent of elderly patients reveal that they will discontinue taking prescribed medications, without seeking the advice of a health care professional, if they do not perceive they are experiencing the beneficial effects of the drug. In other words, if these patients assess that their drug therapy is not being effective, they will discontinue exposing themselves to it.[19]

The pharmacist prioritizes drug therapy problems relative to the amount of risk confronting the patient. Risk is defined by the severity of danger to the patient and the rate at which the problem can do harm. Prioritizing drug therapy problems is essential because of the frequency with which a pharmacist will encounter patients with more than one drug therapy problem at the same time. In the Minnesota Pharmaceutical Care Project, approximately 10 percent of all patients had two or more drug therapy problems when initially assessed by the pharmacist. Some 5 percent of patients had more than four drug therapy problems that required prioritization and resolution.

> Drug therapy problems are prioritized based on the amount of risk confronting the patient.

Once the list of drug therapy problems is prioritized according to risk, the list is reviewed and the following issues are addressed:

1. Which problems must be solved (or prevented) immediately and which can wait
2. Which problems the pharmacist will identify as his or her primary responsibility
3. Which problems can be solved by the pharmacist and patient directly
4. Which problems require the interventions for someone else (perhaps a family member, physician, nurse, or some other specialist)

Once these decisions have been made, the pharmacist is able to determine which resources are necessary to resolve or prevent the patient's drug therapy problems.

COMMON DRUG THERAPY PROBLEMS IN PRACTICE

The identification and classification of drug therapy problems have a major impact on the care a patient requires and receives. Just as a physician's assessment of the patient's disease or diagnosis directs the subsequent medical care, the pharmacist's assessment of the patient's drug-related needs and drug therapy problems directs subsequent pharmaceutical care.

Common things are common. This old adage holds true for many aspects of life, including drug therapy problems. The most frequently encountered drug therapy problems occur in the most commonly encountered patients who are receiving the most commonly used medications. It is seldom that one actually needs to look for the pharmacological "needle in the haystack"; usually we simply need to recognize the hay in the haystack. During the 3 years of the Minnesota Pharmaceutical Care Project, 9399 different individuals received pharmaceutical care that was documented by community pharmacists. Females represented 59 percent of the patient population; 12 percent of patients were 5 years old or less and 12 percent were 65 years old or older. These patients had a total of 5553 drug therapy problems identified and resolved by the pharmacists providing pharmaceutical care. These drug therapy problems were identified in 37 percent of this patient population. Over 1400 patients had multiple drug therapy problems at some time during their care.

The most frequent category of drug therapy problem encountered in patients cared for by community pharmacists is the need for new or additional drug therapies to treat or prevent a variety of medical conditions. Almost 1 in 4 (23 percent) of the drug therapy problems were associated with untreated conditions, conditions requiring additive or synergistic drug regimens to be incorporated into existing therapies, or drug therapies required to prevent a new disorder from occurring. Only through a comprehensive assessment of each patient's drug-related needs can a pharmacist determine the need for additional drug therapies. Simply reviewing an existing patient profile containing only the medications the patient is already taking means that the pharmacist will continue to miss the most common drug therapy problem type occurring in practice—the need for additional drug therapy. These data represent a clear example of how the practice of pharmaceutical care, as a patient-centered practice, is quite different from other traditional pharmacy activities that focus on the drug, prescription, or list of drugs the patient has already purchased.

In this same group of 9399 patients cared for during the Minnesota Pharmaceutical Care Project, 23 percent of the drug therapy problems were identified in patients who were receiving the wrong drug (15 percent) or a drug for which there was no valid medical indication (8 percent). Some drug therapy problems involved doses that were too high for the patient's individual needs (6 percent) and some drug therapy problems (16 percent) were due to underdosage. As one might expect, adverse drug reactions were also common, and were determined to be the primary cause for 21 percent of the drug therapy problems.

These data, which are summarized in Table 3-6, describe the variation in the type and frequency of drug therapy problems patients have when they present to a community pharmacy practitioner for care.

These commonly occurring drug therapy problems are identified in patients who need drug therapy for diseases and illnesses that are very frequently encountered. In fact, 12 of the most frequently encountered indications for drug therapy represent almost half (51.5 percent) of all of the indications seen in general, community-based pharmaceutical care practice. Table 3-7 lists the 25 most frequently encountered indications for drug therapy in patients cared for by their community pharmacist.

TABLE 3-6 SUMMARY OF DRUG THERAPY PROBLEM DATA FROM 9399 PATIENTS		
DRUG THERAPY PROBLEMS	NUMBER OF DRUG THERAPY PROBLEMS	PERCENTAGE OF DRUG THERAPY PROBLEMS, %
Need additional drug therapy	1265	23
Unnecessary drug therapy	453	8
Wrong drug therapy	857	15
Dosage too low	893	16
Adverse drug reaction	1157	21
Dosage too high	332	6
Inappropriate compliance	596	11

TABLE 3-7 THE MOST FREQUENT INDICATIONS FOR DRUG THERAPY

1. Bronchitis
2. Hypertension
3. Sinusitis
4. Otitis media
5. Pain—general
6. Streptococcal sore throat
7. Peptic ulcer disorder (includes esophagitis, peptic ulcer and gastritis)
8. Allergic rhinitis
9. Estrogen replacement therapy (menopausal symptoms and osteoporosis)
10. Skin infection
11. Depression
12. Arthritis (includes rheumatoid arthritis, osteoarthritis, and arthritis pain)
13. Asthma
14. Urinary tract infection
15. Dental infection
16. Conjunctivitis
17. Hyperlipidemia
18. The common cold
19. Rash
20. Hypothyroidism
21. Diabetes
22. Acne
23. Dermatitis
24. Anxiety
25. Vaginitis

TABLE 3-8 THE MOST FREQUENT INDICATIONS FOR DRUG THERAPY IN PATIENTS WITH DRUG THERAPY PROBLEMS	
1. Sinusitis	6. Strep throat
2. Bronchitis	7. Estrogen replacement therapy
3. Otitis media	8. Allergic rhinitis
4. Hypertension	9. Skin infection
5. Pain	10. Depression

TABLE 3-9 THE MOST FREQUENT INDICATIONS FOR DRUG THERAPY IN PATIENTS WITH NO DRUG THERAPY PROBLEMS	
1. Bronchitis	6. Pain
2. Otitis media	7. Allergic rhinitis
3. Sinusitis	8. Estrogen replacement therapy
4. Strep throat	9. Skin infection
5. Hypertension	10. Depression

These 25 indications represent 75 percent of all of the indications for drug therapy in patients who received pharmaceutical care in their communities. It is important that these common indications for drug therapy form the basis of curricula in colleges of pharmacy to ensure that students are familiar with common patient problems they will encounter in practice.

While Table 3-7 lists the most common indications for drug therapy in a general population of patients who present to community practitioners, Table 3-8 lists, in order of frequency of occurrence, the 10 most frequent indications for drug therapy in patients who have at least one drug therapy problem.

For comparison, Table 3-9 lists the most frequent indications for drug therapy in patients who did not have a drug therapy problem.

One can see that the same 10 most frequent indications for drug therapy are the most common ones in patients who had a drug therapy problem and in those who did not. Therefore, using the indication for drug therapy or the disease state itself as a reliable predictor to identify patients who are likely to have a drug therapy problem and who will most likely benefit from pharmaceutical care services will *not* be effective.

Pharmaceutical care is a generalist practice.

These data support the argument for the development of a *general practice* of pharmaceutical care, rather than defining pharmaceutical care as a specialty practice. We found that the majority of the patients have common and relatively straightforward drug therapy problems that can be identified and resolved, thereby optimizing therapeutic outcomes.

In summary, the list of actual and potential drug therapy problems identified for a patient defines the responsibility of the pharmacist to a particular patient. Some drug therapy problems are quite simple and straightforward, while others are complex and can be difficult, dangerous, and time-consuming to resolve. However, the manner in which a drug therapy problem is stated and categorized has a significant impact on the practitioner's ability to resolve it. Therefore, care needs to be taken when constructing the list of drug therapy problems for a patient. Both of the essential components of the drug therapy problem should be described:

1. The patient's medical condition, illness, symptom(s) or risk factor

2. The nature and magnitude of the association with drug therapy

Each drug therapy problem must be stated explicitly. The more specific the information contained in the problem statement, the higher the probability that an effective solution will be realized. The patient needs to be consulted and sometimes also the physician and/or nurse to determine which of the drug therapy problems are most troublesome to the patient or of concern to the prescriber(s). Then, a documented, comprehensive, and prioritized list of drug therapy problems can be made available for the patient, the pharmacist, the physician, the nurse, and others.

With such a documented list of drug therapy problems, the patient, in concert with any and all necessary health care providers, is able to proceed to resolve (or prevent) problems. In addition, the pharmacist now has clearly defined responsibilities as they relate to each drug therapy problem for each patient, and he or she can proceed to work with the patient to resolve (or prevent) problems and ensure that the patient is in fact receiving medications that are appropriately indicated, as effective as possible, safe, and convenient.

REFERENCES

1. Strand, L.M., Morley, P.C., Cipolle, R.J., *et al.* Drug-related problems: Their structure and function. *DICP Ann Pharmacother* 1990; 24:1093–1097.

2. Scott-Levin, Business Barometer. *Drug Topics.* 1996; 140:25.

3. Strand, L.M., Cipolle, R.J., Morley, P.C., Perrier, D.G. Levels of pharmaceutical care: A needs-based approach. *Am J Hosp Pharm* 1991; 48:547–550.

4. Cipolle, R.J., Seifert, R.D., Zaske, D.E., Strate, R.G. Systematically individualizing tobramycin dosage regimens. *J Clin Pharmacol* 1980; 20:570–580.

5. Cipolle, R.J., Seifert, R.D., Zaske, D.E., Strate, R.G. Hospital acquired gram-negative pneumonias:

Response rate and dosage requirements with individualized tobramycin therapy. *Ther Drug Monit* 1980; 2:359–363.

6. Canafax, D.M., Min, D.L., Matas, A.J., *et al.* Effects of initial cyclosporine dose and timing on long-term levels in cadaver renal transplantation. *Clin Transplant* 1990; 4:321–328.

7. Drug interactions and adverse drug reactions, in *AMA Drug Evaluations*, 5th ed. Philadelphia: Saunders; 1983.

8. Rawlins, M.D. Clinical pharmacology: Adverse reaction to drug. *Br Med J* 1981; 282:974–976.

9. Cipolle, R.J., Rodvold, K.A. Heparin, in Evans,

W.E., Schentag, J.J., Jusko, W.J., eds. *Applied Pharmacokinetics: Principles of Therapeutic Drug Monitoring*, 3d ed. Vancouver, WA: Applied Therapeutics Inc; 1992.

10. OBRA Publ No. 101-508 §4401, 1927(g) November 5, 1990.

11. Vanscoy, G.J., Krause, J.R. Warfarin and the international normalized ratio: reducing interlaboratory effect. *DICP Ann Pharmacother* 1991; 25:1190–1192.

12. deTakats, G. Heparin tolerance. *Surg Gynecol Obstet* 1943; 77:31–39.

13. Groce, J.B., Gal, P., Douglas, J.B., *et al.* Heparin dosage adjustment in patients with deep-vein thrombosis using heparin concentrations rather than activated partial thromboplastin time. *Clin Pharm* 1987; 6:216–222.

14. Mungall, D., Floyd, R. Bayesian forecasting of APTT response to continuously infused heparin with and without warfarin administration. *J Clin Pharmacol* 1989; 29:1043–1047.

15. Cipolle, R.J., Uden, D.L., Gruber, S.A., *et al.* Evaluation of a rapid monitoring system to study heparin pharmacokinetics and pharmacodynamics. *Pharmacotherapy* 1990; 10:367–372.

16. Porter, A.M.W. Drug defaulting in a general practice. *Br Med J* 1969, 1:218.

17. Sackett, D.L., Haynes, R.B. *Compliance with Therapeutic Regimens.* Baltimore, MD: Johns Hopkins University Press; 1976.

18. Haynes, R.B., Taylor, D.W., Sackett, D.L. *Compliance in Health Care.* Baltimore, MD: Johns Hopkins University Press; 1979.

19. Eaton, G. Non-compliance, in Mapes, R., ed. *Prescribing Practice and Drug Usage.* London: Croom Helm; 1980.

20. *Drug Store News* 1997; 5:43–45.

21. Descartes, R. *Discourse on Methods and the Meditations.* Harmondsworth, England: Penguin Books; 1968.

RECOMMENDED READINGS

Cutler, P. *Problem Solving in Clinical Medicine: From Data to Diagnosis*, 2d ed. Baltimore: Williams & Wilkins; 1985.

Elstein, A.S., Shulman, L.S., Sprafka, S.A. *Medical Problem Solving: An Analysis of Clinical Reasoning.* Cambridge, MA: Harvard University Press; 1978.

Fincham, J.E., ed. *Advancing Prescription Medicine Compliance: New Paradigms, New Practices.* Binghamton, NY: Haworth Press, Inc.; 1995.

Friedman, H.H., ed. *Problem-Oriented Medical Diagnosis*, 4th ed. Boston: Little, Brown; 1987.

Higgs, J., Jones, M. *Clinical Reasoning in the Health Professions.* Oxford: Butterworth-Heinemann Ltd.; 1995.

Kassirer, J.P., Kopelman, R.I. *Learning Clinical Reasoning.* Baltimore: Williams & Wilkins; 1991.

McClam, T., Woodside, M. *Problem Solving in the Helping Professions.* Pacific Grove, CA: Brooks/Cole; 1994.

Riegelman, R.K. *Minimizing Medical Mistakes.* Boston: Little, Brown, and Co.; 1991.

Schwartz, S., Griffin, T., *Medical Thinking: The Psychology of Medical Judgment and Decision Making.* New York: Springer-Verlag; 1986.

CHAPTER FOUR

THE PATIENT CARE PROCESS

A DESCRIPTION OF THE PATIENT CARE PROCESS

There is only one patient care process in pharmaceutical care, just as there is only one standard process for providing medical care, dental care, or nursing care. It is a rational, systematic, comprehensive, problem-solving process that allows the practitioner to be thorough and consistent, providing a quality service to the patient. Although there is only one patient care process, each practitioner will execute the process slightly differently, allowing for the "art" of professional practice to take shape. The purpose of clearly defining the common patient care process is not to eliminate the freedom of the individual practitioner, but to accomplish a number of positive objectives. A common patient care process allows the process to be described explicitly so it can be consistently practiced by all practitioners. It allows students to be taught the patient care process consistently by all practitioners. It also enables the student/practitioner to practice a process through repetition so he or she is able to become proficient at providing pharmaceutical care. It allows pharmacists the ability to communicate with other health care providers using a consistent vocabulary which is similar to the one used by other practitioners. Also, when practices have multiple pharmacists caring for patients, they are able to communicate easily amongst themselves. Perhaps most importantly, for the benefit of the patient, all pharmacists, regardless of practice setting, are able to use the same patient care process, so continuity of care between ambulatory, hospital, nursing home, and home health care can occur.

Although each patient receives individualized care, the care is delivered in a systematic and consistent manner so that each patient receives the same *standard of care*. Health care professional practice is too complicated, and the risk to the patient too great, to provide care any other way.

The care process is driven by a patient's drug-related needs.

Let us discuss some of the defining characteristics of the patient care process. First, the patient care process is centered on and "driven by" a patient's drug-related needs. Second, the patient care process describes the activities of the practitioner, as he or she interacts with the patient in a standard, systematic manner. And third, the success of the practitioner in meeting the patient's health care needs depends on very strict discipline to accomplish three objectives:

1. Assess the patient's needs.
2. Bring all the practitioner's available resources to meet these needs.
3. Complete a follow-up evaluation to determine the patient's actual outcomes.

These three characteristics are always central to a patient care process.

The patient care process is the heart of the practice. It is that component of professional practice which represents the work of the practitioner. It is what is visible and tangible to the patient, the action portion of the practice. The patient care process is "what occurs between the practitioner and the patient" on a daily basis. It is what the patient sees, what the practitioner does, what becomes tacitly understood as the *practice*. Moreover, the patient care process is that portion of a practice that can be documented in writing and evaluated for quality. It is what the practitioner is paid to do as a patient care provider.

The patient care process can be documented in writing and evaluated for quality.

This chapter presents the patient care process in two different contexts. First we explain the patient care process as a component of the practice of pharmaceutical care, in other words, we explain exactly *what the patient care process is*. Second, we explain *how the patient care process is executed in practice*. We would encourage the reader not to skip over the first explanation, although there is a tendency to want to arrive immediately at how it is actually done. We have found that pharmacists, since they have never had an explicitly defined, common patient care practice as part of their tradition, minimize the need for one, believe they can do without it, and miss the major point of a professional practice—the discipline required when making decisions which can result in life or death consequences in another human being. The patient care process is not to be treated as a list of activities that must be completed by the pharmacist. Instead, it is series of cognitive processes which involve gathering data, integrating it with knowledge, generating information, making decisions and clinical judgments, and documenting the results.

A professional practice demands discipline when making decisions which affect other people.

THE PATIENT CARE PROCESS AS A COMPONENT OF PHARMACEUTICAL CARE PRACTICE

Let us now place the patient care process back into the larger context of the practice of pharmaceutical care. The patient care process is the philosophy of practice acted out on a day-to-day basis. The patient care process is how the pharmacist actually fulfills the responsibilities spelled out in the philosophy of practice. The patient care process, then, can be seen as "descriptive" in that it is what occurs between one practitioner and one patient on a daily basis. Although what occurs in the practice setting will vary with each patient and each practitioner, the variation has to be small enough to remain consistent with the philosophy of pharmaceutical care practice and consistent enough to function as the same patient care process. Furthermore, it must have enough of the common structure and characteristics to be recognized from one day to the next from one patient to the next, from one practitioner to the next as *the* practice of pharmaceutical care.

The patient care process describes what occurs "today" between the patient and the practitioner. These characteristics of the patient care process are summarized and compared to the other components of the practice of pharmaceutical care (Table 4-1).

Just a reminder: all three elements—the philosophy of practice, the patient care process, and the practice management system—must be in place to form a professional practice that will exist in the long term, be recognized by the health care system, and be reimbursed adequately as a patient care service. The characteristics of the practice management system are discussed in Chap. 7.

STEPS OF THE PATIENT CARE PROCESS

It is a privileged few who are granted license by society to care for others when they are in need. Therefore, those who intend to provide care for others must develop the discipline to meet their responsibilities in a consistent and complete manner. The discipline required to provide pharmaceutical care demands that the practitioner use a systematic, comprehensive, and efficient process to achieve the goals of therapy (appropriate, effective, safe, and convenient drug therapy for the patient), to identify, resolve, and prevent any drug therapy problems that might interfere with those goals, and to assure positive patient out-

	PHILOSOPHY OF PRACTICE	PATIENT CARE PROCESS	PRACTICE MANAGEMENT SYSTEM
Purpose	Prescriptive	Descriptive	Predictive
Those influenced	All practitioners, all patients	Individual practitioner Individual patient	A group of practitioners A group of patients
Relevant time frame	Continuous	Present	Future

TABLE 4-1 PRACTICE COMPONENTS AND THEIR CHARACTERISTICS

Establish a Therapeutic Relationship

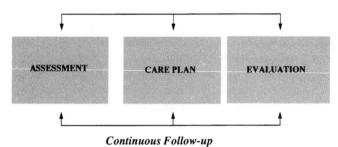

Continuous Follow-up

•**Figure 4-1**   The patient care process.

comes. The patient care process allows the practitioner to accomplish these objectives.

This process is described in Fig. 4-1 and involves three major steps: (1) the practitioner completes an *assessment* of the patient's drug-related needs, including the identification of any drug therapy problems that exist, or need to be prevented in the future. (2) together, the patient and the practitioner construct a *care plan*, complete with goals of drug therapy and appropriate interventions. These goals and interventions are designed to (a) resolve any drug therapy problems present, (b) achieve the individual's goals of therapy; and (c) prevent potential drug therapy problems from occurring in the future. In the last major step (3) the practitioner schedules and conducts a follow-up *evaluation* to determine the actual patient outcomes that have resulted from the care provided.

These three steps of the process occur continuously for a patient. Although the patient is new to the practitioner only once, each time something new occurs involving the patient's drug therapy, the assessment begins again. Just as "you can never step in the same river twice,"[1] you never see the *same patient* twice. Patients change, information is added at each visit and built upon continuously. Therefore the patient and the practitioner will "come in and out of the patient care process" in any order, on numerous occasions over time. Pharmaceutical care is not a static, one-time event. Once care is started, it is ongoing until a patient physically moves away from your practice, seeks out another practitioner to provide pharmaceutical care, or expires.

The continuous nature of this patient care process should be kept in mind, especially since we will now talk about it as though it were a linear process. The steps do occur in order, but as the practitioner internalizes the "cognitive" processes associated with each step, the practitioner will move back and forth from assessment to follow-up evaluation all the time, soon without being consciously aware of doing it. The continuous nature of the patient care process is illustrated below in Fig. 4-2.

Each of the steps is discussed in detail below: the assessment, the care plan, and the follow-up evaluation. For each step, we will discuss its

You never see the same patient twice.

purpose and provide a general outline of the activities involved. A detailed discussion of how to carry out the patient care process can be found at the end of this chapter.

The Assessment

The practitioner always begins to provide pharmaceutical care by making an *assessment* of the patient's drug-related needs at that time. A patient can seek pharmaceutical care directly by asking the pharmacist for help, advice, or input into decisions about his or her drug therapy. A patient might be referred to the pharmacist by another health care provider—for example, a physician, nurse, dentist, veterinarian, or another pharmacist. Or a technician or fellow pharmacist may recognize some need for care during the process of dispensing medications to a patient. Regardless of how a patient is identified as needing care, regardless of the type of patient, the disease (or medical condition) experienced by the patient, and the type of drug therapy involved, the practitioner always begins the care process by making an assessment of the patient's drug-related needs.

> Pharmaceutical care begins with an assessment of the patient's drug-related needs.

An assessment is completed for three different purposes. They are to:

1. Determine that all of a patient's drug therapy is the most appropriate, most effective, safest, and most convenient available.
2. Identify any drug therapy problems that might be interfering with the goals of therapy.
3. Identify any drug therapy problems the patient is at risk of developing in the future—that is to say, any drug therapy problems the pharmacist must help the patient to prevent in the future.

> The primary purpose of the assessment is to identify drug therapy problems.

The assessment step of the patient care process involves extensive communication with the patient to gather information and to integrate this information about the patient with the expert knowledge, skills, and experience of the practitioner. This step is finished when it is decided:

1. That the patient's drug therapy is appropriate, effective, safe, and convenient.
2. If it is not, what drug therapy problems are present at this time.
3. What drug therapy problems need to be prevented in the future.

The answers to these questions establish the basis for a pharmaceutical care plan. However, to answer these questions, the practitioner needs to establish a very good therapeutic relationship with the patient. The therapeutic relationship is described in Chap. 1. As emphasized there, developing the therapeutic relationship takes time, but it develops only during the process of providing quality pharmaceutical care to the patient. This relationship is necessary to successfully complete an assessment of your patient's drug-related needs.

> The assessment ends when the practitioner decides which drug therapy problems are present.

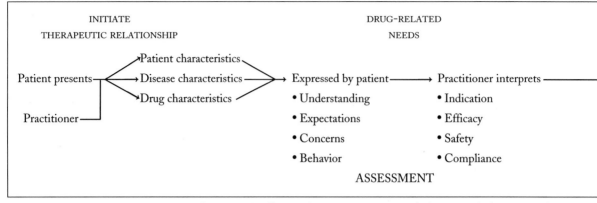

•**Figure 4-2** The continuous care process of pharmaceutical care practice.

A detailed description of how to complete a structured assessment of a patient's drug therapy can be found later in this chapter.

The Care Plan

The *care plan* is an outline of the practitioner's and the patient's responsibilities to meet stated, mutually agreed upon goals and interventions. This care plan represents a joint venture between the patient and the practitioner. It represents a structure for two individuals, the practitioner and the patient, who may have different understanding, different expectations, different concerns, and/or a different value system, to work together to achieve common goals.

The care plan is constructed to define goals, determine appropriate interventions, and to define responsibilities for three different purposes:

1. To resolve the drug therapy problems present at this time, which were identified during the assessment.
2. To meet the goals of therapy for each of the patient's medical conditions, thereby achieving the outcomes desired by the patient.
3. To prevent future drug therapy problems from developing.

The primary purpose of the care plan is to direct the patient's and the practitioner's actions to meet therapeutic goals.

The first and most important step of care planning is establishing goals for each of the purposes just described. These goals need to be clearly stated, measurable, and achievable by the patient. Also, a time frame needs to be associated with each goal so that the patient's expectations about meeting the goals can be realistic. Once the goals have been established, the practitioner must consider the actions to take or choices to be made to successfully meet the patient's drug-related needs. Based on the patient's drug-related needs identified, the care plan will contain *interventions* that are designed to resolve drug therapy problems, achieve therapeutic goals for medical conditions, and prevent new problems from developing. Interventions do not stand by themselves and must be

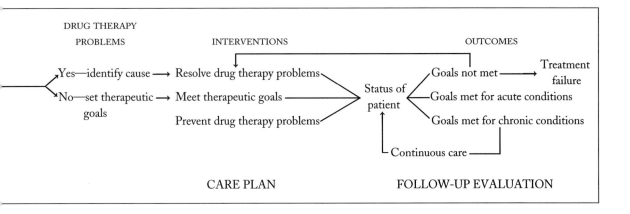

integrated into the patient's care plan. Interventions must be grounded in patient preferences, selected on patient needs, and limited by patient tolerance. All care plans have at least two categories of interventions: the care that needs to be rendered now and what needs to be accomplished at the next follow-up patient encounter.

Interventions are grounded in patient preference, selected according to patient needs, and limited by patient tolerance.

Interventions represent the work that the practitioner performs on behalf of the patient and can include a variety of efforts depending on patient needs and preferences. Interventions in pharmaceutical care might include providing the patient with:

- Information about particular drug therapies
- Information about nondrug therapies
- Changes in drug regimens
- Instructions for drug administration
- Drug product(s) the patient requires
- Assistance with drug administration devices
- Information from other health care agencies
- Referrals to other practitioners

The interventions a practitioner makes must meet the specific drug-related needs of a particular patient. This is why it is difficult for a caring practitioner to use predefined protocols that prescribe certain interventions regardless of individual need. Providing patients with drug products through a dispensing system, mail order, or simply through nonprescription sales is no more and no less than one type of intervention that the practitioner must judge necessary or not for a patient. This is where dispensing products fits within pharmaceutical care. Providing patients with information about nondrug therapies is also an intervention that can be very useful for certain patients, yet not many practitioners would think of defining their practice solely around this particular type of intervention. Therefore, simply providing a patient with drug products cannot drive the care process for an individual

Dispensing drug products is one type of intervention within the patient care process.

patient. Rather, the care process is driven only by patient needs and preferences, both of which go beyond the actual product or any particular means of distribution.

Practitioners want to help their patients. This is most often a good and valuable trait. However, always wanting to help can bias practitioners toward looking only for the good in what might result from their well-meaning interventions. It is imperative that all practitioners who practice pharmaceutical care understand that they are responsible for all of the results (both positive and negative) or outcomes of all of their interventions. This includes not only drug therapies but also information and advice provided to patients. Every intervention has the possibility of helping or hurting the patient. It is the responsibility of the practitioner to be disciplined enough to recognize both of these possibilities and give the probability of negative outcomes the same credence as the possibility of positive outcomes. Patients must understand their commitment, and they must also be willing to assume equal responsibility for their part in the process. In sum, patients cannot be passive recipients of drug therapy; they must participate fully. Communicating this is part of the pharmacist's intervention strategy. And because both positive and negative outcomes will result in almost all patients, it is always necessary to perform a follow-up evaluation.

The care plan is complete when goals have been set, interventions agreed upon, and responsibilities of the patient and the practitioner accepted.

The care plan is complete when goals have been set, interventions agreed upon, and responsibilities of the practitioner and the patient accepted. Then the practitioner is able to establish outcomes (clinical, behavioral, and economic) to be assessed at follow-up. The very last step of the care planning process is to schedule a time to conduct a follow-up evaluation.

The Follow-up Evaluation

The focus of the follow-up evaluation is actual patient outcomes.

The final step in the patient care process is the follow-up *evaluation* of the patient. A follow-up evaluation is a patient encounter, either in person or by telephone, which allows the practitioner to collect necessary information to determine whether the decisions made and actions taken during the assessment and care planning produced positive results. Follow-up evaluations are an active process. Times must be scheduled with the patient, since expecting that patients will call or stop by if something is not working is neither effective nor efficient. Conversely, assuming that everything must be satisfactory with their drug therapy because patients did not call or stop by with further complaints is neither appropriate nor ethical in pharmaceutical care practice. In order to determine patient outcomes, the practitioner must follow up and document what actually happened to the patient. This means actively doing everything reasonable to contact the patient.

And, since drug therapy can produce both positive and negative results, a follow-up evaluation is necessary to fulfill one's responsibilities to the patient.

A follow-up evaluation is conducted for two different purposes:

1. To determine progress toward meeting the established goals of therapy for each of the patient's medical conditions by evaluating the actual outcomes a patient experiences against these stated goals

2. To assess whether any new drug therapy problems have developed or whether any new drug therapy problems need to be prevented in the future

The follow-up evaluation process ensures continuity of care. In practice, many patients have chronic disorders and require continuous care and serial follow-up evaluations in order to compare previously stated goals with progress or status to date. Documented, serial determinations of a patient's progress serve practitioners to evaluate therapeutic approaches designed to help patients make slow but steady positive progress toward long-term goals.

The follow-up evaluation ensures continuity of care.

When the practitioner accomplishes the second purpose for doing a follow-up evaluation (to assess whether any new drug therapy problems have developed or any new ones need to be prevented), the practitioner has come full circle in the patient care process, back to the assessment process once again. This is the only way we can know that we have provided care to a patient, that we have been complete in our care, and that we are able to hold ourselves accountable for our actions.

If you do not follow-up, you do not care.

In summary, the patient care process allows the practitioner to put the philosophy of practice into action for the patient's benefit. It consists of three inseparable steps: the assessment, the care plan, and the follow-up evaluation. The steps of the pharmaceutical care process are summarized in Fig. 4-3.

Although each step of the patient care process is a joint venture between the patient and the practitioner, the amount and type of work required at each step varies with the particular step and the specific needs of a patient. For example, in practice, it appears that a thorough assessment of a patient's drug-related needs requires the majority of

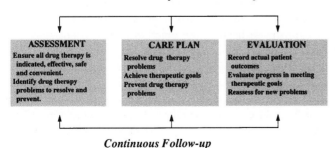

Establish a Therapeutic Relationship

ASSESSMENT	CARE PLAN	EVALUATION
Ensure all drug therapy is indicated, effective, safe and convenient. Identify drug therapy problems to resolve and prevent.	Resolve drug therapy problems Achieve therapeutic goals Prevent drug therapy problems	Record actual patient outcomes Evaluate progress in meeting therapeutic goals Reassess for new problems

Continuous Follow-up

•**Figure 4-3**   The pharmaceutical care process—assessment, care plan, evaluation.

effort on the part of the practitioner. The care plan, in comparison, requires a true fifty-fifty joint venture between the practitioner and the patient. The care plan must represent a course of action that has the acceptance and accountability of the patient. Follow-up evaluations of patient status and outcomes require substantial patient input and effort if they are to truly represent and describe the actual patient experiences and outcome of drug therapies. To ensure that follow-up evaluations reflect actual patient outcomes, the majority of the input must come from the patient.

Practitioners who provide pharmaceutical care impose on them-selves the self-discipline required to make a comprehensive assessment, individualize a care plan, and rigorously follow-up to evaluate the outcomes of the care provided. These three fundamental steps essential to the pharmaceutical care process must be mastered by the practitioner. All three must always be completed, and during each episode of care, the assessment, care planning, and evaluation steps must be addressed in order and fully documented. We have developed a learning aid that will help the pharmacist to master the cognitive processes involved in the patient care process. This aid is called the Pharmacist's Workup of Drug Therapy,[2] and it is used to illustrate how the patient care process is internalized by the practitioner and is executed in practice.

THE PHARMACIST'S WORKUP OF DRUG THERAPY

The Pharmacist's Workup of Drug Therapy is the practitioner's cognitive map to provide pharmaceutical care.

The Pharmacist's Workup of Drug Therapy is a description of the prac-titioner's cognitive thought processes when he or she provides pharma-ceutical care for a patient. The Pharmacist's Workup of Drug Therapy also serves as the outline for what the practitioner must write down, or document, in practice. Each section of the Pharmacist's Workup of Drug Therapy is discussed in detail below, and a complete copy is located at the end of the chapter.

The thought processes involved in the Pharmacist's Workup of Drug Therapy will eventually become internalized as "tacit" knowledge. However, for this to happen, the practitioner must understand exactly what these thought processes are and engage in extensive practice with each process. This can take a practitioner already in practice from 2 months to 2 years. It will take a student up to 4 years, through the for-mal educational process, to become a pharmacist. The exact time it takes usually depends on the number of patients taken care of by the practitioner. The more patients, the steeper the learning curve and the shorter the time it takes to internalize the Pharmacist's Workup of Drug Therapy and become highly proficient at providing pharmaceuti-cal care.

The Pharmacist's Workup of Drug Therapy is the result of extensive research designed to create a rational decision-making process for drug therapy. It became clear early in this research process that the decisions about drug therapy require the same level of disciplined thought and intellectual focus as those required to make rational and appropriate medical diagnoses and nursing care decisions. The standard medical workup[3] serves the medical student, intern, resident, and physician as a standardized format for the efficient gathering and integrating of patient- and disease-specific information for the purpose of practicing good medicine—that is, arriving at the appropriate medical diagnosis and medical care plan. Likewise, nurses utilize a similar standard, problem-oriented format for the purpose of practicing nursing care.[4]

When these approaches are studied, it is easy to identify the common decision-making processes in each and to apply these important steps to the work of the pharmacist when providing pharmaceutical care. The similarity between the professions is extensive and understandable, since all of the health care professions are trying to identify and care for a unique set of patient needs before these become serious health problems. Whether dealing with medical problems, nursing care problems, or drug therapy problems, it is logical that the problem-solving *process* is very similar, only the specific focus and content differ. For this reason, the Pharmacist's Workup of Drug Therapy, as a problem-solving process, parallels the standard medical workup and the nursing care workup. These problem-solving approaches to patient care represent common approaches to slightly different work, many times for the same patient.

All patient care providers use a similar problem-solving process.

These similarities in the way health professionals fulfill their responsibilities (a standard workup of their patients with an assessment, care plan, and follow-up evaluation) are important and can be used to everyone's advantage. First, it allows the various professions to communicate when working to care for a patient. The common approaches to the different work, similar vocabulary, and common understandings of responsibilities, all aid in the communication between different professionals. This should make it easier to integrate specific responsibilities, and helps individuals to function as a "team," to meet the patient's needs.

Another advantage of clearly stating the work of the pharmacist in terms of the Pharmacist's Workup of Drug Therapy is that it makes teaching the student a much more coherent and manageable task. As we have repeatedly emphasized, the work to be completed can be complex. Without explicitly conceptualizing a process by which this patient-specific work can be organized, understood, and managed, it is extremely difficult for the practitioner to teach the student at a consistent, comprehensible level. Moreover, with common approaches to the practice of medicine, nursing, and pharmacy, practitioners can support each other in the process of helping the student and the patient. Learning to constructively work together must occur at all levels from student through to the experienced practitioner.

In addition to guiding the practitioner through the patient care process, the Pharmacist's Workup of Drug Therapy also serves as the framework for the documentation that is required to establish and maintain a viable pharmaceutical care practice. The Pharmacist's Workup of Drug Therapy and its associated documentation generate information and decisions which the practitioner and patient will use repeatedly to solve therapeutic problems. In this sense, as stated earlier, it is similar to the medical record utilized by medical practitioners.

The following section describes the Pharmacist's Workup of Drug Therapy in sufficient detail to permit an inexperienced practitioner to understand this instrument as an aid to the disciplined thought process required to provide pharmaceutical care. A detailed discussion of documentation can be found in Chap. 5.

ASSESSMENT

To carry out a comprehensive assessment of the drug-related needs of a patient, the practitioner must accomplish two objectives: (1) to collect, collate, and integrate several categories of patient-specific data and (2) to make the following decisions.

1. Determine that all of a patient's drug therapy is the most appropriate, most effective, the safest, and the most convenient that is available for the patient
2. Identify any drug therapy problems that might be interfering with the goals of therapy
3. Identify any drug therapy problems the pharmacist must help the patient to prevent in the future

Each component of the assessment is described below in significant detail. However, to make the detail meaningful, we first discuss an overview of how the assessment is done in practice. This should make the section that follows much more useful.

Practitioners and students, in the beginning stages of developing their pharmaceutical care practice skills, must understand that there is a structure to the patient assessment or patient interview. The dialogue between the patient and the practitioner must be designed to determine how to best meet the patient's needs. Given that the primary goal of the assessment is to identify drug-related needs and to identify any drug therapy problems, it makes sense to begin the assessment by asking patients what they want. All patients have some idea of what they want. They may not know how best to achieve their desired outcomes or those outcomes might not be achievable, but through dialogue they can and will express personal goals. Patients may not always have the ability to describe exactly what they need; therefore the pharmacist must develop the skills to apply an organized problem-solving process designed to determine all of the patient's drug-related needs. Only by ascertaining what a patient wants can the practitioner ensure that the services provided will meet the patient's expressed needs and therefore be valued.

Assessment questions such as "What can I do for you today?" or "How can I help you today?" or "What do you need today?" serve to open dialogue with patients, thereby facilitating a description of patient needs. This is very important because the practice of pharmaceutical care is driven by patient needs.

If the first step is to identify patient wants and expectations, then the next logical area to assess is what the patient does not want. Is the patient concerned about whether drugs can really help the particular condition? How concerned is the patient about drug therapy harming him or her? Is the patient concerned about a drug regimen becoming habit-forming?

A practitioner's knowledge of drugs (empirical/objective) is essential to know what concerns a patient should have, but only the patient can provide information revealing subjective concerns. For instance, many patients do not know whether the drug therapy they are expected to take can be habit-forming or not. Without determining if this is a concern of the patient, a pharmacist is not very likely to reassure the patient that the prednisone, fluoxentine (Prozac), sulindac (Clinoril), or conjugated estrogens (Premarin) does not have addictive characteristics and will not be habit-forming even when taken to treat a chronic disorder.

Assessment questions such as "What concerns do you have that I can address for you today?" or "Are there any issues or questions about your medications or your condition that you would like me to answer today?" or "Is there anything that concerns you or that you are worried about before starting this new drug therapy?" can serve to allow your patient to describe personal concerns. Just as your patient's wants and needs will be responded to in the care plan, your patient's concerns must also be directly addressed. Patient concerns that are not discovered, discussed, and addressed will only add to confusion, lack of patient confidence, and noncompliance.

Patients must be encouraged to "tell their story" in order to fully express understanding of their medical condition and related drug therapies, their expectations of treatment and/or recovery, and their awareness of the risks associated with particular drug products. Patients' narratives seldom proceed in a nice, "neat," rational order of providing information to the practitioner. Generally, patient narratives have a beginning, a middle, and an end, often told in a sequence, which is often combined with experiences/observations taken from another point in time, or by portions of the story that are of immediate concern or priority to the patient. For example, in response to "How may I help you?" a

The success of pharmaceutical care is dependent on the quality of the therapeutic relationship.

patient could offer a discursive response such as the following: "My allergies have been really bothering me for the past week—not as bad as my mom's—but a lot worse than last year when I missed almost two weeks of school during the fall. I took some of my mom's Benadryl on Tuesday and that helped some but made me feel sleepy all of the time. Do you have anything I can take that won't bother me so much? I have final exams next week, and I need to do as well as I can to keep my scholarship."

The practitioner must be thoroughly familiar with the Pharmacist's Workup of Drug Therapy to properly interpret and organize all of the patient's narrative. Some of this patient's story about her allergic rhinitis was chronological (last fall it was worse), some family history was included (mother also suffers from allergic rhinitis), patient's concerns were expressed (not wanting to miss school), and we see that the patient's goals include relief of symptoms within a few days, without causing drowsiness. Consistently placing such valuable information within an organized, coherent, conceptual framework clarifies problems and facilitates appropriate action for both patient and practitioner.

The information acquired from the patient then must be integrated with the knowledge and experience of the practitioner. Patients may not know how to recognize potential problem areas, may not know what the pharmacist knows, and so may not be able to articulate all of their drug-related needs themselves. This is the point at which the expertise of the practitioner should drive the assessment process. This makes the collection of patient information essential.

Patient data become useful clinical information once integrated with the knowledge and experience of the practitioner.

To this point the patient assessment has focused on two primary areas: what the patient wants (expectations) and what the patient does not want (concerns). In order for the practitioner to determine how best to respond to meet individual patient needs, the practitioner must develop an individualized response based on each patient's unique aspects and characteristics. The patient's uniqueness is drawn from collecting and incorporating patient demographic information. The purpose of collecting patient demographic data is to provide the practitioner with information to modify the response to the patient's needs and concerns. In other words, patient demographic data are used to modify how the practitioner responds to a given patient's needs. Demographic data such as age, gender, weight, occupation, and allergies are used by the practitioner to develop and continually modify (personalize) the response to the patient's original needs and concerns. Developing a response (care plan) to treat a cough might differ considerably in a patient who is 3 years old versus one who is 93 years old. Similarly, developing a care plan to treat a cough in a 35-year-old pregnant woman might differ from the plan to treat a cough in a 35-year-old commercial airline pilot.

Therefore, the patient data required for the practitioner's assessment of drug therapy must include patient needs, demographics and sociocultural background, diseases and illnesses, alerts, medications, and a systematic review of systems. The extent to which each and every portion of these data are required or useful in the patient-specific pharmaceutical care process depends on a particular patient's clinical situation at the time the assessment is being conducted.

In addition to patient demographic information, the assessment process also includes a review of systems. This comprehensive review is where the pharmacist adds new information to the patient's case. The purpose of this systematic review is to collect and assess other problems or needs the patient might have that may not have been previously identified. Through the review of systems, the pharmacist both expands the information describing the patient's primary problem and can identify new problems that must be addressed now or at some time in the future. Reviews of the patient's vital signs, cardiovascular status or history, and/or renal function allows the pharmacist to ensure that other problems or risk factors are taken into account in developing a personalized care plan. Additionally, information from the review of systems is often essential as baseline data to be used for comparison later to evaluate the impact (positive or negative) of newly initiated drug therapies.

It is through the constant incorporation of individual patient demographics and review of systems information, that the practitioner modifies the "standard protocol" response to ensure that the patient's needs, expectations, and concerns are being met. With only drug and disease information, one cannot individualize care to meet the unique needs of the patient. Furthermore, with only drug and disease information in hand, one can only provide impersonal, general information and generic "patient counseling." In these situations the pharmacist's work and energies, by default, must be directed toward the drug product or in some situations solely on the disease state. Computers, books, package inserts, and even the internet contain this type of drug product-focused information. Armed with only a prescription for amoxicillin to treat otitis media, a pharmacist can only provide general drug information. In order to provide a valuable, unique, patient-focused service, the pharmacist must incorporate patient demographic information through the structured assessment process to modify "general" information, develop a personalized response and plan to meet the patient's needs.

The assessment personalizes the care process.

During the patient assessment process, the pharmacist is constantly collecting and analyzing data to address two fundamental questions. "What are the patient's drug-related needs?" and "Does the patient have any drug therapy problems?" Both of these questions must be asked in order to develop a personalized care plan for the patient. Responsible, competent, clinical, decisions and judgments cannot be made without data!

The first step in deciding what the patient's drug-related needs are is to ask: "What indications for drug therapy does the patient have?" In order to answer this question, the practitioner must combine patient, disease, and drug information. All three are necessary. Usually the question that must first be asked for any patient with a new prescription is: "Is this drug therapy appropriately indicated for this person at this time?" Also, the practitioner must assess what the patient understands about drug therapy and the disorder. The more the patient understands, the less time and effort is required in patient education or patient counseling. The less the patient understands the more effort, time, and resources will be required to ensure that he or she can and will comply with the medication directions and instructions in the care plan being developed.

The Pharmacist's Workup of Drug Therapy is a fluid process and can be expanded as necessary. In practice, the collection of data is cumulative. Moreover, experienced practitioners become highly efficient at gathering the information necessary to identify a patient's drug-related needs. On the other hand, inexperienced practitioners are less certain and frequently less confident regarding the nature and type of information that will actually assist them in their decision making tasks. Thus, we find that inexperienced practitioners all too frequently tend to develop a "shotgun" approach to information gathering thereby producing quite discursive, and less than useful, data. In either case, it is crucial that practitioners internalize all the components of the Pharmacist's Workup of Drug Therapy in order to collect and reassemble patient responses and "medication narratives" into a succinct, effective document.

There must be a purpose for each item of patient data collected.

Data are never gathered as an end in themselves. Each item that is gathered from the patient is collected for a purpose. Before any data are collected, the practitioner must determine (1) that they are necessary, (2) why are they necessary, and (3) how will they be used. Do not waste the patient's time. When the information is collected, it must be used immediately to determine if more information is required and to make decisions about the patient's drug therapy.

The assessment must determine what the patient wants (expectations), what the patient does not want (concerns), and what the patient knows (understands) about drug therapy.

In summary, the assessment process represents a structured data- and information-gathering dialogue between the patient and the pharmacist and is designed to determine very specific, essential information in order to allow a patient-specific care plan to be developed to respond to the patient's unique needs, expectations, and concerns. What the patient wants (expectations), what the patient does not want (concerns), and what the patient knows (understanding) are the three essential topics that must drive the assessment dialogue. Additionally, patient demographic information is then used to modify and personalize the pharmacist's response to the patient's drug-related needs and drug therapy problems.

We are now ready to approach the detail of the Pharmacist's Workup of Drug Therapy. We will do this by discussing how the practitioner works through each of the sections of the assessment.

Patient Needs

As described in detail above, the assessment always begins with the needs of the patient. The pharmacist begins by collecting the following data from the patient.

The assessment always begins with the needs of the patient.

PATIENT NEEDS

Patient Understanding of Drug Therapy: What is your patient's level of understanding of his or her diseases, drug therapies, and instructions? Does your patient understand that it will be necessary to actively participate in his or her care?

Patient Expectations: What does your patient want? What are your patient's expectations of his or her drug therapies? Are they realistic, achievable? Does your patient expect to be an active participant in his or her care?

Patient Concerns: What concerns does your patient have about his or her health in general, medical conditions, or drug therapies? Side effects, toxicity, allergies, costs?

These needs should be the basis for all the following information collected. It is important to remind oneself that these needs are the most important of all, since they reflect how the patient sees the situation.

Patient Demographics and Background

Following is the material included in the patient demographics and background. The pharmacist will need this information about a patient to make his/her assessment of the patient's drug-related needs.

PATIENT DEMOGRAPHICS AND BACKGROUND:

Age:____ **Gender:**____ **Race:**____ **Ht:**____ **Wt:**____ **LBW:**____
Male = 50 kg + [2.3 × (no. inches > 5′0″)]
Female = 45 kg + [2.3 × (no. inches > 5′0″)]

Health Plan:_____ **Primary Physician:**_____

Family: Describe your patient's family. If an adult, married? Children? How many? Ages? Does your patient live with his/her parents? Does your patient have a family history of certain diseases, conditions, or risk factors for drug therapy problems?

Living Arrangements: Who lives with your patient? Who cares for your patient? Does your patient live alone? Who administers medications?

Occupation: Socioeconomic status of your patient? Does employment put your patient at risk for certain diseases or drug therapy problems? Insurance plan and coverage.

(continued)

PATIENT DEMOGRAPHICS AND BACKGROUND (*continued*):

Special Needs: What unique needs does your patient have that will need to be accommodated when designing a personalized pharmaceutical care plan? Physical abilities, allergies, cultural traits, health care beliefs, labeled instructions, childproof tops, drug administration devices, compliance reminders, taking medications at work/school?

History of Present Condition and Past Medical History: When did the present primary condition(s) begin, and what has been the course of the disease over the recent past? Has the present medical problem been treated with drugs previously? What was the outcome? Describe other important past medical events that may impact your patient's present or future care. Is there anything in the patient's history or background to suggest a risk factor to develop a serious condition or that would represent a contraindication to drug therapy?

The *patient demographics* portion of the Pharmacist's Workup of Drug Therapy includes name, gender (to assess risk factors including pregnancy), and ethnicity/cultural origin (to assess certain risk factors and/or health care beliefs, occupation, religion, marital status, etc.). The patient's age is required for dosing guidelines and is identified and documented as birth date, so that age can be continuously updated. Each patient's height and weight are noted and can be used for dosage individualization. Lean body weight is estimated when required for dosage individualization of specific medications. The patient's address is documented for billing purposes or to mail drug supplies or health information of interest to the patient. Each patient's, or parent(s), preferred phone numbers are recorded and are to be used for follow-up evaluations. Primary prescriber(s) are documented for referrals or consultation, and the patient's health care plan(s) information assists in determining formulary restrictions and payment. Except for frequent changes in some health care plans and noteworthy restrictions, most patient demographic information involves a one-time collection and documentation. However, as with all sections of the Pharmacist's Workup of Drug Therapy, the patient demographics are to be changed and updated when circumstances require such attention.

In order to identify all of a patient's drug-related needs, the *patient's background information* should be incorporated into the assessment process. Most often the background information that is instrumental in making drug therapy decisions includes descriptions of the patient's family situation, living arrangements, understanding, concern, and expectations of drug therapy and any other unique needs the individual might have. The patient's family situation is often very important in determining drug-related needs. Does the patient have children who live at home, and is their age important to consider for safety purposes? (Childproof tops, storage of medications) Do other family members have a history of certain diseases, illnesses, or other risk factors that may negatively affect drug therapy? (Heart disease, depression, allergies) Does the patient live with his or her parents, spouse, or significant other? Does he or she live alone? Who is responsible for administering medications and making health care decisions? Who lives with the patient, and who cares for the patient? The patient's occupation and socioeconomic status can have a dramatic influence on drug-related needs and outcomes. Does the patient's occupation put him or her at risk for certain diseases, injuries, or drug therapy problems?

Important patient-specific information required to make an assessment of a patient's drug-related needs includes the patient's general understanding of therapy, concerns about it, and expressed expectations of therapeutic outcomes. Are these expectations realistic? Are they achievable? In order to reach realistic conclusions practitioners may ask:

- What is the patient's level of understanding of his or her disease or illness, drug therapies, and therapeutic instructions?
- Does the patient understand what it means to actively participate in his or her personal health care?
- Are the patient's expectations realistic and achievable?
- What concerns does the patient have about his or her health in general or medical conditions and drug therapies in particular?
- What concerns does the patient have about side effects, toxicities, allergies?
- To what degree is the cost of drug therapy, clinic visits, hospitalizations, or treatment failures, a concern for the patient?
- What does the patient dislike about his or her drug therapies?
- To what extent does the patient want to be an active participant in his or her care?

These are important questions asked to provide the scope of patient information necessary to familiarize the practitioner with the patient (via their therapeutic relationship) and provide essential background information to contextualize decision making.

Every patient has some special or unique needs that must be identified and incorporated in the assessment of specific drug therapy requirements. These often include physical limitations such as sight and/or hearing impairment which might require larger than usual print for instructions, or written follow-up rather than telephone communications. Patients requiring contact lenses or eyeglasses for vision correction may appreciate larger or bolder print for their instructions and may be very interested in new products or advances in contact lens technologies or lens care products as they become available. They may also benefit from referral to other health care providers to meet these special non-drug-related needs. Other physical limitations—including the need for a cane, walker, or wheelchair—must be documented and might require home visits by the practitioner, delivery services, or mail services for medication and supplies to ensure that the patient receives all of the support and care required.

Optimal patient outcomes require the practitioner be sensitive to a patient's health beliefs, culture, and language.

Language difficulties or barriers are a particularly important problem area. Patients with diverse cultural backgrounds, health beliefs, and values that may differ from those of the practitioner require special attention. Such cultural contexts and the languages used to represent them can, and do, build barriers and prevent positive therapeutic outcomes.

Many patients require drug administration devices to assist in the drug delivery process or to assist with adherence difficulties, and their record should document these special needs. Children who must take some of their medication supplies to school or day care may have special needs for extra containers or special labeling as well as separate drug administration instructions for the teachers and/or nurses in the school. Similarly, adults who take medications to the workplace may have special needs for extra supplies or containers to simplify integrating multiple daily dosing regimens into their otherwise busy lifestyles.

Current Medical Problem List

Here is a look at what information is required, how to understand the information, and how to comprehend the current medical problem list:

> **Current Medical Problem List** (Diagnoses, Complaints, Conditions): What is your patient's primary medical problem and its associated drug therapy? List all of your patient's other current (active) medical conditions and their associated drug therapies. Are these medical conditions being treated with drug therapy? Are all medical problems being appropriately treated? Do any of these medical problems suggest an indication for additional or new drug therapy? Are any of these conditions the result of drug therapy, or could they affect the way drugs are absorbed, distributed, metabolized, or eliminated by your patient?

The *current medical problem list* in the Pharmacist's Workup of Drug Therapy includes the patient's current complaints, diagnoses, conditions, and illnesses. For each of these current problems, if and how they are being treated is described. Additionally, the practitioner must assess whether all of the patient's current, active problems are being appropriately treated, or if any are actually the result of drug therapy the patient is presently receiving. Finally, an assessment is made to determine to what extent, if any, the patient's morbidity is affecting drug absorption, distribution, metabolism, and elimination.

The *history of present condition* section of the Pharmacist's Workup of Drug Therapy describes the present primary problem, when it began, previous attempts to treat it and the results or outcomes of any previous therapeutic approaches. Here is a complete look at the necessary information:

> **History of Present Condition and Past Medical History:** When did the present primary condition(s) begin, and what has been the course of the disease over the recent past? Has the present medical problem been treated with drugs previously? What was the outcome? Describe other important past medical events that may impact your patient's present or future care. Is there anything in the patient's history or background to suggest a risk factor to develop a serious condition or that would represent a contraindication to drug therapy?

Any information in the patient's history or background that suggests a high risk predisposition to develop a serious condition or that would represent a contraindication to future drug therapies should be described as part of the patient's *past medical history*. It is important to note that past successful or failed drug therapies are often the best predictors of future drug therapy outcomes for individual patients. Without an adequate documentation of patient history, practitioners are destined to repeat old mistakes and reinstitute therapeutic approaches that have failed in the past. A failure to document previous therapeutic approaches not only wastes time and resources but also places the patient at risk for repeated treatment failures and continued drug-related morbidity.

Every assessment of a patient's drug-related needs must contain a comprehensive description and analysis of any patient *allergies* and *alerts* that the practitioner must use to prevent future drug therapy problems. Here is a comprehensive description:

> **ALLERGIES AND ALERTS**
>
> **ALLERGIES AND ADVERSE DRUG REACTIONS:**
> Have any allergic reactions occurred in the past? What is the nature and significance of past allergic reactions? Do potential allergies exist (drug, food, preservatives, additives, etc.)? Is there evidence that the patient could not tolerate a medication or dosage form in the past due to an adverse drug reaction? What concerns does your patient have about their drug allergies or reactions? Pay particular attention to allergic symptoms that are common during infancy and childhood, including eczema, urticaria, perennial rhinitis, and reactions to insect bites.
>
> **SMOKING/ALCOHOL/RECREATIONAL DRUG USE:**
> Describe the tobacco, alcohol, or caffeine, or recreational use of your patient. Does it contribute to the patient's medical problems of health risks in general? Does it affect drug absorption, distribution, metabolism, or elimination?
>
> **COMPLIANCE HISTORY:**
> Who is responsible for medication administration for your patient? Is there evidence that your patient has any difficulty understanding and complying with medication instructions?
>
> *(continued)*

ALLERGIES AND ALERTS (*continued*):

IMMUNIZATION HISTORY:

Is your patient's immunization protection up to date including diphtheria, tetanus, pertussis, *Haemophilus influenzae* type B, poliovirus, measles, mumps, rubella, , Hepatitis B, Varicella zoster?

To meet the responsibility of preventing drug therapy problems, it is essential that practitioners be in a position to make a complete and comprehensive assessment of therapeutic risk. Clearly, not "red-flagging" a patient who is allergic to a drug product can, and often does, produce a devastating outcome. Exposing a patient who is aspirin-intolerant to aspirin or one of the ever-expanding number of other non-steroidal anti-inflammatory agents is both dangerous and unnecessary. Reexposing a patient who is allergic to penicillin to a penicillin-containing product can be life-threatening. Such observations should generate no controversy. Most often these high-risk situations are the result of poor documentation or a failure to critically use the documentation at hand, and make responsible judgments/decisions. In contrast, rechallenging a patient who experienced nausea from an erythromycin product in the past does not usually preclude the use of this efficacious antimicrobial agent. In far too many patient care documentation systems, allergic reactions, and almost any adverse reaction or side effect that might have occurred during a drug therapy treatment, is classified as a "drug allergy." However, in the practice of pharmaceutical care, allergic reactions to medications and adverse reactions to medications are classified and documented separately because they have different meanings in the context of the rational drug therapy decision-making process of pharmaceutical care.

Allergies to drugs, in most cases, require that the patient not be exposed to the offending drug or drug product at any time in the future. However, if a patient experiences an adverse effect or predictable side effect from a drug or drug product, that information is important to the patient and practitioner, so that the future use of the offending agent can be critically examined should it again be considered. Erythromycin might certainly be considered a viable treatment in a patient who experienced nausea from erythromycin as long as the first episode was appropriately assessed and documented as an adverse effect and not as an allergic response.

To distinguish between an allergic and an adverse reaction that is not of allergic origin, the practitioner must not only conduct a comprehensive history of the event but also be familiar with the nature and significance of past allergic reactions and be able to identify common presenting signs and symptoms of allergic reactions to drugs. The practitioner must also pay particular attention to allergic symptoms that are common during infancy and childhood. These include, for example:

- Eczema
- Urticaria
- Perennial allergic rhinitis
- Reactions to insect bites and stings

In the case of adverse reactions to drug products, the practitioner must assess whether the patient could tolerate the medication or a particular dosage form and what reservations the patient might have about being reexposed to this particular medication.

In most societies, tobacco use, alcohol consumption, even occasional use of "drugs of abuse" are placed in a unique context and very often are not recognized as influencing the drug-related needs of patients. Also, the use of these frequently potent drugs is almost ignored by most standard patient care documentation systems and therefore not incorporated into most patient care plan decisions. When providing pharmaceutical care, the practitioner must assess the patient's use or exposure to these ubiquitous drugs and determine the impact this exposure has on the health and well-being of the patient. Products that have proven to be very effective in supporting patients who want to stop smoking are widely available without a prescription and can have a dramatically positive influence on the patient's quality of life and outcomes. Moreover, poor outcomes from comorbidities, especially respiratory and cardiovascular, can often be prevented through a comprehensive assessment of a patient's smoking and alcohol history. Similarly, constant exposure to drugs of abuse and the associated addictive behaviors of tolerance, withdrawal symptoms, self-deception, loss of will power, and distortion of attention can place a patient at risk to experience serious medical, financial, compliance, or other drug therapy problems.

The literature on compliance problems certainly establishes the enormous need for practitioners to make comprehensive assessments of each patient's ability and willingness to understand and follow instructions for care plans and medication use.[5,6] Recall, the pharmacist must understand that there is always a reason for noncompliance. Too often well meaning pharmacists reach the conclusion that noncompliance is *the* problem if a patient is not responding to therapy. However, the disciplined thought process and problem-solving approaches that serve as foundations for pharmaceutical care practice call for a systematic assessment, which must deal with the appropriateness of the indication for drug therapy first, followed by effectiveness and safety. Only when these responsibilities are fully addressed in the assessment should compliance be considered a likely reason for the problem at hand.

Many of the reports of noncompliance rates of 40 to 60 percent include cases in which there was not an adequate assessment of other (often more common) drug therapy problems. People do not take drug

Compliance cannot become a drug therapy problem until inappropriate, ineffective, and unsafe drug therapies are eliminated from the patient's regimen.

therapy if they do not understand the indication or believe it is in their best interest. People also do not take drug therapy that makes them feel miserable or if they have concerns of toxicity or harm that have not been adequately addressed.

However, as we noted earlier, compliance remains a major challenge in the practice of pharmaceutical care. Therefore, for some patients, the assessment should identify the individual responsible for medication administration and assess any difficulty understanding instructions. The following questions will elicit this information:

- Does the patient understand how to administer the medications?
- Can the patient physically manipulate the prescription container, the inhaler, the dropper, the unit-dose packaging?
- What language does the patient speak?
- What language, if any, does the patient read?
- Can the patient see the written instructions?
- Does the patient understand what you said?
- Did the patient even hear what the practitioner said?
- Does the patient understand the directions?
- Do directions that state "every 4 to 6 hours" mean the patient is required to wake up just to take a dose on time?
- Does the patient understand the purpose of all these numbers, initials, and abbreviations on the prescription label?
- Is the purpose of refills clearly understood by the patient?
- Has the patient been told why the color of the pills might change?
- What is the patient's interpretation of "as needed" or "as directed"?
- What does "twice a day" mean to the patient?
- Does the patient know what kind of food is required/recommended when the label says "take with food"?

Noncompliance is a communication problem between the patient and the practitioner.

It has been our experience that noncompliance is a communication issue and that compliance with care plan instructions, as well as instructions for medications, is directly related to the quality of the therapeutic relationship between the patient and the practitioner. It is very important to always keep in mind that the patient needs clear, concise, and complete understanding of his or her medical condition as well as medications. Patients whose concerns are not adequately addressed are unlikely to comply with instructions. If the patient does not believe that his or her expectations are going to be met or respected, then compliance with drug therapy, referrals, and health care advice will be minimal. It is essential that the practitioner takes seriously the need to do all of the necessary work required to ensure that the patient experiences positive drug therapy outcomes, before patient noncompliance is considered a primary drug therapy problem.

With the exceptions of clean water, sanitation, and nutrition, the most effective mechanism that modern health care has developed to prevent disease and human suffering is immunization. Diseases such as polio, mumps, tuberculosis, diphtheria, tetanus, pertussis, rubella, and many forms of hepatitis and influenza can be effectively prevented if patients are properly immunized.[7] Unfortunately, most patient care documentation systems—and, in fact, many health care record systems in general—do not adequately address individual immunization records. In the United States, "tracking" vulnerable children to ascertain their immunization status is largely left to school systems. However, because a primary responsibility of pharmaceutical care practitioners is prevention, *immunization history* is an essential part of the Pharmacist's Workup of Drug Therapy and must be considered in the assessment of every patient's drug-related needs. Immunization standards vary throughout the world, but they are commonly designed to ensure adequate protection against diseases that can reach epidemic proportions. Ensuring that patients are adequately immunized is certainly a primary health care priority, and pharmaceutical care practice is designed to directly improve our ability to meet this important need.

Medication Record

The patient's *medication record* functions as that section of the Pharmacist's Workup of Drug Therapy where the indication for drug therapy, and all of the drugs a patient is actually taking, are organized in a meaningful context.

Here is the format most frequently used for gathering this information:

MEDICATION RECORD: Identify **all** medications presently taken by your patient as well as those taken during the past 6 months. Prescription (Rx), samples (S), nonprescription (OTC), as well as herbal remedies (H).

Indication	Drug Product	Dosage Instructions	Goals of Therapy & Progress

---

This includes prescription medications, nonprescription products, professional samples, medications obtained from friends or family members, home remedies, natural and homeopathic remedies, and drugs of abuse. Indeed, it includes *all* things considered drugs! Estab-

Herbal medicines, home remedies, vitamins, samples, nonprescription, and prescription products, can all cause drug therapy problems.

lishing the appropriate indication or "connection" between each and every drug the patient uses and the medical condition, disease, or illness is an absolute necessity in the provision of pharmaceutical care. For many patients, this will be the first time that any practitioner has put forth the effort to collect and document all indications and associated drug therapies. These data are invaluable, not only to the pharmaceutical care practitioner but also to medical, nursing, emergency, and dental practitioners, as well as other care providers. In addition to the list of indications and drug therapies, the current "problem list" section is used to document the assessment of whether or not the patient has any indications that are presently not being adequately treated with drug therapy, or if any of the patient's present condition(s) might be the result of medications taken. The problem section is also used to assess if any of the patient's conditions might adversely influence the manner, or extent, to which drugs are absorbed, distributed, metabolized, or eliminated.

The indication represents the actual reason a patient requires drug therapy.

In order to provide pharmaceutical care it is essential to establish and document the *indication* for every medication the patient is taking. Indication is a critically reflexive category. The concept of "indication for drug therapy" is intended to encompass *all* of the possible reasons that drug therapy might be required by a patient. Therefore, indication reaches well beyond disease or medical diagnosis and in general includes curative, preventive, palliative, and diagnostic purposes.

An indication for drug therapy is designed to:

- Cure a disease or illness
- Prevent a disease or illness
- Provide comfort and temporary relief from signs and symptoms of a disorder
- Assist in the diagnostic process
- Correct abnormal laboratory values

It is vital during the assessment that the *intended* indication for each medication the patient is taking is described, associated with the appropriate medication(s), and documented.

All of the *drug products* that a patient is taking (or is expected to take) are documented on the medication record. Whether the medication is a prescription filled at some other pharmacy, a mail-order item, a nonprescription product purchased at a grocery store, gas station, or from some other source, it must be included in the medication record in order to make a comprehensive assessment of the patient's unique drug-related needs. The practitioner must be able to assess the appropriateness of the entire dosage regimen, including the dosage form, the dose the patient is expected to take, the intended route of administration, and the frequency of actual drug administration. When the patient began the particular drug regimen and, if applicable, when it was discontinued, is also important to consider and document. Lastly, this portion of the Pharmacist's Workup of Drug Therapy also considers goals of therapy and any evidence as to the progress in meeting those goals, and associated side effects. In many situations the single most influential determinant a practitioner will use in the drug therapy decision-making process is this type of direct, patient-specific evidence as to the actual effectiveness, or toxicity, of a particular drug regimen(s). Therefore, to reiterate, each workup of a patient should document any evidence of drug therapy outcomes, be they successes or failures.

In summary, the medication record lists and makes the associations (and cause-and-effect relationships when appropriate) between the patient's indication for drug therapy, the drug product and dosage regimen, and the patient's response to his or her particular drug therapy. This stage of the Pharmacist's Workup of Drug Therapy assists the practitioner to identify and document the fundamental connections linking the most important information in the pharmaceutical care process, that of patient, disease, and drug. All three types of information are absolutely necessary in order to make rational decisions about a patient's drug-related needs. A medication record, such as that described here, contains highly individualized, specific information essential for the provision of patient care. A comprehensive medication record consistently organized by therapeutic indications for the patient, including clinical evidence of outcomes, rarely exist in any other place in the health care system in any meaningful way. It is an extremely valuable instrument, not only to the pharmaceutical care practitioner but to other health care practitioners who care for the patient. Also, patients express a need and voice appreciation for this type of information, and our research indicates that they respond very positively when this record is made available to them as part of their personalized pharmaceutical care plan.

Review of Systems

All of the information included in the review of systems, along with all the decisions that need to be made with the information, are described below.

The Pharmacist's Workup of Drug Therapy facilitates and structures the practitioner's efforts to collect and document patient, disease, and drug data. The workup presents an organized review of systems for the purpose of identifying additional drug-related needs of the patient. The review of systems is used to organize new findings and the practitioner's interpretation of any abnormal or unexpected values to ensure that a comprehensive review has been conducted. As described earlier, patients do not always have the ability to identify or describe all of their drug-related needs, therefore the pharmacist must systematically investigate and assess the patient's medical conditions, complaints, and concerns.

This process is completed through the review of systems. The review of systems includes physical findings, descriptions and experi-

The review of systems is a secondary level of inquiry designed to identify additional drug-related needs.

ences offered by the patient, and laboratory values, in addition to base-line information required for later comparison to evaluate effectiveness and/or toxicity. The specific order of the sections in the review of systems has been developed through clinical and research experience to represent the most common and useful sequence for practitioners. However, in practice some patients will have extensive information, and even numerous laboratory findings in some sections, and they may have very little that requires consideration in other sections. Obviously, in the Pharmacist's Workup of Drug Therapy for a patient with a seizure disorder, the neurological section of the review of systems might contain considerably more information than the gastrointestinal section. However, the discipline that is required of a pharmaceutical care practitioner demands that each and every section of the review of systems be considered in a comprehensive assessment. Only with this type of professional discipline and serious attention to detail, can patients be confident that all of their drug-related needs are being addressed, and the practitioner can also be reasonably confident that errors of omission are avoided.

Useful sources of information to supplement direct patient information include medication profiles. In practice these often lack important information about many medications that people use on a daily basis. Most prescription profile systems do not record prescription medications purchased from other pharmacies, physician samples, medications from friends or relatives, drugs of abuse, natural or home remedies. Our experience indicates that these nonprofiled drugs represent up to 20 percent of the drugs patients actually take. In addition, most traditional pharmacy dispensing profile systems do not include nonprescription medications, which are more common than prescription drugs in most countries. The patient's medical chart or medical record is also a useful source of information that can be used to supplement the direct patient information. The difficulties in obtaining a current copy of a patient's medical record in a timely fashion are well known to most health care practitioners. And because the original purpose of the medical record was to support the provision of medical care and not pharmaceutical care, these records are most often lacking in drug and patient information required by the pharmaceutical care practitioner. Within the review of systems, laboratory test results can be very useful to supplement direct patient information. Again the patient's medical record is often an effective source for these data. However, sometimes it is more efficient to directly involve the patient in the collection of test results that are useful in the provision of pharmaceutical care.

The pharmaceutical care practitioner must determine if abnormal findings are caused by drug therapy or can be treated with drug therapy.

It is important to consider not only the more objective, empirical data, but also to record the practitioner's and the patient's interpretations of the therapeutic experience. Simply inserting laboratory data into the Pharmacist's Workup of Drug Therapy is of very little use without the practitioner's interpretation of specific findings as they present in the patient who frequently has a specific set of disorders, and who is often taking a variety of drug products. Again, each new finding considered in the review of systems section of the Pharmacist's Workup of Drug Therapy should be accompanied by a concise interpretation of the patient's status or laboratory test results at a specific time. The practitioner's interpretation is most useful if it consistently addresses two important questions:

1. Are there deviations from normal or expected which could be due to any particular drug therapy the patient is receiving?
2. Are there deviations from normal or expected which can be treated or corrected using drug therapy?

In other words, is the identified problem caused by a drug, or can it be treated with a drug? It is of little value to merely copy laboratory test results from one computer system to another or even from one piece of paper to another without interpreting those findings in the actual context of a patient taking drugs for specific therapeutic purposes. In this section the practitioner can also establish and document cause-and-effect relationships such as an elevation in blood glucose caused by an antihypertensive agent taken by the patient. Similarly, if the patient suffers from confusion and is going to be started on a particular drug that is known to cause cognitive difficulties, then this baseline status is pertinent in order to effectively evaluate the impact this medication has on the patient.

The review of systems section of the Pharmacist's Workup of Drug Therapy most often begins with the patient's vital signs. Every patient has a temperature, a pulse, a systolic and diastolic blood pressure, and a respiratory rate. These data are always available, can be collected at very little or no cost, and are often important in drug therapy decision-making and subsequent monitoring. The practitioner's interpretation transform these data into information that can be useful in the provision of pharmaceutical care. Remember, many of the most commonly used medications can cause undesirable increases or decreases in a patient's vital signs. Additionally, these most important monitoring parameters are used to evaluate the outcome of drug therapies in almost all patients. For example, change in patient temperature is a hallmark indicator for almost every type of infectious disease process from sinusitis to malaria. Heart rate and blood pressure are greatly influenced by most commonly used medications taken to treat and prevent cardiovascular diseases ranging from hypertension to congestive heart failure. Similarly, there are no protocols or critical pathways developed to treat asthma patients that do not use respiratory status of the patient to evaluated the success or failure of drug regimens.

For each section in the review of systems within the Pharmacist's Workup of Drug Therapy we have developed key questions, or areas of patient-specific information, that are useful and should be documented to permit efficient retrieval at a later date, either by the practitioner initially providing care for the patient or by colleagues who subsequently participate in the care of the patient. These questions are by no means exhaustive, but they are examples of important probes focused on identifying and solving problems at the patient-specific level.

REVIEW OF SYSTEMS:

The primary purpose of the review of systems is to identify any other or additional drug-related needs. Make your own observations and include your findings, your interpretation of any abnormal or unexpected findings, as well as any required baseline values to be used as comparisons for later follow-up evaluations

VITAL SIGNS Are there deviations from normal which could be drug-related? Are there deviations from normal which should be incorporated into the plan for follow-up evaluations of drug therapy?
Temperature: Heart Rate: Blood Pressure: Respiratory Rate:

CARDIOVASCULAR Is the patient experiencing side effects from drugs manifested in the cardiovascular system (hypertension, dysrhythmias, tachycardia, bradycardia, angina pectoris, congestive heart failure, hyperlipidemia)? Is the patient's cardiovascular dysfunction affecting drug absorption, distribution, metabolism, or elimination? Is your patient receiving drug therapy that might cause orthostatic hypotension, dizziness, or falling?

PULMONARY Does the patient have pulmonary dysfunction (asthma, pneumonia, bronchitis, sinusitis, influenza, COPD, pulmonary embolism) which may contraindicate the use of certain drugs? Is the pulmonary function compromised by drugs the patient is receiving?

FLUID/ELECTROLYTE STATUS Does the patient require vitamin or nutritional supplements? Is the patient experiencing side effects from certain drugs manifested as fluid & electrolyte disturbances? Does your patient need potassium supplements? Calcium supplements?

RENAL Does the patient have a urinary tract infection? Is the patient receiving drug(s) that can alter renal function? Is the patient's renal function affecting the elimination of certain drugs? Do you need to adjust drug dosing due to poor renal function?
Creatinine clearance calculations (CrCl):
$$CrCl = \frac{(140\text{-age}) \times LBW}{SCr \times 72} = mL/min$$
{CrCl females estimated as CrCl males $\times$ 0.85}

HEPATIC Are any drugs producing toxic effects in the liver? Is the patient's hepatic function affecting drug metabolism or elimination?

ENDOCRINE Does the patient have diabetes, hypothyroidism, hyperthyroidism? Does the patient's glucose require frequent evaluation? Are any of the drugs the patient is taking affecting endocrine functions (glucose, thyroid, menstrual bleeding/menopause, glucose control?

REVIEW OF SYSTEMS (*continued*):

HEMATOLOGY Does the patient have anemia? Are there abnormalities in red blood cell, white blood cell, or serum proteins that may be caused by drugs the patient is receiving? Are any hematological parameters abnormal requiring follow-up evaluation? Are coagulation studies needed to determine liver function and/or therapeutic end points for anticoagulation (baseline stauts)? Does your patient require iron and or folic acid supplements?

GASTROINTESTINAL Does the patient have a peptic ulcer disorder? Is the condition of the patient's GI system suggesting an indication for drug therapy (ulcer, stress ulcer, esophagitis, gastritis, diarrhea, constipation, Crohn's disease, ulcerative colitis)? Is the patient's GI dysfunction (nausea, vomiting, diarrhea) drug-related or affecting drug absorption or bioavailability?

GU/REPRODUCTIVE Does the patient have a yeast infection? Does the patient require estrogen replacement therapy? Is the condition of the patient's GU system suggesting an indication for drug therapy (prostatitis, vaginitis, endometriosis, dysmenorrhea, osteoporosis, incontinence)? Do culture results indicate the need for drug therapy? Is the patient experiencing impotence secondary to drug therapy? Are drugs being taken during pregnancy or lactation? Could your patient benefit from contraceptive therapy, advice, or estrogen replacement therapy?

MUSCULOSKELETAL Does the patient have pain requiring drug therapy (back pain, tendinitis, sports injury, muscle spasm)? What is the type and location of pain? What medication(s) does the patient take for pain, arthritis pain, rheumatoid arthritis, osteoarthritis, or headaches? Does the patient suffer from multiple sclerosis? Does the patient have gout? Could the patient benefit from external analgesics, ice packs, or heating pads?

NEUROLOGICAL Does the patient have a seizure disorder, epilepsy, migraines, stroke, TIA, disorientation to person-place-time, memory loss, dementia, Alzheimer's disease, dizziness? Does this condition compromise your ability to evaluate outcomes of drug therapy or adverse drug reactions? Is the patient experiencing a neurologic abnormality (confusion, drowsiness) resulting from drug therapy? Is the patient's neurologic status affecting his or her ability to understand or adhere to required drug regimens?

PSYCHOLOGICAL Does the patient have depression requiring drug therapy? Does the patient suffer from anxiety, schizophrenia, panic disorder, attention deficit disorder? Is the patient experiencing a psychological abnormality resulting from drug therapy? Is the patient's psychological status affecting his or her ability to adhere to required drug regimens? Does your patient's history or background include a psychological condition (memory loss, thought content, mood, anxiety, depression, confusion, delirium, insomnia) that might compromise your ability to evaluate outcomes of drug therapy or adverse drug reactions?

(continued)

REVIEW OF SYSTEMS (*continued*):

SKIN Does the patient have dermatitis, eczema, psoriasis, acne, wound infection, skin infection, rash? Is the patient using any topical medications? Is the dermatologic disorder being caused by drugs the patient is receiving? Determine the patient's baseline status so potential side effects may be identified. Would the patient benefit from sunscreen protection?

EENT Does the patient have a streptococcal sore throat, cough, cold, otitis media, allergic rhinitis, conjunctivitis, cold sores, glaucoma, hearing loss, thrush, dental infection, dental pain? Are abnormalities caused by drug therapy? Does the patient need vision correction? Does the patient have difficulties with contact lenses, ophthalmic drops, or ointments? Would the patient benefit from a vaporizer or humidifier?

Making Decisions about Drug Therapy Problems

The initial data collection portion of the Pharmacist's Workup of Drug Therapy is now complete. At this point the practitioner can make an assessment of the patient's drug-related needs. This step is a decision-making step. At this point the pharmacist must decide if the patient is experiencing any *drug therapy problems* now or if there are any that need to be prevented in the future. It would be highly irresponsible to define this exercise as mere ritual, since this is the unique contribution made by the pharmacist. The pharmaceutical care practitioner has the responsibility to make therapeutic decisions, or refer the patient to another practitioner who has the knowledge and skills to make the needed assessment (see the table "Drug Therapy Problem(s) to Be Resolved or Prevented").

A statement describing a patient's drug therapy problems has three components and includes the following:

1. The patient's problem or condition
2. The drug-therapy involved
3. The association between the drug(s) and the patient's condition(s)

How the drug therapy problem is described by the practitioner is of paramount importance. Indeed, how the patient's drug therapy problem is described will direct all subsequent care, interventions, and evaluations. In the context of a single patient, the identification of a drug therapy problem establishes the practitioner's responsibilities to that patient.

Identifying drug therapy problems requires clinical judgment, discipline, a thorough understanding of the patient as a whole person, drug, and disease knowledge, communication skills, and a systematic approach to the patient care process. Just as a medical diagnosis is sometimes tentative pending further information, the decision as to whether or not a patient has a drug therapy problem is also sometimes tentative.

DRUG THERAPY PROBLEM(S) TO BE RESOLVED OR PREVENTED			
ASSESSMENT	DRUG THERAPY PROBLEM	ASSESSMENT	DRUG THERAPY PROBLEM
Appropriate indication	***Needs Additional Drug Therapy*** __Untreated condition __Synergistic/potentiating __Preventive/prophylactic ***Unnecessary Drug Therapy*** __No medical indication __Addictive/recreational __Nondrug therapy indicated __Duplicate therapy __Treating avoidable ADR	**Safety**	***Adverse Drug Reaction*** __Unsafe drug for patient __Alergic reaction __Incorrect administration __Drug interaction __Dosage change too rapid __Undesirable effect ***Dosage Too High*** __Wrong Dose __Frequency inappropriate __Duration inappropriate __Drug interaction
Effectiveness	***Wrong Drug*** __Dosage form inapporpriate __Contraindications present __Condition refractory to drug __Not indicated for condition __More effective drug available ***Dosage Too Low*** __Wrong dose __Frequency inappropriate __Duration inappropriate __Incorrect storage __Incorrect administration __Drug interaction	**Appropriate compliance**	***Not Following Instructions*** __Drug product not available __Cannot afford drug product __Cannot swallow/administer __Directions not understood __Patient prefers not to take __Other reasons

__**Patient has no drug therapy problems at this time.**

However, at this point in the care process, it is the practitioner's responsibility to identify any and all drug therapy problems that the patient could have. Or, if the case warrants, conclude, with solid substantive evidence, that the patient does not have any drug therapy problems at present.

A conclusion that no drug therapy problems exist at present can and will be interpreted to mean that all the patient's drug therapies are appropriately indicated and that the dosage regimens are producing the desired therapeutic goals and are not causing any unwanted side effects. This category of decision within the assessment indicates that all of the patient's drug-related needs are being met and no additional drug therapy is required. Finally, a conclusion that there are no drug therapy problems present should also indicate that the patient understands, agrees with, and is able to be compliant with all of his or her drug regimens. Practitioner-patient dialogue is essential to this process.

The sequence of how the seven drug therapy problems are assessed is important to the pharmaceutical care process. The order of decision making is of the utmost importance to ensure that this process is both systematic and rational. Remember, in the practice of pharmaceutical care, decisions concerning an *indication* must be made first. Then, decisions concerning *effectiveness* can be established, followed by *safety* considerations.

The discipline and thought required to practice pharmaceutical care require the pharmacist to first make certain that all of the patient's indications for drug therapy are being appropriately treated. Then, and only then, does the practitioner consider product selection and dosage to maximize the effectiveness of the medication. Note that there is no reason to individualize drug dosage regimens to maximize effectiveness for a medication that is not even indicated for the patient. The practitioner must then make certain that all drug therapy will be as safe as possible for the patient. It is important to reemphasize that only after these first three primary drug-related needs have been fully addressed can issues of compliance, cost, and convenience be considered. In this context, causes of negative compliance problems include, among others, product availability, cost considerations, patient preferences, and drug administration difficulties. Our research and clinical experience indicate that the vast majority (80 to 90 percent) of drug therapy problems generally involve problems with indication, effectiveness, and/or safety. When these drug-related needs have been met, and only after these types of drug therapy problems have been identified and resolved can the remaining 10 to 20 percent of drug therapy problems that interfere with patient compliance be addressed.

THE CARE PLAN

The care plan is a structure for two people (the patient and the practitioner) with different value systems to work together to achieve a common goal.

The care plan functions as a structure for working together with individuals who may have different levels of drug awareness and different values, expectations, and understanding of the pharmaceutical care process and its responsibilities. Most often the care plan serves as an agreement or a "joint venture" between the patient and the practitioner. In the case where care is provided using a team approach, the team functions as a single entity when negotiating a care plan. When family members, guardians, friends or other caregivers act on the patient's behalf, or in conjunction with the patient, it is helpful if this "group" represents a single patient when negotiating the details of a care plan with the practitioner. The structure of a care plan functions as a framework for the cooperative efforts of all those involved in patient care.

All care planning activities and negotiations involve at least two major decision steps. During the care planning portion of the pharmaceutical care process patient-specific goals are established, and decisions concerning which interventions are appropriate for the patient are made. As a blueprint for pharmaceutical care, the care plan includes what must be accomplished to meet the patient's drug-related needs, when this should be accomplished, and how specific goals will be achieved in terms of interventions.

The practitioner will know that the care plan is complete when he or she has worked with the patient to establish a plan to:

1. Resolve all existing drug therapy problems
2. Achieve the goals of therapy intended for each active medical condition
3. Prevent any future problems that have a potential to develop

The resolution of drug therapy problems is given high priority within the pharmaceutical care plan because the presence of drug therapy problems interferes with, or inhibits, patients from realizing their desired therapeutic goals. For example, if a patient is not realizing the full effectiveness from a certain prescribed drug regimen because the dose of medication is too low, the dosage regimen must be increased before there is any realistic hope of actually achieving positive patient outcomes. Similarly, if a patient is experiencing dose-dependent side effects, the dosage regimen must be decreased in order for the patient to be receiving appropriately indicated drug therapy that is both effective and safe. Therefore, in most cases, the patient's drug therapy problems must be dealt with first and then specific interventions and individualized drug therapy regimens to achieve the desired therapeutic goals for each of the patient's medical problems or conditions can be designed, implemented, and evaluated. Pharmaceutical care plans must also address the prevention needs of each patient in order to avoid the development of new drug therapy problems and to minimize the patient's risk of developing new medical conditions or illnesses.

Following is the *care plan* portion of the Pharmacist's Workup of Drug Therapy:

II. THE CARE PLAN

MEDICAL CONDITION: In the care plan, organization is important, therefore each medical condition is to be addressed completely and separately. It is useful to number or letter your patient's medical problems in order to keep associated drug therapy problems, goals, alternatives and interventions organized appropriately.

(continued)

II. THE CARE PLAN (*continued*):

DRUG THERAPY PROBLEMS
Statement of the drug therapy problems to be resolved (and/or prevented)

> State your patient's drug therapy problem. Drug therapy problems include (1) the patient's problem or condition, (2) the drug involved, and (3) the association between the drug and the patient's problem.

Alternatives to resolve (or prevent) your patient's drug therapy problem

> For each drug therapy problem, list the drug regimen(s) or changes in your patient's drug regimens that might be expected to resolve the drug therapy problem(s).

Interventions to resolve (or prevent) your patient's drug therapy problems

> List the pharmacist's intervention designed to resolve your patient's drug therapy problems. For each drug therapy problem document recommendations made to the patient (or patient's caregiver) or on the behalf of the patient to the prescriber (physician, dentist, nurse practitioner).

GOALS OF THERAPY

> Establish therapeutic goals for each of your patient's medical conditions: Format: Goals are stated in the future tense . . .. i.e., "The patient will achieve, maintain . . ." or "Infection will be cured," or "Disease, signs or symptoms will be eliminated or reduced." Therapeutic goals should be measurable, observable, specific, and have a definite time frame.

PHARMACIST'S AND/OR PATIENT'S INTERVENTIONS

> For each medical condition, document recommendations made to the patient (or patient's caregiver) or on the behalf of the patient to the prescriber (physician, dentist, nurse practitioner). Format: Interventions are stated in the past or present tense, and document the work actually done by the pharmacist to achieve the therapeutic goals previously established. These can be routine interventions addressing the patient's medical problem.

FOLLOW-UP PLAN AND SCHEDULE

> Follow-up consists of a scheduled (*when*) patient interaction (face to face or telephone) that is agreed upon by the patient and the pharmacist and which is designed to gather information directly from the patient as well as other sources to ensure that the recommended care plan is producing the desired effects and not resulting in undesirable or intolerable side effects.

The care plan, which is designed to meet all of the drug-related needs of patients, is organized by medical condition. Actually, in the practice of pharmaceutical care, the patient's care plan is organized by indications for drug therapy (i.e., hypertension, sinusitis, prevention of osteoporosis). Within each medical condition, the care plan must address drug therapy problems that need to be resolved and prevented, alternative methods to resolve and prevent each drug therapy problem, and the interventions that have actually been chosen to resolve and prevent the drug therapy problem. In this sense, a problem-solving approach is applied to the drug therapy problem first (if one is identified), then a problem-solving approach is applied to the primary medical condition.

Goals of Therapy

Once the drug therapy problem is fully addressed in the patient's care plan (i.e., change the dose, change the drug, etc.), the therapeutic goal of the primary condition (indication for drug therapy) is considered. The intent of a goal is to provide an integrating purpose or intelligent direction to a variety of activities. The therapeutic goal becomes the agreed upon target of the prescriber's drug therapy, the patient's nonprescription drug therapy, the pharmacist's interventions, and the patient's interventions and compliance behavior. In general, each medical condition is associated with a set of *therapeutic goals* that have been established in the literature and verified in practice. These include such parameters as goals for blood pressure in patients with hypertension and goals for serum lipids in patients with hyperlipidemia. However, the patient's presenting signs and symptoms most often form the foundation for the patient-specific goals within the care plan. For example, for a patient who suffers from allergic rhinitis and presents with nasal congestion, runny nose, and eye itching but no cough or loss of taste, the patient-specific goals of therapy will include the relief of the patient's complaints of nasal congestion, runny nose, and eye itching in a certain time frame. Given this type of patient-specific goal, a rational approach to patient-specific drug therapy is possible.

The intent of therapeutic goals provides an integrating purpose to a variety of interactions and activities.

Whereas therapeutic goals for diseases and other medical problems are generally established using population data or by a group of practitioners and researchers who have specialized in the treatment of a particular disorder, patient-specific goals must be established and agreed upon between the individual patient and the individual practitioner. Patient-specific goals should be realistic and observable or measurable if possible. They will include the patient's presenting concerns, problems, complaints, signs, symptoms, and/or abnormal laboratory test results. Patient-specific goals have a futuristic time frame describing when each goal should be met. This time frame is important to patients as it lets them know what to expect and when to expect it. The time course for achieving patient-specific goals also serves as a guide to establishing an appropriate time for the practitioner and the patient to evaluate the impact or actual outcome of drug therapy decisions. Determining what

The patient's signs and symptoms often form the foundation for therapeutic goals within the care plan.

interventions are best suited to achieve the therapeutic goals is an essential function of the care planning process.

The patient's care plan then lists the interventions that have been determined will best help the patient to realize the therapeutic goal. These interventions include what the patient will do and what interventions the pharmacist will provide on behalf of the patient. Additionally, any interventions that are required to prevent future drug therapy problems are incorporated into the care plan. Finally, all care plans must contain a scheduled plan for the follow-up evaluation.

Practitioner Interventions

The *interventions* section of the care plan represents the most creative portion of the care planning process. Based on the patient's value system and the patient's sense of what is truly important, the practitioner and the patient collaborate to establish a prioritized list of activities designed to effectively and efficiently address all drug-related needs. Interventions chosen to specifically address the unique drug-related needs of individual patients, in addition to empirical considerations, are by definition grounded in patient preferences, selected according to patient needs, and limited by patient tolerance. Therefore, the higher the level of patient participation and the more creative the practitioner becomes at individualizing the care plan to meet the patient's unique needs, the higher the success rate will be. This success is not only measured as compliant behavior but also in terms of positive actual patient outcomes of therapy measured objectively and subjectively.

Interventions represent the work that must be performed by the practitioner and by the patient now in order to ensure that drug therapies will be as effective and safe as possible. In general interventions can include what drug regimen(s) the patient should receive, changes in drug therapy that are required, patient-specific information, referrals that might serve to meet specialized patient needs, instructions on how to take prescription drug products and nonpreprescription drug products and how to use other remedies, products and devices, and the provision of the drug products themselves. The provision of drug products is an important type of intervention in a patient's care plan. However, the provision of drug product is nothing more and nothing less than one of the many types of patient-specific interventions that must be considered for each patient's care plan. Interventions also represent the work that needs to be performed at some later date to ensure the continued effectiveness and safety of drug therapies. The final intervention that must be planned during the care planning process is to schedule and plan for follow-up evaluation. The appropriate time for the patient and the practitioner to meet again in order to evaluate the progress, or lack thereof, of all of the interventions must be negotiated.

The interventions section of the care plan represents its most creative portion.

Disease and illness treatment cues the practitioner to select certain interventions based on the unique constellation of the patient's presenting signs and symptoms. Preventive interventions are different. These require a comprehensive, disciplined assessment to identify patient risk factors that indicate the need for preventive interventions. The delay in observable results or outcomes make interventions designed solely to prevent problems less prevalent in most factions of the health care industry. In health care systems where acute treatment and therapies designed to cure illness and reduce symptomatology are the primary focus, preventive measures often are relegated to a second priority status and do not always become fully integrated into a patient's care plan. In the United States during the height of the health care industry's focus on high technology and expensive, curative medical interventions, the immunization rate among 2-year-olds for measles, mumps, rubella, polio, diphtheria, tetanus, pertussis was only about 50 percent.[7] During this time, as we stated earlier, the primary responsibility to ensure that children received proper immunizations was relegated to the school systems.

The delay in observable positive patient outcomes is often accompanied by a more immediate negative risk and/or cost of the preventive intervention itself. Interventions designed to prevent the development of a drug therapy problem can take the form of the initiation of drug therapies, vitamins, diets, immunizations, exercise programs, or counseling patients (directly or the patient's caregiver) or recommendations made on behalf of the patient to the prescriber (physician, dentist, nurse practitioner, optometrist, etc.).

Common interventions designed to prevent the development of future drug therapy problems, new diseases or illnesses, include the following:

- Estrogen replacement therapy and calcium supplements in postmenopausal females
- Subcutaneous heparin or low molecular weight heparin to prevent pulmonary emboli and deep venous thrombosis
- Aspirin to prevent recurrent myocardial infarction or stroke
- The use of lipid-lowering agents to prevent cardiovascular disease
- Maternal folic acid supplements to prevent neural tube defects and congenital orofacial clefts[8]
- Misoprostol use to prevent gastrointestinal erosions and ulcers associated with nonsteroidal anti-inflammatory drugs[9]
- Smoking cessation approaches to prevent pulmonary disease, cardiovascular disease, or cancer
- Antibiotics used to prevent infections during surgical or dental procedures
- The need to prevent the flu using influenza immunizations in an elderly patient with chronic diseases

- The need for allergy or "bee sting" kits for a patient with a history of severe allergic reactions

Many prevention types of interventions have very little to do with drug therapies themselves. For the millions of patients who suffer from allergic rhinitis or seasonal allergies, it is often helpful to avoid or minimize the exposure to the allergens by keeping windows closed and using air conditioning if available. Instructing these patients not to hang clothes outside to dry, as allergy-causing materials can collect on clothing, can help a great deal. Additionally, some people who suffer from "house dust" allergies find it helpful to cover the mattress and pillows with plastic or other special materials to avoid contact with house dust mites. Vacuuming mattress, pillows, and bedding weekly and the use of synthetic pillows so they can be washed weekly can greatly reduce a patient's symptoms. For heavy exposure activities like raking leaves, cutting grass, or housecleaning, wearing a mask to filter the air may be very beneficial and is less expensive than many drug therapies. All of these preventive interventions can supplement antihistamine and decongestant drug therapies and result in substantially improved patient outcomes.

Every well-meaning, well-designed intervention in a pharmaceutical care plan may have a positive impact on the patient, a negative impact, or no demonstrable impact at all. Only through a planned, comprehensive follow-up evaluation can the practitioner and the patient really learn whether the services, products and information provided have actually met the patient's drug-related needs and resulted in the intended positive patient outcomes.

THE FOLLOW-UP EVALUATION

The purpose of the follow-up evaluation is to compare actual patient outcomes with intended therapeutic goals.

An essential step in the provision of pharmaceutical care is the *follow-up evaluation* portion of the care process. The evaluation is used to compare the desired therapeutic goals with the patient's present status. For acute disorders, the follow-up evaluations can serve to evaluate the actual (final) patient outcomes; however, for patients with chronic conditions, follow-up evaluations can only establish the present status of the patient and the progress or lack of progress in achieving desired therapeutic goals. Following below are all the components of the follow-up evaluation.

During the evaluation, actual patient outcomes are recorded, progress in meeting therapeutic goals is evaluated, and an assessment is made to determine whether new problems have developed.

The follow-up evaluation not only serves to determine if the patient is experiencing the desired effectiveness from the drug therapy but also serves as the mechanism to determine whether the patient's drug therapy is in fact safe and not causing any harmful or uncomfortable side

FOLLOW-UP EVALUATION: Evaluate actual patient outcomes. This section contains the pharmacist's professional evaluation of how effective the care plan and the associated drug therapies have been in achieving the desired therapeutic goals for each of your patient's medical conditions. From the information gathered at the follow-up evaluation, the pharmacist evaluates and documents the progress (or lack of progress) in achieving the desired outcomes. The status of each medical condition and/or the status of the overall patient at the time of each follow-up evaluation can be described as *resolved, stable, improved, partial improvement, unimproved, worsened, failure,* or *expired.*

STATUS	DEFINITION
Resolved	Goals achieved, therapy completed
Stable	Goals achieved, continue same therapy
Improved	Progress being made, continue same therapy
Partial Improvement	Progress being made, minor adjustments required
Unimproved	No progress yet, but continue same therapy
Worsened	Decline in health, adjust therapy
Failure	Goals not achieved, initiate new therapy
Expired	Patient died while receiving drug therapy

Patient's Medical Conditions/Medications _____
_____
_____

Actual Outcome/Status/Progress _____
_____
_____

New Drug Therapy Problems:
Evaluate patient for new drug therapy problems. This section contains the pharmacist's clinical assessment of whether the patient has developed new drug therapy problems since the previous evaluation.

effects. Another purpose of the follow-up evaluation is to identify new medical conditions that require treatment with drug therapy or recognize new drug therapy problems that have developed since the last evaluation. The evaluations are the critical points at which the actual effectiveness and safety of the patient's care plan and associated drug therapies are determined, balanced against one another, and where decisions concerning changes in drug therapy are made. Although the evaluations represent the practitioner's clinical judgment of the patient's progress or status, they are based almost entirely on direct patient input combined with sound clinical judgment.

The follow-up evaluation step is a proactive level of practitioner involvement in the provision of drug therapy. That is to say, it is here that the practitioner assertively assumes the responsibility to reach out to the patient and demonstrate caring behavior. To conduct a complete,

Outcomes are what the patient
actually experiences as a result of
drug therapies.

adequate follow-up evaluation the practitioner must be highly motivated to actively communicate with the patient and seek feedback concerning any problems associated with his or her well-being. Such feedback either validates the care plan or questions its appropriateness, thereby leading to modifications.

In addition to supporting the caring portion of the patient-practitioner relationship, the follow-up evaluation is the only method available to determine actual patient outcomes. Outcomes are what the patient actually experiences as a result of specific drug therapies circumscribed by drug information, advice, counseling, and other pharmaceutical care interventions. Although all practitioners provide drug therapy, advice, and instructions with the best of intentions, these well-meaning interventions do not always have positive outcomes. In order to determine what impact pharmaceutical care services of any type actually had on an individual patient, the practitioner must accept the responsibility to follow up and determine the current status of the patient and, in so doing, clarify the extent to which pharmaceutical care services are meeting the intended goals of therapy.

The optimal timing for the next follow-up evaluation is often difficult for practitioners to determine. The time should be based on the most likely period for the desired benefits to manifest themselves, balanced with the most likely time for harm or side effects to appear. The optimal timing for the next follow-up evaluation might be as soon as you expect to be able to observe demonstrable improvement versus waiting until the end of the treatment course. For example, it might only require two to four weeks of anti-depressant therapy to observe the onset of antidepressant effects, but require a full three to four months or longer to be able to fully evaluate the effectiveness of a specific antidepressant drug regimen. Similarly, an initial reduction in fever and otalgia should be expected within 24–72 hours of antibiotic therapy for acute otitis media in children, however, another evaluation at the end of the ten day course of antibiotics is often required to evaluate the success of therapy. In general, the more confident the practitioner is that the care plan will result in positive outcomes and not result in undesired toxicity, the longer the time interval between follow-up evaluations. On the other hand, the less supportive evidence, data, information, and confidence that the practitioner and the patient have in the care plan, the sooner and more frequent the follow-up evaluations must be scheduled.

Much has been written about "outcome" evaluations and the positive outcomes that will result from pharmacist's providing pharmaceutical care. However, most of this discourse is somewhat hollow. In fact, much of what is described as outcomes of drug therapy or pharmaceutical care has little to do with patient outcomes at all. Much of this energy is misdirected toward counting and measuring outputs of pharmacist activities (such as doses changed or number of prescriptions substituted with a formulary approved generic product) and totally disregards the pharmacist's impact on patient care.

Dictionaries define *outcome* as the final result, or consequence. As applied to pharmaceutical care, *outcome* would refer to that which is a direct consequence of the collaborative efforts of practitioner and patient. This is particularly important when the patient's physical and sociopsychological experiences are examined. Patient outcomes do not include whether or not the prescriber followed the pharmacist's recommendation to change a dose. Patient outcomes do not include successfully substituting a less expensive drug product for another. It is also important to note that patient outcomes do not include implementing a disease-state management protocol for a group of patients with a particular disorder, and outcomes do not include counseling patients on how to properly administer medications. Each of these well-meaning and frequently useful pharmacist interventions may or may not have a positive impact on patients. To determine the actual positive and negative impact on patients, the effects of drug therapy on the patient must be central to all outcome measurements.

There are no shortcuts to positive patient outcomes. Actual patient outcomes resulting from drug therapy and associated pharmaceutical care cannot be determined from a distance. Outcomes cannot be measured from the board room, they cannot be measured from the hallway, and they most certainly cannot be measured by a computer program. If one is truly concerned with the impact that drug therapy and pharmaceutical care have on patients, there is no other method available to determine this than by personally contacting each and every patient at appropriately planned intervals and eliciting information directly from the patient. Only then will the impact drug therapy is actually having be understood. These identifiable and measurable actual patient outcomes must be documented in order to compare them with the desired goals of therapy and to evaluate progress and failures that the patient has experienced. The performance of this responsibility is essential to the practice of pharmaceutical care.

> There are no short cuts to positive patient outcomes.

To fully accept responsibility for patient outcomes associated with drug therapy, the practitioner must be prepared to recognize not only what positive outcomes can be anticipated but also what negative outcomes the patient might experience from drug therapy decisions that are made. It is important to keep in mind that even the most carefully designed care plans and associated drug therapies cannot be expected to always result in positive patient outcomes. In light of this, the practitioner must be willing to engage in critical (self-critical) reviews rather than affirming incorrect judgments or simply placing responsibility elsewhere. This often means that the practitioner admits to mistakes and works diligently toward modifications. When good rapport exists between patient and practitioner (a good therapeutic relationship), such modifications are "worked out" between partners rather than mani-

Actual patient outcomes are unpredictable because patients represent a complex biological system influenced by exogenous drug therapy.

festing themselves as "confessionals" that undermine confidence and threaten the security of both parties. All related activities must involve continuous dialogue and an understanding that changes/modifications may occur.

Unfortunately, we tend to teach students and each other about pharmacotherapy as if it consists entirely of a physical system in which, if one understands the drug and understands the patient's disease, the intended positive outcome should be expected. But in actuality, drug therapy represents a classic example of a biological system in which, when one introduces an exogenous influence (drug) into a living complex biological system (patient), the outcome is certainly not always consistent and therefore not universally predictable. Pharmaceutical care practice requires, as do all health care practices, that the practitioner and the patient make decisions in areas of uncertainty. In practice, some 10 to 30 percent of actual patient outcomes are not positive, and pharmacist's who accept the professional and ethical mandates associated with the practice of pharmaceutical care must effectively and efficiently address negative patient outcomes. In the pharmaceutical care practice model, negative patient outcomes are resolved in the same way that other patient-specific, drug-related needs are addressed. A negative patient outcome is considered a drug therapy problem and must be prioritized as such and resolved as expeditiously as possible. For example, if a certain drug therapy has failed to produce the desired effects, then the patient still has an indication for drug therapy that is not adequately being met by the present drug regimen. Corrective action is required.

In order to evaluate and communicate patient outcomes resulting from the pharmaceutical care process in a consistent and comprehensive manner, we found it necessary to develop a glossary of terms to describe the status of the patient, the patient's medical conditions, and the comparative evaluation of that status with the previously determined therapeutic goals. This common vocabulary becomes noticeably important when we consider the irreducible complexity of conditions found in practice. Some patients, for example, have acute or self-limiting problems or conditions that might be expected to be totally resolved by appropriate drug therapy. Patients with acute bacterial infections represent common examples in which one might establish a realistic goal to "resolve" the infection within ten days. However, the vast majority of patients suffer from chronic disorders such as hypertension, depression, hyperlipidemia, asthma, and arthritis, for which desired patient therapeutic goals do not include the complete resolution, but rather include interim (palliative) goals such as stabilizing or improving the condition by reducing severity and frequency of signs and symptoms, correcting abnormal test results, and/or improving the patient's endurance or ability to ambulate. In practice, many patients actually have multiple conditions and require drug therapy for both acute and chronic conditions simultaneously. Therefore, as asserted in Chap. 1, pharmacists require a working vocabulary of terms that can be used to effectively describe as well as document the outcome and status of any and all patient conditions.

To be most useful, documented patient outcomes must depict both status and time. Toward this end, the following eight terms and their associated definitions were developed to describe patient outcomes resulting from drug therapies and pharmaceutical care. Each of these outcome evaluation terms are intended to describe the practitioner's clinical evaluation of how effective the drug therapy has been in producing the desired therapeutic outcomes for each of the patient's conditions at the time the particular follow-up evaluation is made and documented.

Documented patient outcomes must depict both status and time.

RESOLVED: In this situation, the patient's desired goals of therapy have all been successfully achieved and drug therapy can be discontinued. The evaluation of resolved issues is intended to represent the final positive patient outcome, and is most often applicable to acute problems or conditions. The action taken, in this case discontinuing the drug therapy, should be documented in the patient's pharmaceutical care records. An example of such a resolution would be a case of acute otitis media in a 3-year-old patient with a 10-day course of oral amoxicillin therapy. No additional follow-up is indicated beyond day ten if the specific condition has a positive outcome.

STABLE: In this situation, the patient's desired therapeutic goals have been realized (at present) therefore the same drug therapy will be continued. In these cases, stabilizing the patient's condition, or test results, was in fact the predetermined, desired achievable goal. An example would be stabilizing a patient's blood pressure within the desired range of 110-120/70-80 within 2 months with a pharmaceutical care plan that recommends 50mg of hydrochlorothiazde every day, a sodium-restricted diet, and a low impact exercise program. The next follow-up might be planned to occur in 90 days to reevaluate the entire care plan.

IMPROVED: In this situation, positive progress is being realized in meeting the patient's desired goals of therapy and therefore no substantial changes in drug therapy will be implemented at this time. Consider a patient whose depressive sign and symptoms of disturbances in normal sleep, and eating patterns have improved following the initial three weeks of antidepressive drug therapy with fluoxetine (Prozac) 10 mg daily, and note that the dosage regimen will not be changed at this time. In such a case the practitioner might follow up in another 4 weeks to determine the patient's status.

PARTIAL IMPROVEMENT: In this situation, the practitioner's evaluation indicates that some positive progress is being made in achieving the patient's desired therapeutic goals, but some minor adjustments in the patient's care plan are indicated at this time in order to more fully meet all of the goals of therapy by the next follow-up evaluation. For example, a 58-
(continued)

PARTIAL IMPROVEMENT (*continued*):

year-old patient, whose arthritic pain has been somewhat relieved following 2 weeks of therapy with ketoprofen 12.5 mg four times daily, desires considerably more relief from her discomfort, and the practitioner's evaluation indicates that greater effectiveness might be realized by increasing the daily dosage of ketoprofen to 75 mg taken as 25 mg three times daily. The next follow-up evaluation is to occur in two weeks to determine if this adjustment in the dosage regimen of the nonsteroidal anti-inflammatory medication produces continued and/or additional relief for the patient without intolerable stomach irritation, headache, or fluid retention.

UNIMPROVED: In this situation, the practitioner's evaluation is that little or no positive progress has been made in achieving the patient's therapeutic goals at this time, but further improvement is expected. Therefore, the patient's care plan will not be substantially altered. Thus, the unimproved status evaluation is very dependent on the timing of the evaluation. An example of this situation would be an adult male patient who is allergic to penicillin is started on erythromycin 250 mg orally four times a day for the treatment of a localized soft tissue infection following a work-related injury to the right forearm. Twenty-four hours after initiating erythromycin therapy the patient experiences some nausea from the antibiotic, and the injured area on the arm is still inflamed and slightly swollen. The practitioner reassures the patient about the nausea, provides him or her with suggestions as to how to minimize this undesirable effect associated with erythromycin, and documents an evaluation of the current effectiveness of therapy. The practitioner reports that although the arm is unimproved at this early stage in therapy, no dosage changes are indicated, and that 3 to 5 days would be an appropriate time to make another evaluation of the effectiveness of the erythromycin therapy.

WORSENED: In this situation, the practitioner's evaluation describes a decline in the health of the patient despite what was considered to be the best possible care plan for this individual. Because the therapeutic goals are not being achieved, changes in the patient's drug therapies are considered to be useful at this time. A future follow-up evaluation is planned to examine the status to the patient's conditions and once again consider whether changes in the care plan would be appropriate. For example, a teenage athlete whose elbow stiffness and muscle pain have progressively become more bothersome over the previous 2 weeks despite the use of acetaminophen 325 mg three (3) times a day and ice packs. This worsening condition might call for increasing the acetaminophen dosage and adding a topical analgesic such as capsicum.

FAILURE: In this situation, the practitioner's evaluation indicates that the present care plan, and associated drug therapy approaches have now been given full consideration and have not helped the patient achieve desirable therapeutic goals. Therefore, the present therapy should be discontinued, and new drug therapy initiated. In these situations, the desired outcomes have not been met and the treatment is considered to have failed. An example would be a patient whose symptoms of seasonal allergic rhinitis have not

---

FAILURE: (*continued*)

improved with two weeks of continuous chlorpheniramine therapy, therefore it should be discontinued, and new drug therapy initiated using a combination of astemizole (Hismanal) and pseudoephedrine. The next follow-up evaluation is planned in 3 days.

EXPIRED: In this situation, the fact that the patient dies while receiving drug therapy is documented in the pharmaceutical care chart. In addition, any important observations about contributing factors in the patient's demise, especially if they are drug-related, should be recorded.

It is important to note that each of these definitions not only describes the patient's status with respect to the medical or drug therapy problem but also indicates whether any changes in the patient's drug therapies were recommended and/or implemented. For example, using the term *resolved* as outcome documentation of a medical condition in the patient's pharmaceutical care chart should record that the associated drug therapy was completed and discontinued, thus accurately depicting the length of therapy. Similarly, in the case of a patient whose condition or status was evaluated as having "improved" would indicate that there would be no changes in the associated drug therapies documented in the patient's pharmaceutical care chart at that time.

As indicated earlier, using terminology such as described above can be a powerful tool in analyzing and improving one's ability to care for patients and maintain a viable practice. Carefully documented follow-up evaluations can provide important summary data to address vital questions such as "How long does it take my patients with hypertension to become stable on their new antihypertensive drug therapies?" Also we must address questions, such as "Which of my patients receiving antidepressants are unimproved or only partially improved after 60 to 90 days of therapy?" Outcome data supporting the positive contributions of pharmaceutical care require person-to-person follow-up evaluations and systematic, explicit documentation of actual patient outcomes over time.

Finally, it is essential that the practitioner who conducts the follow-up evaluation record the actual patient outcomes, determine the status of the patient, and sign the evaluation. This step, in essence, completes the circle of care, at least at this point in time. Furthermore, patients and payers must be able to identify with the individual practitioner, not the pharmacy or the clinic building. Care represents a people process, therefore, take responsibility and sign your work.

We have just described a very detailed process which must appear overwhelming to the new pharmaceutical care provider. We want to make a number of points about the patient care process generally and the Pharmacists Workup of Drug Therapy specifically. First, it is not an easy assignment to accept responsibility for making decisions which

have consequences, in this case potentially life-threatening consequences, for another human being. This responsibility should not be
accepted lightly, nor should it be executed frivolously. Therefore, it
should come as no surprise that to successfully assume this responsibility
requires discipline, hard work, and time.

Second, because the process is described explicitly it is now possible
to learn it, practice it, and become adept at making these important decisions. This should be incredibly encouraging to pharmacists who have
wondered for so many years what their unique contribution to patient
care is and how to execute it.

Third, pharmacists now are able to be recognized and rewarded for
their contributions because they can describe the practice, document,
evaluate, teach, discuss, and critique it. This means the practice can be
changed, but most importantly, it can be improved, which means pharmaceutical care practice will endure.

The patient care process is arguably the most important component
of pharmaceutical care practice. It is what allows the practitioner to
meet the patient's drug-related needs. What could be more important
than that?

THE PHARMACIST'S WORKUP OF DRUG THERAPY

I. PHARMACIST'S ASSESSMENT OF THE PATIENT'S DRUG-RELATED NEEDS

PATIENT NEEDS

Patient Understanding of Drug Therapy: What is your patient's level of understanding of his or her diseases, drug therapies, and instructions? Does your patient understand that it will be necessary to actively participate in his or her care?

Patient Expectations: What does your patient want? What are your patient's expectations of his or her drug therapies? Are they realistic, achievable? Does your patient expect to be an active participant in his/her care?

Patient Concerns: What concerns does your patient have about his or her health in general, medical conditions, or drug therapies? Side effects, toxicity, allergies, costs?

PATIENT DEMOGRAPHICS AND BACKGROUND

Age_____   Gender_____   Race_____   Ht_____   Wt_____   LBW_____
Male = 50 kg + [2.3 × (no. inches > than 5′0″)]   Female = 45 kg + [2.3 × (no. inches > than 5′0″)]

Health Plan: What type of payment system does the patient have? How will this affect my decisions about the patient's drug therapy?

Primary physician: Is there one primary physician? More? What type of relationship does patient have with physician? What does patient share with physician about drug therapy?

Family: Describe your patient's family, children? how many? ages? Does your patient live with his or her parents? Does your patient have a family history of certain diseases, conditions, or risk factors for drug therapy problems?

Living Arrangements: Who lives with your patient? Who cares for your patient? Does your patient live alone? Who administers medications?

Occupation: Socioeconomic status of your patient. Does employment put your patient at risk for certain diseases or drug therapy problems? Insurance plan and coverage.

Special needs: What unique needs does your patient have that will need to be accommodated when designing a personalized pharmaceutical care plan? Physical abilities, allergies, cultural traits, health care beliefs, labeled instructions, child-proof tops, drug administration devices, compliance reminders, taking medications at work/school?

Current Medical Problem List (Diagnoses, Complaints, Conditions): What is your patient's primary medical problem and its associated drug therapies? List all of your patient's other current (active) medical conditions and their associated drug therapies. Are these medical conditions being treated with drug therapy? Are all medical problems being appropriately treated? Do any of these medical problems suggest an indication for additional or new drug therapy? Are any of these conditions the result of drug therapy, or could they affect the way drugs are absorbed, distributed, metabolized, or eliminated by your patient?

History of Present Condition and Past Medical History: When did the present primary condition(s) begin and what has been the course of the disease over the recent past? Has the present medical problem been treated with drugs previously? What was the outcome? Describe other important past medical events that may impact your patient's present or future care. Is there anything in the patient's history or background to suggest a risk factor to develop a serious condition or that would represent a contraindication to drug therapy?

THE PHARMACIST'S WORKUP OF DRUG THERAPY *(continued)*

ALLERGIES AND ALERTS

ALLERGIES AND ADVERSE DRUG REACTIONS:

Have any allergic reactions occurred in the past? What is the nature and significance of past allergic reactions? Do potential allergies exist (drug, food, preservatives, additives, etc.)? Is there evidence that the patient could not tolerate a medication or dosage form in the past due to an adverse drug reaction? What concerns does your patient have about their drug allergies or reactions? Pay particular attention to allergic symptoms that are common during infancy and childhood including: eczema, urticaria, perennial rhinitis and reactions to insect bites.

SMOKING/ALCOHOL/RECREATIONAL DRUG USE:

Describe the tobacco, alcohol, or caffeine, or recreational drug use of your patient. Does it contribute to the patient's medical problems of health risks in general? Does it affect drug absorption, distribution, metabolism, or elimination?

COMPLIANCE HISTORY

Who is responsible for medication administration for your patient? Is there evidence that your patient has any difficulty understanding and complying with medication instructions?

IMMUNIZATION HISTORY

Is your patient's immunization protection up to date including diphtheria, tetanus, pertussis, *Haemophilus Influenzae* type B, poliovirus, measles, mumps, rubella, Hepatitis B, Varicella zoster?

MEDICATION RECORD: Identify **all** medications presently taken by your patient as well as those taken during the past six months. Prescription (Rx), samples (S), nonprescription (OTC), as well as home remedies (H).

Indication	Drug Product	Dosage Instructions	Goals of Therapy & Progress

REVIEW OF SYSTEMS: The primary purpose of the review of systems is to identify any other or additional drug-related needs. Make your own observations and include your findings, your interpretation of any abnormal or unexpected findings, as well as any required baseline values to be used as comparisons for later follow-up evaluations

VITAL SIGNS Are there deviations from normal which could be drug-related? Are there deviations from normal which should be incorporated into the plan for follow-up evaluations of drug therapy?

Temperature_____   Heart Rate_____   Blood Pressure_____   Respiratory Rate_____

CARDIOVASCULAR Is the patient experiencing side effects from drugs manifested in the cardiovascular system (hypertension, dysrhythmias, tachycardia, bradycardia, angina pectoris, congestive heart failure, hyperlipidemia)? Is the patient's cardiovascular dysfunction affecting drug absorption, distribution, metabolism, or elimination? Is your patient receiving drug therapy that might cause orthostatic hypotension, dizziness, or falling?

PULMONARY Does the patient have pulmonary dysfunction (asthma, pneumonia, bronchitis, sinusitis, influenza, COPD, pulmonary embolism) which may contraindicate the use of certain drugs? Is the pulmonary function compromised by drugs the patient is receiving?

THE PHARMACIST'S WORKUP OF DRUG THERAPY *(continued)*

FLUID/ELECTROLYTE STATUS   Does the patient require vitamin or nutritional supplements? Is the patient experiencing side effects from certain drugs manifested as fluid & electrolyte disturbances? Does your patient need potassium supplements? Calcium supplements?

RENAL   Does the patient have a urinary tract infection? Is the patient receiving drug(s) that can alter renal function? Is the patient's renal function affecting the elimination of certain drugs? Do you need to adjust drug dosing due to poor renal function?
Creatinine clearance calculations (CrCl):

$$\text{CrCl} = \frac{(140\text{-age}) \times \text{LBW}}{\text{SCr} \times 72} = \text{mL/min} \qquad \{\text{CrCl females estimated as CrCl males} \times 0.85\}$$

HEPATIC   Are any drugs producing toxic effects in the liver? Is the patient's hepatic function affecting drug metabolism or elimination?

ENDOCRINE   Does the patient have diabetes, hypothyroidism, hyperthyroidism? Does the patient's glucose require frequent evaluation? Are any of the drugs the patient is taking affecting endocrine functions (glucose, thyroid, menstrual bleeding/menopause, glucose control)?

HEMATOLOGY   Does the patient have anemia? Are there abnormalities in red blood cell, white blood cell, or serum proteins that may be caused by drugs the patient is receiving? Are any hematological parameters abnormal requiring follow-up evaluation? Are coagulation studies needed to determine liver function and/or therapeutic endpoints for anticoagulation [baseline status]? Does your patient require iron and or folic acid supplements?

GASTROINTESTINAL   Does the patient have a peptic ulcer disorder? Is the condition of the patient's GI system suggesting an indication for drug therapy (ulcer, stress ulcer, esophagitis, gastritis, diarrhea, constipation, Crohn's disease, ulcerative colitis)? Is the patient's GI dysfunction (nausea, vomiting, diarrhea) drug-related or affecting drug absorption or bioavailability?

GU/REPRODUCTIVE   Does the patient have a yeast infection? Does the patient require estrogen replacement therapy? Is the condition of the patient's GU system suggesting an indication for drug therapy (prostatitis, vaginitis, endometriosis, dysmenorrhea, osteoporosis, incontinence)? Do culture results indicate the need for drug therapy? Is the patient experiencing impotence secondary to drug therapy? Are drugs being taken during pregnancy or lactation? Could your patient benefit from contraceptive therapy, advice or estrogen replacement therapy?

MUSCULOSKELETAL   Does the patient have gout? Does the patient have pain requiring drug therapy (back pain, tendonitis, sports injury, muscle spasm)? What is the type and location of pain? What medication(s) does the patient take for pain, arthritis pain, rheumatoid arthritis, osteoarthritis, or headaches? Does the patient suffer from multiple sclerosis?

NEUROLOGICAL   Does the patient have a seizure disorder, epilepsy, migraines, stroke, TIA, disorientation to person-place-time, memory loss, dementia, Alzheimer's disease, dizziness? Does this condition compromise your ability to evaluate outcomes of drug therapy or adverse drug reactions? Is the patient experiencing a neurologic abnormality (confusion, drowsiness) resulting from drug therapy? Is the patient's neurologic status affecting his or her ability to understand or adhere to required drug regimens?

PSYCHOLOGICAL   Does the patient have depression requiring drug therapy? Does the patient suffer from anxiety, schizophrenia, panic disorder, attention deficit disorder? Is the patient experiencing a psychological abnormality resulting from drug therapy? Is the patient's psychological status affecting his or her ability to adhere to required drug regimens? Does your patient's history or background include a psychological condition (memory loss, thought content, mood, anxiety, depression, confusion, delirium, insomnia) that might compromise your ability to evaluate outcomes of drug therapy or adverse drug reactions?

SKIN   Does the patient have dermatitis, eczema, psoriasis, acne, wound infection, skin infection, rash? Is the patient receiving any topical medications? Is the dermatologic disorder being caused by drugs the patient is receiving? Determine the patient's baseline status so potential side effects may be identified.

EENT   Does the patient have a streptococcal sore throat, cough, cold, otitis media, allergic rhinitis, conjunctivitis, cold sores, glaucoma, hearing loss, thrush, dental infection, dental pain? Are abnormalities caused by drug therapy? Does the patient need vision correction? Does the patient have difficulties with contact lenses, ophthalmic drops, or ointments? Would the patient benefit from a vaporizer or humidifier?

DRUG THERAPY PROBLEM(S) TO BE RESOLVED OR PREVENTED			
ASSESSMENT	DRUG THERAPY PROBLEM	ASSESSMENT	DRUG THERAPY PROBLEM
Appropriate indication	***Needs Additional Drug Therapy*** __Untreated condition __Synergistic/potentiating __Preventive/prophylactic ***Unnecessary Drug Therapy*** __No medical indication __Addictive/recreational __Nondrug therapy indicated __Duplicate therapy __Treating avoidable ADR	**Safety**	***Adverse Drug Reaction*** __Unsafe drug for patient __Alergic reaction __Incorrect administration __Drug interaction __Dosage change too rapid __Undesirable effect ***Dosage Too High*** __Wrong Dose __Frequency inappropriate __Duration inappropriate __Drug interaction
Effectiveness	***Wrong Drug*** __Dosage form inapporriate __Contraindications present __Condition refractory to drug __Not indicated for condition __More effective drug available ***Dosage Too Low*** __Wrong dose __Frequency inappropriate __Duration inappropriate __Incorrect storage __Incorrect administration __Drug interaction	**Appropriate compliance**	***Not Following Instructions*** __Drug product not available __Cannot afford drug product __Cannot swallow/administer __Directions not understood __Patient prefers not to take __Other reasons

__**Patient has no drug therapy problems at this time.**

THE PHARMACIST'S WORKUP OF DRUG THERAPY *(continued)*

II. THE CARE PLAN

MEDICAL CONDITION: In the care plan, organization is important, therefore each medical condition is to be addressed completely and separately. It is useful to number or letter your patient's medical problems in order to keep associated drug therapy problems, goals, alternatives, and interventions organized appropriately.

DRUG THERAPY PROBLEMS
Statement of the drug therapy problems to be resolved (and/or prevented)
State your patient's drug therapy problem. Drug therapy problems include: 1) the patient's problem or condition 2) the drug involved and 3) the association between the drug and the patient's problem.

Alternatives to resolve (or prevent) your patient's drug therapy problem
For each drug therapy problem, list the drug regimen(s) or changes in your patient's drug regimens that might be expected to resolve the drug therapy problem(s).

Interventions to resolve (or prevent) your patient's drug therapy problems
List the pharmacist's intervention designed to resolve your patient's drug therapy problems. For each drug therapy problem document recommendations made to the patient (or patient's caregiver) or on the behalf of the patient to the prescriber (physician, dentist, nurse practitioner)

GOALS OF THERAPY
Establish therapeutic goals for each of your patient's medical conditions: Format: Goals are stated in the future tense. . . . i.e. "the patient will achieve, maintain . . ." or "infection will be cured", or "disease, signs or symptoms will be eliminated or reduced". Therapeutic goals should be measurable, observable, specific, and have a definite time frame.

PHARMACIST'S AND/OR PATIENT'S INTERVENTIONS
For each medical condition document recommendations made to the patient (or patient's caregiver) or on the behalf of the patient to the prescriber (physician, dentist, nurse practitioner) Format: Interventions are stated in the past or present tense, and document the work actually done by the pharmacist to achieve the therapeutic goals previously established. These can be routine interventions addressing the patient's medical problem.

FOLLOW-UP PLAN AND SCHEDULE
Follow-up consists of a scheduled (*when*) patient interaction (face to face or telephone) which is agreed upon by the patient and the pharmacist and which is designed to gather information directly from the patient as well as other sources to ensure that the recommended care plan is producing the desired effect(s) and not resulting in undesirable or intolerable side effects.

THE PHARMACIST'S WORKUP OF DRUG THERAPY *(continued)*

III. FOLLOW-UP EVALUATION

Evaluate actual patient outcomes. This section contains the practitioner's clinical evaluation of how effective the care plan and the associated drug therapies have been in achieving the desired therapeutic goals for each of your patient's medical conditions. From the information gathered at the follow-up evaluation, the pharmacist evaluates and documents the progress (or lack of progress) in achieving the desired outcomes. The status of each medical condition and/or the status of the overall patient at the time of each follow-up evaluation can be described as *resolved, stable, improved, partial improvement, unimproved, worsened, failure,* or *expired.*

STATUS	DEFINITION
Resolved	Goals achieved, therapy completed
Stable	Goals achieved, continue same therapy
Improved	Progress being made, continue same therapy
Partial Improvement	Progress being made, minor adjustments required
Unimproved	No progress yet, but continue same therapy
Worsened	Decline in health, adjust therapy
Failure	Goals not achieved, initiate new therapy
Expired	Patient died while receiving drug therapy

Patient's Medical Conditions/Medications _____

_____

_____

Actual Outcome/Status/Progress _____

_____

_____

NEW DRUG THERAPY PROBLEMS

Evaluate patient for new drug therapy problems. This section contains the practitioner's clinical assessment of whether the patient has developed new drug therapy problems since the previous evaluation.

REFERENCES

1. Bender, T.B. *Don't Squat With yer Spurs On! A Cowboy's Guide to Life*. Salt Lake City, UT: Gibbs-Smith Publisher; 1992.

2. Strand, L.M., Cipolle, R.J., Morley, P.C. Documenting clinical pharmacy services: Back to basics. *Drug Intell Clin Phar*, 1988; 22:63–67.

3. Weed, L.L. Medical education and patient care. *Medical Records*. Cleveland OH: Case Western Reserve University Press; 1971.

4. Woolley, F.R., Warnick, M.W., Kane, R.L., Dyer, E.D. *Problem-Oriented Nursing*. New York: Springer-Verlag; 1974.

5. Sackett, D.L., Haynes, R.B. *Compliance with Therapeutic Regimens*. Baltimore, MD:The Johns Hopkins University Press; 1976.

6. Haynes, R.B., Taylor, D.W., Sackett, D.L. *Compliance in Health Care*. Baltimore, MD: The Johns Hopkins University Press; 1979.

7. Shalala, D.E. Giving pediatric immunizations the priority they deserve. *JAMA* 1993; 269:1844–1845.

8. Shaw G.M., Lammer, E.J., Wasserman, C.R., et al. Risks of orofacial clefts in children born to women using multivitamins containing folic acid periconceptionally. *Lancet* 1995; 346:393–396.

9. Levine, J.S. Misoprostol and nonsteroidal anti-inflammatory drugs: A tale of effects, outcomes, and costs. *Ann Intern Med* 1995; 123:309–310.

RECOMMENDED READINGS

Annas, G.J. *Standard of Care.* New York, NY: Oxford University Press; 1993.

Barrows, H.S., Pickell, G.C. *Developing Clinical Problem Solving Skills.* New York: Norton; 1991.

Blenkinsopp, A., Paxton, P. *Symptoms in the Pharmacy.* Oxford, England: Blackwell; 1992.

Galant G.A. *Caring for Patients from Different Cultures.* Philadelphia: University of Pennsylvania, 1991.

Hahn, R.A. *Sickness and Healing: An Anthropological Perspective.* New Haven, CT: Yale University Press; 1995.

Helman, C.G. *Culture, Health and Illness*, 3d ed. Oxford, England: Butterworth-Heinemann; 1994.

Higgs, J., Jones, M., eds. *Clinical Reasoning in the Health Professions.* Oxford, England: Butterworth, 1995.

Kassirer, J.P., Kopelman, R.I. *Learning Clinical Reasoning.* Baltimore: Williams & Wilkins; 1991.

Lyons, R.F., Sullivan, M., Ritro, P.G., Coyne, J.C. *Relationships in Chronic Illness and Disability.* Thousand Oaks, CA: Sage; 1995.

Veatch, R.M. *The Patient-Physician Relation: the Patient as Partner, Part 2.* Bloomington, IN: Indiana University Press; 1991.

CHAPTER FIVE

DOCUMENTING A PRACTICE

The provision of pharmaceutical care for a prolonged period of time requires a documentation system that adequately supports the practice. Such a system must generate three different types of output. The most important of the three is the *Pharmaceutical Care Patient Chart*, created primarily for the practitioner's use. Pharmaceutical care cannot be provided without this chart. The data in the patient chart also serve as the source of information necessary to generate other important reports, one for the patient's use and the other for the practice manager's use.

The *Patient's Personalized Pharmaceutical Care Plan* is generated for the patient's use. This care plan is printed and presented to the patient at each pharmaceutical care encounter. It is the tangible evidence that the patient is receiving pharmaceutical care. It includes all the information required by the patient to successfully address all drug-related needs. Although this plan is designed for the primary use of the patient, we have found it to be extremely useful to physicians and other prescribers. This will become clear when we discuss each of these reports in detail.

To manage a practice and support the work that must be done, a number of different reports must be generated. These *management reports* are used by the practice manager to make decisions about workload, workflow, reimbursement levels, and performance reports, to list just a few. Although the Pharmaceutical Care Patient Chart and the Patient's Personalized Pharmaceutical Care Plan are generated on a patient specific basis, management reports are summaries of the practice activities across the entire patient database.

These three forms of documentation derive from the patient care process and record the cognitive processes described in the Pharmacist's Workup of Drug Therapy. These relationships are depicted in Table 5-1.

TABLE 5-1 ALL ASPECTS OF THE PATIENT CARE PROCESS			
	THE THERAPEUTIC RELATIONSHIP		
THE PATIENT CARE PROCESS	ASSESSMENT OF DRUG THERAPY	CARE PLANNING	FOLLOW-UP EVALUATION
THE PHARMACIST'S WORKUP OF DRUG THERAPY	• Data collection	• Resolve drug therapy problems	• Determine actual patient outcomes
	• Determine the patient's drug-related needs	• Establish therapeutic goals	• Reassess patient's drug therapy
	• Identify drug therapy problems	• Prevent drug therapy problems	
DOCUMENTATION	• Pharmaceutical Care Patient Chart • Patient's Personalized Pharmaceutical Care Plan • Practice management reports		

The documentation of a service, specifically a health care service, is very different from the documentation required to dispense a medication. If one asks a physician, nurse, or other health care practitioner to describe documentation, it is commonly understood that reference is being made to the patient care records containing specific treatment recommendations and assorted clinical observations, all directed toward complete patient care. The pharmacist's response to this request will usually be to describe the record related to dispensing a prescription, commonly called *the patient profile*. Although this patient profile does have limited value in terms of providing a record of the prescription drug products dispensed at a particular pharmacy, the profile is constructed in such a static manner that its use is very limited in pharmaceutical care practice. Therefore we will dispense with the patient profile and introduce a new approach to documentation for pharmaceutical care. The term *documentation* is used here to refer to all material recorded for long-term use. This includes everything written down in longhand or entered into a computer software program, which becomes data for the practitioner, the patient, or the practice itself.

Documentation of pharmaceutical care, in all three forms just described, is so important that it is not an exaggeration to suggest that, without a documentation system, a practice does not exist.

A frequently expressed concern about documentation is whether to do it in written form or with computer software. Although all three forms of documentation can be done in writing on a small scale, and hard copies may be a logical place to start the practice, it will not take long before the written documentation needed to practice pharmaceutical care becomes unmanageable. The amount of information needed to provide care, the need to generate a care plan for the patient, and the necessity to create management reports on an ongoing basis makes computerization essential once the practice begins to grow. We will discuss both approaches to documentation, first the written and the task of computerizing the functions.

THE PHARMACEUTICAL CARE PATIENT CHART

The term *formative documentation* refers to the recording of certain activities at the time they are performed, describing what is done when a physician, nurse, or pharmacist is caring for a patient.[1] The medical record is created in a formative manner. This document is a record of the information collected by the practitioner, the decisions made, and the actions taken at the time these events occur. It is created one patient at a time. This documentation is recorded at the same level it is used— at a patient-specific level. The output of this type of documentation is, optimally, the generation of a database describing patient, disease, and drug information. Also included are decisions related to drug choice, dose determinations, and modalities of administration, parameters for patient monitoring, and patient outcomes in terms of efficacy, length of treatment, incidence of side effects, toxicity, and other drug-related events. This type of documentation serves a formative function, which is to improve the care the patients receive and to develop the skills and knowledge of the practitioners through repeated practice and the collection and analysis of patient care information. It is performed concurrently with the practitioner's activities and decisions and accommodates changes when additional data become available. A distinct advantage of the formative type of documentation is the interactive nature of the process. Corrections can be made and adjustments recorded, which is consistent with any changing patient status.

> Documentation is created one patient at a time.

The creation of a Pharmaceutical Care Patient Chart is important for many different reasons. Perhaps the most obvious one today, and the one that comes to mind first, is legal liability. It is unfortunate but truly the case that all activities performed for another need to be documented so that if, in the future, legal action is brought against the practitioner, appropriate documentation is available. It is clearly the case that the more comprehensive the documentation, the "safer" the practitioner. But let us concern ourselves with other, more patient-centered reasons for documenting the pharmaceutical care provided to patients.

We would like to think that the most important reason for creating the Pharmaceutical Care Patient Chart is to provide quality care to the patient. Documenting patient care activities and patient care decisions is a vital responsibility of every practitioner providing pharmaceutical care. Documentation is essential because the patient's condition, needs, and outcomes are constantly changing. And the amount of information required to provide pharmaceutical care is so voluminous as to necessitate recording the information. No one is able to remember all the vital, clinically relevant information about an individual, and, as the practitioner sees the patient repeatedly and the practice grows, it is unrealistic to think that quality care can be provided without complete documentation. In the practice of pharmaceutical care, you never see the "same patient" twice. Records must report decisions made, on a continuous basis, and reflect input from multiple practitioners. Each patient care decision made is based on accumulated data and results derived from all of the previous decisions and outcomes. Therefore patient care documentation must be a chronological record that can be constantly updated and evaluated to improve patient care.

> It is unrealistic to think that quality care can be provided without complete documentation.

Also, it will seldom be the case that a practitioner works entirely alone. Technicians, support personnel, other pharmacists, and other health care providers may require access to the written patient record. Therefore it must be complete, consistent, easily retrievable, and up to date.

There are other reasons to record what is done in practice. It is not possible for the practitioner to learn about his or her practice without being able to "look" at the practice over time. It is difficult for a practitioner to "improve" if he or she is not able to critically examine the decisions and clinical judgments rendered and even review the mistakes made. This requires written patient charts. Additionally, if a practitioner wishes to teach students or other practitioners, written patient charts are necessary. Reimbursement for patient care is necessary if the practice is to survive in the long term. The patient chart serves as the database for generating the Personalized Pharmaceutical Care Plan as well as the management reports. All are necessary outputs of a pharmaceutical care practice.

The Pharmaceutical Care Patient Chart is important to the practice in the long term since it serves as the basis for reimbursement. Third-party payers have taken the position that "if it is not documented, it was not done." Therefore reimbursement is not possible without this documentation.

THE STRUCTURE OF THE PHARMACEUTICAL CARE PATIENT CHART

The Pharmaceutical Care Patient Chart (Fig. 5-1) is a record of the outcomes of the cognitive activities described in the Pharmacist's Workup of Drug Therapy.

The Pharmacist's Workup of Drug Therapy prescribes the nature of the problem solving that must occur between the pharmacist and the patient. The pharmacist records what transpired during this interaction in the patient chart. During the workup, the pharmacist collects general and specific information and makes connections between the patient and his or her diseases and drug therapies. During the documentation process, the pharmacist records these connections. For example, recall that during the workup the pharmacist assesses the patient to determine whether any of the seven types of drug therapy problems are present. This requires a logical, disciplined process and calls for many different decisions to assess appropriate indications, including the patient's medical condition or signs and symptoms and the time of onset and nature of the illness. Effectiveness is assessed by the reduction of pain and suffering or the resolution of illness; safety is assessed by exploring the presence of predictable side effects and known adverse reactions associated with the medication taken by the patient. If the patient does have a drug therapy problem, the pharmacist gathers another set of data to determine the most likely cause. Documentation in the patient chart will contain only the final decisions made. In other words, the patient care chart will record only the drug therapy problem and its cause. The primary difference between the Pharmacist's Workup of Drug Therapy and the patient care chart is that the Pharmacist's Workup of Drug Therapy is a system that assists the pharmacist in gathering all of the necessary clinical information required to make patient care decisions, while the Pharmaceutical Care Patient Chart is primarily designed to record and communicate those decisions so they can be used to continually evaluate and improve the patient's health status.

The patient chart is a living document.

A computerized patient care documentation system is needed to provide pharmaceutical care to numerous patients on an ongoing basis and to build and maintain a successful practice. However, to learn and become proficient at providing pharmaceutical care for a limited number of patients, a paper system can be quite useful. The following Pharmaceutical Care Patient Chart (Fig. 5-1) (printed with permission from Mike Frakes, Pharm.D., Health Outcomes Management, Inc.) was developed to record patient care decisions and activities. All of the data and information contained in the Pharmaceutical Care Patient Chart are described in detail in Chap. 4.

The Pharmaceutical Care Patient Chart contributes significantly to your practice. The unique aspects of this record include the fol-lowing:

- The structure of the document is similar to records maintained by physicians, nurses, and other health care providers; therefore it can be shared, used jointly, and others can easily contribute to it.
- It serves as the basis for reimbursement, so it will be necessary to include financial information, insurance details, and family information.

(*Text continues on page 184*)

PHARMACEUTICAL CARE PATIENT CHART

PETERS INSTITUTE OF PHARMACEUTICAL CARE   10/14/97   14:01

Patient ID: 100026   **Name:**   John Doe
Phone # :   (612) 555-5187 WORK
Weight :   195 lbs   **Height:** 6' 0"
Age :   46 years
Gender :   Male
Carrier :   Self Pay

Allergies and Adverse Reactions:
Allergies: ASPIRIN - Lips swell with ASA and NSAIDs, IBUPROFEN.
Alerts:
Tobacco Use: No tobacco use, Alcohol Consumption: 2–6 drinks per week, Caffeine Use: More than 2 cans/cups per day, Patient requires eye glasses

Problem: BACK PAIN 10/14/97 Back pain
Description:
Lower back pain, similar to episode last year. Will try to reduce weight and resume jogging, which helped in the past.

Drug	Sts	Dose	Freq	Start	Stop	Physician	Type	Rx Number
ACETAMINOPHEN EXTRA STRENGTH TABS, 500MG	A	1000MG	QID	10/14/97	12/14/97		0	

Associated Drug Therapy Problems

Type	Description	Eff Date	Res Date	Resolution Description
2B	Contraindication present ACETAMINOPHEN EXTRA STRENGTH _CLINORIL TABS, 200 MG_	10/14/97	10/14/97	MD changed product MD Initiated New Therapy

Interv. Type	Intervention Text	To-Do Date
FOLLOW-UP	Determine effectiveness of the acetaminophen therapy for back pain. Question about exercises if recommended by the MD.	10/24/97
AGENCY	Educational materials are available from the Back Pain Hotline at 1-800-247-2225	

Problem: DEPRESSION 09/14/97 Depressive Disorder
Description:
Not eating well and unable to sleep. He has complaints of feeling tired, lack of energy, and less able to concentrate at work.

Drug	Sts	Dose	Freq	Start	Stop	Physician	Type	Rx Number
PROZAC PULVULES, 20MG	A	20MG	QAM	09/14/97		Ralph Hutchinson	P	246899

•**Figure 5-1** An example of a Computerized Pharmaceutical Care Patient Chart.

Patient ID : 100026　　　　　　　　　**Name :** John Doe　　　　　　　10/14/97　　　14:01

DEPRESSION　(continued)

Interv. Type	Intervention Text	To-Do Date
FOLLOW-UP	Determine effectiveness of Prozac therapy including changes in energy levels (2-6 weeks), sleeping & eating, and ability to concentrate (2-6 months)	10/24/97
AGENCY	Educational materials are available from the National Foundation for Depressive Illness at 1-800-248-4344	

Evaluations

Evaluation Text	Related Problem	Date
RJC　　IMPROVED Eating now somewhat improved. Will continue exercise program.	DEPRESSION	10/14/97
RJC　　INITIAL Initial Clinoril prescription changed to acetaminophen due to ASA and NSAID allergy. Back pain similar to last episode.	BACK PAIN	10/14/97
RJC　　IMPROVED After 3 weeks of therapy, energy level improved, but still has difficulty eating and sleeping well.	DEPRESSION	10/06/97

_____　　　　_____
　　　　　　　Pharmacist's Signature　　　　　　　　　　　Date

•**Figure 5-1**　(Continued).

- This chart is the source of truly unique information that no other health care provider generates or collects. For example,

  —The drug therapies, complete with National Drug Code (NDC) codes, are linked to a specific medical indication for the drug, complete with International Classification of Diseases, 9th Revision, Clinically Modified (ICD-9-CM) codes.

  —Drug therapy problems and their resolutions are associated with causes within a medical condition and an outcome. No one else has these data about ambulatory patients in terms of their total care.

  —Goals of therapy are established for each medical condition, and drug therapy goals are associated with actual patient status and outcomes.

The paper version of the Pharmaceutical Care Patient Chart consists of two pages that the pharmacist fills out and a third page upon which the drug therapy problem codes and resolution codes used in the chart are found. The first page (Fig. 5-2) summarizes the patient's demographic and pharmacotherapeutic information, including the indication and goals for all forms of drug therapies the patient is taking. A standard insurance release and signature are included to allow the Pharmaceutical Care Patient Chart to be available to other care providers and payer's as needed.

The second page of the Pharmaceutical Care Patient Chart allows the practitioner to describe the patient's progress at each follow-up evaluation. However to facilitate initial data collection needs, the left column allows coded data to be recorded for easy review and summary. The patient care data that can easily be recorded in coded format include which indication or indications were evaluated at each follow-up evaluation, the category and cause of any drug therapy problems identified, the resolution code describing the intervention employed to solve the problem, the patient's status at time of the follow-up, and the date of the next scheduled follow-up evaluation. As with all paper systems, additional pages need to be added for patients who require many visits and/or who have numerous complex drug-related needs.

Numeric codes for drug therapy problems, resolution codes, and outcome status are presented in Table 5-2. The list of resolution codes is designed to allow the practitioner to document how the drug therapy problem was resolved and describe any savings or costs realized by this intervention. For instance, "pt.dose" is used to indicate that the practitioner dealt directly with the patient, and the dose was changed. Similarly, "SV.UR" is intended to indicate that a visit to an urgent care center was avoided because of the pharmaceutical care provided.

Pharmaceutical Care Patient Chart

Last Name: _____ First Name: _____ MI: _____

Address: _____ City: _____ ST: _____ Zip: _____

Home Phone: _____ Work Phone: _____ Employer: _____

Primary Physician: _____ Phone: _____ Occupation: _____

Birth Date: _____ Age: _____ Gender: _____ Due Date: _____ Height: _____ Weight: _____

Marital Status: _____ Race: _____ Patient ID: _____

Allergies	Reaction	Adverse Reactions	Reaction

Special Alerts or Devices

Past Medical Background

Tobacco	Past History	None	0-1 pack/day	> 1 pack/day	
Caffeine	Past History	None	1-2 bev/day	> 2 bev/day	
Alcohol	Past History	None	< 2 drinks/week	2-6 drinks/week	> 6 drinks/week

Current Medical Indications (including approximate dates)	Drug Therapies, how taken, dates, goals of therapy (including non-prescription medications, vitamins and herbals)

Insurance: _____ Group: _____ ID# _____

I authorize this pharmacy to release to insurance carriers and other health care providers any medical or other information about me which is needed to assure continuity of care or determine benefits for health related claims. I permit a copy of this authorization to be used in place of the original, and request payment or medical insurance benefits either to myself of the party who accepts this assignment. Regulations pertaining to Medicare assignment of benefits apply.

Signature: _____ Date: _____

•**Figure 5-2** The Pharmaceutical Care Patient Chart. Reprinted with permission from Mike Frakes, Pharm.D., Health Outcomes Management © 1998 Health Outcomes Management, Inc. ALL RIGHTS RESERVED.

Patient Name: **Patient ID**

	Progress Note and Drugs Involved:
Date/Pharmacist:	
Indications:	
Drug therapy problems:	
Resolution codes:	
Status:	
Follow-up date:	
Date/Pharmacist:	
Indications:	
Drug therapy problems:	
Resolution codes:	
Status:	
Follow-up date:	
Date/Pharmacist:	
Indications:	
Drug therapy problems:	
Resolution codes:	
Status:	
Follow-up date:	
Date/Pharmacist:	
Indications:	
Drug therapy problems:	
Resolution codes:	
Status:	
Follow-up date:	
Date/Pharmacist:	
Indications:	
Drug therapy problems:	
Resolution codes:	
Status:	
Follow-up date:	

•**Figure 5-2**   (Continued).

TABLE 5-2 NUMERIC CODES FOR DRUG THERAPY PROBLEMS, RESOLUTION CODES, AND OUTCOME STATUS

I: Drug Therapy Problem Codes

Code	Type	Cause
0		None known at this time
1A	**Indication**	Untreated condition
1B	Needs	Synergistic therapy
1C	therapy	Prophylactic therapy
2A	**Indication**	No medical indication
2B	Unnecessary	Addiction/recreational drug use
2C	drug	Non-drug therapy appropriate
2D	therapy	Duplicate therapy
2E		Treat avoidable ADR
3A	**Efficacy**	Dosage form inappropriate
3B	Wrong	Contraindication present
3C	Drug	Condition refractory to drug
3D		Drug not indicated for condition
3E		More effective drug available
4A	**Efficacy**	Wrong dose
4B	Dosage	Frequency inappropriate
4C	too low	Duration inappropriate
4D		Incorrect storage
4E		Incorrect administration
4F		Drug interaction
5A	**Safety**	Unsafe drug for patient
5B	Adverse	Allergic reaction
5C	drug	Incorrect administration
5D	reaction	Drug interaction
5E		Dose increase/decrease too fast
5F		Undesirable effect
6A	**Safety**	Wrong dose
6B	Dosage	Frequency inappropriate
6C	too high	Duration inappropriate
6D		Drug interaction
7A	**Compliance**	Drug product not available
7B		Cannot afford drug product
7C		Cannot swallow/administer
7D		Does not understand
7E		Patient prefers not to take

(continued)

II: Resolution Codes (who & what)

#	Code	Description
1	pt.device	PT Given **Reminder Device**
2	pt.dose	PT Changed **Dose**
3	pt.form	PT Changed **Dosage Form**
4	pt.qty	PT Changed **Quantity**
5	pt.int	PT Changed **Interval**
6	pt.prod	PT Changed **Product**
7	pt.filled	PT **Filled As Is**
8	pt.unfilled	PT Said **Do Not Fill**
9	pt.disc	PT **Discontinued**
10	pt.init	PT Initiated **New Therapy**
11	pt.generic	PT **Generic Substitution**
12	pt.otc	PT **Started OTC**
13	pt.barrier	**Eliminated** Patient **Barrier**
14	pt.no.otc	PT **Did Not Buy OTC**
15	pt.ed	PT **Education Beyond OBRA**
16	pt.nores	PT Problem **Not Resolvable**
17	md.dose	MD Changed **Dose**
18	md.form	MD Changed **Dosage Form**
19	md.qty	MD Changed **Quantity**
20	md.int	MD Changed **Interval**
21	md.prod	MD Changed **Product**
22	md.filled	MD Said **Fill As Is**
23	md.unfilled	MD Said **Do Not Fill**
24	md.disc.	MD **Discontinued**
25	md.ther	MD **Therapeutic Interchange**
26	md.generic	MD **Generic Substitution**
27	md.init	MD Initiated **New Therapy**
28	md.nores	MD Problem **Not Resolvable**
29	cr.cover	Carrier **Does Not Cover**
30	cr.ther	Carrier **Therapeutic Interchange**
31	cr. generic	Carrier **Generic Substitution**

Race	**Marital Status**
Indian/Alaskan	Divorced
Asian/Pacific Islands	Married
Black	Never Married
Hispanic	Separated
Caucasian	Unknown
	Widowed

TABLE 5-2 (CONTINUED) NUMERIC CODES FOR DRUG THERAPY PROBLEMS, RESOLUTION CODES, AND OUTCOME STATUS

III: Resolution Codes (savings & costs)

#	Code	Description
32	SV.10	**$10 OR LESS Rx** net saved 90 days
33	SV.25	**$11-25 Rx** net saved 90 days
34	SV.50	**$26-50 Rx** net saved 90 days
35	SV.100	**$51-100 Rx** net saved 90 days
36	SV.200	**$101-200 Rx** net saved 90 days
37	SV.400	**$201-400 Rx** net saved 90 days
38	SV.401	**Over $400 Rx** net saved 90 days
39	SV.OF	**Office visit** saved
40	SV.MOF	**Multiple office visits** saved
41	SV.UR	**Urgent Care** visit saved
42	SV.ER	**ER Visit** saved
43	SV.RN	**Nursing visits** saved
44	SV.HOS	**Hospital stay** saved
45	SV.LTC	**LTC stay** saved
46	CS.10	**$10 OR LESS Rx** net cost 90 days
47	CS.25	**$11-25 Rx** net cost 90 days
48	CS.50	**$26-50 Rx** net cost 90 days
49	CS.100	**$51-100 Rx** net cost 90 days
50	CS.200	**$101-200 Rx** net cost 90 days
51	CS.400	**$201-400 Rx** net cost 90 days
52	CS.401	**Over $400 Rx** net cost 90 days
53	CS.OF	**Additional Office visit** incurred
54	CS.MOF	**Multiple Office visits** cost incurred
55	CS.UR	**Urgent Care visit** cost incurred
56	CS.ER	**ER visit** cost incurred
57	CS.RN	**Nursing visits** cost incurred
58	CS.HOS	**Hospital stay** cost incurred
59	CS.LTC	**LTC stay** cost incurred

Status: Patient Outcome at Follow-up	
Goals Met	**Goals Not Met**
Resolved	Unimproved
Stable	Worsened
Improved	Failure
Partial Improvement	Expired
Initial	

THE PATIENT'S PERSONALIZED PHARMACEAUTICAL CARE PLAN

The Patient's Personalized Pharmaceutical Care Plan encourages active participation by the patient.

The patient is central to all therapeutic decisions and pharmacist interventions, therefore it is important to design documentation to support the patient's active participation in the care process. The Patient's Personalized Pharmaceutical Care Plan serves this purpose. The Patient's Personalized Pharmaceutical Care Plan represents the integration and culmination of the knowledge, experience, and skills of both the pharmacist and the patient applied for the benefit of the patient. The patient takes this document home and uses it to actively participate in his or her own care. The Patient's Personalized Pharmaceutical Care Plan was designed after extensive examination of the information patients actually write down, carry with them, and use to ensure that their drug therapy is safe and effective.

Historically, medical personnel have kept the public relatively uninformed about its health or lack thereof. It is unrealistic to assume that patients have the necessary resources or are empowered to care for themselves after being subjected to the paternalistic approaches of the health care industry. The patient is certainly capable of actively participating in his or her health care, more so if appropriate information and resources are made available. The Patient's Personalized Care Plan attempts to accomplish this objective by empowering the patient to become and stay actively involved in his or her drug therapy.

This form of documentation is designed to be used to record the patient's questions, observations, or findings related to the outcomes resulting from drug therapy. This record will provide the patient with the information needed to discuss important issues with his or her pharmacist, physician, dentist, or other health care provider. It will also legitimize the input of the patient into decisions made by these providers. This is a very important step to the meaningful participation in the care process.

The Patient's Personalized Care Plan is of use to others in addition to the patient. It will help care givers understand the drug therapy of the patient, and, as is illustrated below, provides unique information which can help prescribers, nursing personnel, and other support personnel to fulfill their responsibilities more comprehensively and more easily. This is a very important advantage.

THE STRUCTURE OF THE PATIENT'S PERSONALIZED PHARMACEUTICAL CARE PLAN

Figure 5-3 shows the Patient's Personalized Pharmaceutical Care Plan. This printed document is often referred to by patients as their "list." It is quite common for elderly patients to keep such a list with them in their purse or wallet. Also, spouses who care for their partners and parents who care for children requiring drug therapy often keep such lists to help them "keep everything straight." These lists not only explain what the patient is supposed to take but also, often, point out what the patient is not supposed to take.[1]

Summary of All of Your Medications

The *Summary of All of Your Medications*, for the first time, puts all of a patient's drug therapies and their associated uses and directions for use in one place. This section connects four pieces of information for the patient: the indication or medical condition being treated, the medication, the directions for use, and the prescriber or pharmacist who recommended the medication. The Patient's Personalized Pharmaceutical Care Plan can and should be updated continuously so that it can truly represent the patient's current therapies, indications, and directions.

If a patient is taking two of three medications for the same indication, all three are organized and associated with the single indication. For instance, a patient taking conjugated estrogens (Premarin), calcium supplements, and a multiple-vitamin supplement for the prevention of osteoporosis would have all three of these therapies related to the same primary indication. Similarly, the Patient's Personalized Pharmaceutical Care Plan for a patient who is being treated for high blood pressure with enalapril maleate (Vasotec) and hydrochlorothiazide would have these two medications related to the same "hypertension" indication. Such an association may seem trivial on the surface but can have a significant impact on how a patient comes to understand his or her medical condition and drug therapy.

> The personalized plan makes the connections between medical condition (indication), drug therapies, and directions for use, for the patient.

All the information on the Patient's Personalized Pharmaceutical Care Plan should be clearly stated (avoid as much technical jargon as possible) and should be as "user friendly" as possible. The indications for drug therapy should be in terms the patient understands. If you have discussed hypertension in terms of *high blood pressure*, then the indication on the Patient's Personalized Pharmaceutical Care Plan should use the term *high blood pressure*. Similarly, if the patient refers to episodes of gastritis as *heartburn*, then this term might best serve as the indication for the patient's ranitidine (Zantac). Allergic rhinitis might be recognized by the patient as *hay fever* or *seasonal allergies*.

There are no legal labeling requirements for the Patient's Personalized Pharmaceutical Care Plan. Thus, medications can be listed by generic, trade name, or both, whichever is most helpful to the patient. A description of the tablet or capsule is often useful for the patient to distinguish one medication from another. For example, omeprazole (Prilosec, purple capsule), amoxicillin/clavulanate potassium (Augmentin, yellow round tablet), clarithromycin (Biaxin, yellow tablet) serve the patient as useful descriptions. The "Directions for Use" should indicate how the patient is actually going to take the medication. In

(*Text continues on page 194*)

PATIENT'S PERSONALIZED PHARMACEUTICAL CARE PLAN:
Name:
Address: Date:

SUMMARY OF ALL OF YOUR MEDICATIONS

Indication or Medical Condition	Medications	Directions for use	Prescriber (Source)

MEDICATION RELATED NEEDS

	Special instructions for you
Unique needs/preferences:	
Medication allergies:	
Adverse reactions:	

NEW CONCERNS/QUESTIONS/EXPECTATIONS: (note your questions or concerns here)

Date	Concerns/Questions/Expectations

•**Figure 5-3** The format for a Patient's Personalized Pharmaceutical Care Plan. Copyright© 1996 Peters Institute of Pharmaceutical Care. With permission.

INFORMATION FOR EACH OF YOUR MEDICATIONS AND INSTRUCTIONS

Medical Condition or Indication for drug therapy

Health Advice

Medication	Goals of Therapy	How to Take This Medication	Common Side Effects
	Follow-up Checkpoints	Follow-up Checkpoints	Follow-up Checkpoints
Medication	Goals of Therapy	How to Take This Medication	Common Side Effects
	Follow-up Checkpoints	Follow-up Checkpoints	Follow-up Checkpoints

SIGNATURE _____   DATE _____

•**Figure 5-3**   (Continued).

most cases the legal prescription requires the directions to read as the prescriber wrote them, even if these directions are not clear or directly relevant to what the patient is actually going to do. For instance, common prescription directions such as "Take 1 TID with meals and HS" might appear on the legal prescription label as "Take one (1) tablet three (3) times each day with meals and one (1) at bedtime." However, for the millions of people who do not eat the customary three meals a day, the directions for use on the Patient's Personalized Pharmaceutical Care Plan might read "Take one (1) tablet four (4) times a day. Take in the morning, at midday, in the evening, and at bedtime with some food to prevent stomach upset." In this situation the prevention of nausea with food is made explicit on the Patient's Personalized Pharmaceutical Care Plan, while it remains implicit on the legal prescription label. It is important for the Patient's Personalized Pharmaceutical Care Plan to translate or interpret complex and often confusing directions into meaningful, comprehensible language and to communicate a realistic, attainable set of goals and directions to patients. In this sense the plan becomes a "cognitive map" for patients to locate solutions and follow pathways to effective drug therapy.

It might also be useful to list drug therapies that the patient is no longer taking in a Patient's Personalized Pharmaceutical Care Plan. If the patient has been using an antihistamine preparation for several days with no relief of symptoms of the common cold, and is advised to begin therapy with a decongestant nasal spray to control nasal congestion, it might be very helpful to use the *Summary of All Your Medications* section of the Patient's Personalized Pharmaceutical Care Plan to remind the patient not to use the antihistamine for her cold.

Medication-Related Needs

This section describes any unique patient needs or preferences that might influence drug therapy. Medication allergies and adverse reactions the patient may have experienced in the past that should be used to guide future drug therapy decisions should be noted. Information describing patient preferences—such as liquid dosage forms or medication during the school day, requiring an extra bottle to be left with the school nurse—can help patients receive the care they expect. Medication allergies noted on the Patient's Personalized Pharmaceutical Care Plan do not merely refer to the offending drug but also include special instructions such as "Allergic to penicillin and should avoid penicillin and related antibiotics such as amoxicillin, ampicillin, and amoxicillin/ clavulanate potassium." Similarly, patients who are allergic to aspirin might be instructed to avoid other nonsteroidal anti-inflammatory drugs (NSAIDs) such as ibuprofen (Motrin), ketoprofen (Orudis), and sulindac (Clinoril).

Consistent with the Pharmacist's Workup of Drug Therapy, the Patient's Personalized Pharmaceutical Care Plan distinguishes adverse reactions to medications from true drug allergies. The patient can see that a past adverse reaction to a drug, such as nausea from erythromycin taken for acute bronchitis 2 years earlier, might influence the choice of antibiotics in the future but not necessarily rule out the future use of some other erythromycin product. Another example is sunburn associated with tetracycline therapy, which can be avoided with proper precautions in the future. Such precautions would, of course, be noted and brought to the attention of the patient.

New Concerns/Questions/Expectations

The Patient's Personalized Pharmaceutical Care Plan also includes a very important section to be used by patients to record concerns, questions, or other important issues that they want to discuss with the pharmacist or prescriber during their next visit. This "New Concerns/Questions/Expectations" section of the Patient's Personalized Pharmaceutical Care Plan serves to not only allow but also to encourage patients to have all of their questions addressed. Often, patients think of additional questions or have new concerns after they have left the pharmacy or prescriber's office. This portion of the Patient's Personalized Pharmaceutical Care Plan makes it convenient to record these questions within the context of all of the patient's medical indications and associated drug therapies. Since this is likely to be a new experience for the patient, it may be necessary to explain how best to utilize this section.

The personalized plan allows the patient to record concerns, questions, or comments about drug therapy.

Information for Each of Your Medications and Instructions

The Patient's Personalized Pharmaceutical Care Plan contains the summarized information mentioned above, but in addition, for each medical indication for drug therapy, the patient receives expanded, more detailed information. The medical condition is described, including common terminology, signs and symptoms, causes, and common approaches to treatment. The Patient's Personalized Pharmaceutical Care Plan also includes other health advice the patient might find useful to assist in meeting expected outcomes. Advice about nondrug approaches, diet, exercise, foods or beverages to avoid, and methods to prevent the condition from recurring are useful forms of health advice and make up the final part of this section.

The more detailed information in the Patient's Personalized Pharmaceutical Care Plan describes the medication(s) for each medical condition or indication for drug therapy as well as the goals of therapy, so the patient can understand what benefit to expect from the medications. Again, for each medication or drug product, specific, detailed instructions are written, including times of day, length of therapy, and use with or without food are included. Also associated with each medication are the common side effects of which the patient should be made aware. Here the judgment of the pharmacist is needed to keep the Patient's

Personalized Pharmaceutical Care Plan useful to the patient and avoid making it just another long list of side effects that the manufacturer must list for medical legal purposes. Rather, the contents of the "Common Side Effects" section of the Patient's Personalized Pharmaceutical Care Plan reflect the discussion the pharmacist and the patient had about the patient's specific drug therapy. The therapeutic relationship between the patient and the pharmacist has a substantial influence on how much detail needs to be contained in any given Patient's Personalized Pharmaceutical Care Plan.

By contrast to a hand-generated list of drugs a patient is taking, the Patient's Personalized Pharmaceutical Care Plan serves as a summary record of what the patient has agreed to undertake as personal responsibility for the care process ("How to Take the Medication" and "Follow-up Checkpoints"), what should happen ("Goals of Therapy"), and what might happen ("Common Side Effects").

Follow-up Checkpoints

A key section of the Patient's Personalized Pharmaceutical Care Plan is the listing and description of the "Follow-up Checkpoints". This section includes dates when the patient and/or pharmacist will have follow-up encounters to monitor progress of therapy. The Patient's Personalized Pharmaceutical Care Plan might suggest different follow-up checkpoints to monitor side effects as opposed to monitoring measurable improvement in the patient's health status. The follow-up checkpoints cover not only the agreed upon time and date that the patient and the pharmacist have agreed on to monitor benefits and side effects but also what the patient should look for when evaluating the success or failure of therapy. Conversely, the follow-up checkpoints should describe how the patient can tell if the drug is causing any unwanted side effects. Here the patient's information should be as detailed and useful as possible and indicate how patients will recognize that they are experiencing side effects.

Finally, the Patient's Personalized Pharmaceutical Care Plan is signed and dated by the pharmacist who prepares it for the patient. This is done after the pharmacist and patient agree that the content and its implications are understood by both.

PRACTICE MANAGEMENT REPORTS

Summative or practice-level documentation is created by combining the formative pharmaceutical care records described above and summarizing different aspects of a practice—not necessarily for the purpose of caring for a specific patient but for the purpose of better caring for all patients in a practice. This type of documentation usually takes on the form of management reports. The management reports will focus on such issues as how many patients are seen daily and how much time, on average, practitioners spend with patients. What types of problems are most common in the practice? What types of resources are most frequently required for patient care? Such issues can be addressed from the data generated from summative documentation, which are essential to the effective management of any practice.

Because most management reports represent work and services performed in the past and reflect the interventions or outcomes of several individuals providing care for many different patients, summative data in the form of management reports are not used to improve the care of an individual patient. However, summative data and management reports generally are often useful to assist practitioners to determine which services are most effective and should be continued and which are less valuable and should be modified or discontinued. Most importantly, the documentation system for pharmaceutical care, generated on a patient-by-patient basis, must be summarized to help the practitioner better understand his or her practice, and, in effect, improve performance and quality. The generation of these reports will be much easier if your patient care charts are computerized. This is discussed later in the chapter.

Managing a practice is different than managing a patient.

Management reports have many uses. Perhaps the most basic and important use of management reports is to understand the nature of the practice. Summary data are compiled to present a composite picture of the number of patients, the patients' characteristics, the number and type of medical conditions, and the nature of the drug therapy used in the practice. They help to describe the types of resources required to meet patient needs, and they summarize the quality of the work performed to achieve positive patient outcomes. A word of caution here. We have found that few software programs facilitate understanding the "whole" patient. Most programs dissect the patient into diseases, drugs, demographics, consumption of resources, and outcomes before an understanding of the patient, per se, can be realized. It is important to be aware of this when evaluating programs that generate management reports.

Practice management must improve the way practitioners deliver patient care.

Management reports can generate data about how efficient a service is (how much time is spent with each type of patient), how effective personnel are at managing workload, and how satisfied patients are with the services provided. They can describe the financial health of a practice, and they can help identify inefficiencies at each step of the practice process. However, to benefit from management reports, it is necessary to first generate the raw data used to create the report. It is necessary to spend time reviewing the reports and interpreting their meaning in the context of the specific practice. Finally, the reports need to be acted upon in a timely manner. Without taking all of these steps it is not necessary to generate management reports, since their use will be very limited.

THE STRUCTURE OF MANAGEMENT REPORTS

The capacity to integrate patient data from selected groups or populations with similar characteristics to make management, protocol-development, marketing, staffing, and staff-development decisions is essential to the provision of quality pharmaceutical care services. The patient variables and combination of patient variables frequently used to select patient populations for this type of summative management report include:

- Age, body weight, gender, pregnancy status, race, marital status, tobacco use, alcohol use, caffeine use
- Insurance carrier, employer
- Occupation
- Address
- Indication for drug therapy, ICD-9 code
- Medication classification, drug product (NDC), type and number of drug therapy problems
- Practitioner interventions
- Patient outcome, patient status at last follow-up evaluation
- Complexity of the patient drug-related needs, service date(s)
- Practitioner providing care
- Billing amount(s)

This is by no means an all-inclusive list of all the information needed to generate management reports. It more closely represents the minimum amount of data required to manage a practice. It will become necessary to computerize the documentation function to create and generate Pharmaceutical Care Patient Charts, Patient's Personalized Pharmaceutical Care Plans, and management reports.

COMPUTER PROGRAMS FOR PHARMACEUTICAL CARE

Pharmacists who have provided pharmaceutical care agree that a computer software program for documentation is essential. When discussing the software programs, we will refer to the formative documentation as the patient chart and the summative documentation as management reports. Early in the development of the practice of pharmaceutical care described in this text, we found that in order to care for many patients on a continuous basis, paper records could not adequately support the pharmacist or provide the useful summative reports to manage busy practices.

To aid pharmacists participating in the Minnesota Pharmaceutical Care Project,[2] we worked with Health Outcomes Management, Inc. (2331 University Avenue S.E., Minneapolis, MN 55414), to develop a computerized pharmaceutical care documentation system now marketed worldwide as the Assurance Coordinated Pharmaceutical Care System. This computerized documentation system is based on the practice of pharmaceutical care as described in this text and is designed to assist pharmaceutical care practitioners to provide care for many patients over time. The Health Outcomes Management, Inc. computer support system is presently available in DOS and Windows format and is used by pharmacists in several countries as well as to teach pharmacy students in the Pharmaceutical Care Teaching Laboratory at the University of Minnesota. In addition, all of the patient data analyses presented in this text were made possible because of this software.

The pharmaceutical care documentation system specifically developed to support the practice of pharmaceutical care uses a relational database to create and maintain a patient-centered, longitudinal, complete record of the patient's drug-related needs, the care provided, and patient outcomes. Being patient-centered means the patient's charts are always kept together as a whole record with the patient as the central identifying unit (rather than the drug or the disease). The relational database allows the practitioner to "relate," compare, or contrast any and all patient, drug, and disease information. This can be accomplished within an individual patient, among a selected group of patients, or across the entire patient population. This form of patient care documentation supports keeping longitudinal records of patient progress toward achieving desired therapeutic goals and positive outcomes.

Figures 5-4 through 5-8 describe the core information maintained in a pharmaceutical care documentation system and the relationships that must be maintained among the various data elements in order to be of maximal use to the pharmaceutical care practitioner and patient. It is important for multiple pharmacies in networks, health maintenance organizations, chains, and franchises to be able to share information and compile data. This requires the use of a similar data structure for patient care charts. Complete patient demographic information is needed to assist the pharmacist in assessing all of the patient's drug-related needs. Allergies, alerts, and special needs of the patient are vital in the assessment of a patient's drug-related needs.

Patient care plans can be standardized for all patients across an entire network or individualized care plans can be created to meet unique patient needs. Industry-standardized protocols can also be implemented for patients who meet the clinical criteria. Medical conditions, their associated ICD-9-CM codes, goals of therapy, and the drug or drugs being used to treat or prevent the condition are maintained as part of the relational database.

Drug therapy problems as well as how and when they were resolved are documented within the appropriate care plan for the patient. Interventions designed to achieve the therapeutic goals and those designed to prevent new problems are documented.

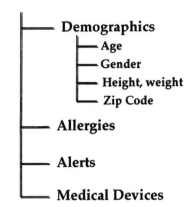

•**Figure 5-4**   Pharmaceutical care database—patient assessment.

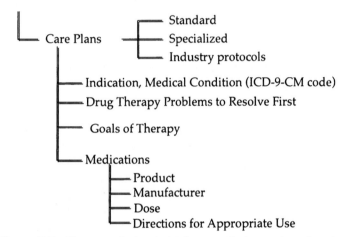

•**Figure 5-5**   Pharmaceutical care database—patient care plans: Overview.

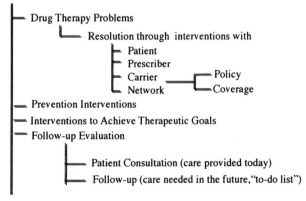

•**Figure 5-6**   Pharmaceutical care database—patient care plans: Drug therapy problems.

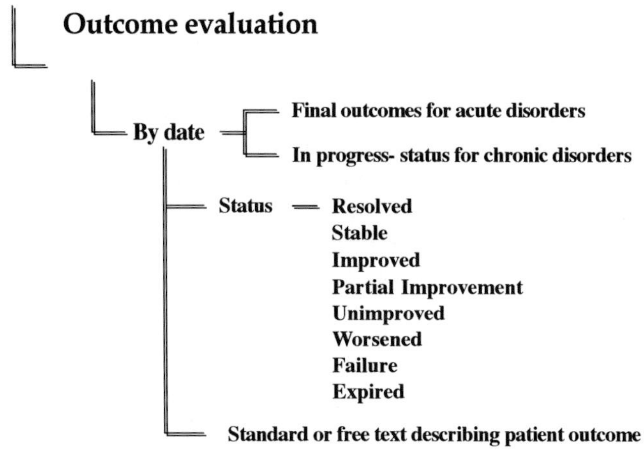

Outcome evaluation

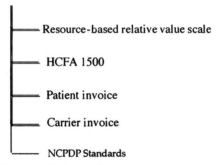

By date
— Final outcomes for acute disorders
— In progress- status for chronic disorders

Status — Resolved
Stable
Improved
Partial Improvement
Unimproved
Worsened
Failure
Expired

Standard or free text describing patient outcome

•**Figure 5-7** Pharmaceutical care database—follow-up evaluation of patient care outcomes.

— Resource-based relative value scale

— HCFA 1500

— Patient invoice

— Carrier invoice

— NCPDP Standards

•**Figure 5-8** Pharmaceutical care database—billing for pharmaceutical care services.

Follow-up evaluations of the patient's status at each encounter and actual patient outcomes associated with drug therapy are documented, described, and compared to the goals of therapy to establish progress toward meeting these goals.

All commonly used billing mechanisms must be supported by the pharmaceutical care software. These include invoices using a resource-based relative value scale to determine the ability to generate standardized forms such as the HCFA 1500 (Health Care Finance Administration) as well as an individualized invoice for private, self-pay patients.

Practitioners and managers need to evaluate software as to how best it can support their patient care services, ensure that appropriate billing records exist, and generate required management reports.

Unlike commonly used dispensing computer systems, in which the primary concerns are speed and simplicity of data input, patient care systems should be primarily evaluated on their output capacities. In this

Patient care documentation systems should be evaluated by their output (patient chart, care plans, and management reports, billing process).

context, output capacities include the Pharmaceutical Care Patient Charts for the pharmacist's use, Patient's Personalized Pharmaceutical Care Plans for the patient's use, and practice management reports for use by managers. Pharmaceutical care software systems should also facilitate communication between pharmacists, physicians, dentists, nurses, and other health care providers. Furthermore, pharmaceutical care software systems must have the capacity to generate reimbursement information and billing for private-pay patients, commercial third-party payers, pharmacy benefit management companies, and governmental agencies.

The following is a list of important questions to ask when evaluating software to support the practice of pharmaceutical care.

- Does the software system support the specific practice of pharmaceutical care as described here or does it direct the pharmacist to perform activities or gather patient information arbitrarily-without a practice process explicitly articulated?
- Does the program allow access to other clinical databases without exiting the pharmaceutical care documentation system?
- Is the system sufficiently comprehensive to support numerous patients with diverse medical conditions, diseases, and illnesses?
- How much free text input is required? Remember, free text input is time-consuming and not very useful when combined or integrated into summative management reports.
- Can the software system accommodate the continuous addition of data and updating of patient records required to provide continuous care to patients with chronic medical conditions?
- Can the system support the use of drug therapy protocols from numerous sources such as physician clinics, health maintenance organizations, insurance carriers, pharmacy benefits management companies, the pharmaceutical industry, governmental agencies, and research institutes?
- Does the program use a *relational database* to support the association of each drug product with its unique indication, drug therapy problems, resolutions, interventions, and outcomes?
- Does the program's database permit integrating data from numerous patients into useful management reports?
- Can it track cost savings?
- Can the program support searching patient records by multiple patient, drug, and/or disease characteristics?
- Can the software support several terminals in busy practice settings?
- Can the software system integrate large sets of patient data from numerous pharmacies into a single large databank to support network, franchise, or chain pharmacy operations?
- Does the software system have on-line tutorials and "help" screens to facilitate new employees as they begin to use the patient care documentation system?

Because many pharmacies have computerized their prescription dispensing systems, it would seem logical to try to interface the pharmaceutical care documentation system and the prescription dispensing system. The primary objective would be to reduce the need for double entries for data such as patient name, address, and insurance information. Also, an interface might reduce some double entries for prescription medications. However, when one examines specific data that could actually be useful to both systems, the real benefit of such an interface is unimpressive.

Most dispensing computer systems organize patient profiles by date of the prescription or the last refill rather than the onset of the therapy. The essential connection between the appropriate indication and the medication is absent from the majority of dispensing computer systems. Family relationships are difficult or impossible to track in dispensing systems because the files are organized by prescription rather than by patient. Hence, because most dispensing systems actually function as label generators and third-party billing systems, they do not contain any records of prescription medications that the patient obtained from some other pharmacy, clinic, or mail-order supplier. Most dispensing systems do not keep track of non-prescription products or any physician samples the patient is taking. In many communities, legal requirements mandate giving long-term medications a "new" prescription number each time continued prescriber authorization is granted. Although this may legally be a new prescription, it is not a new medication for the patient. Also, dispensing systems rarely maintain records of discontinued drugs or products that were prescribed but not actually dispensed or taken by the patient. Thus, in addition to all of the patient, care plan, and follow-up outcome evaluation information that is not available in most dispensing systems, much of the drug information contained in these systems is not accurate or complete enough to be useful in the provision of pharmaceutical care. An inclusive system could be of value in reducing duplicate entries for new patients, and some new prescription medications. These data would be transfered in a report form from the dispensing computer to the pharmaceutical care documentation system, on an "on-demand-only" basis.

The computer program is not your practice. At the beginning of this chapter we emphasized the importance of differentiating between the description of the patient care process, the cognitive activities within the process, and what is recorded in the practice. The greatest risk comes from pharmacists who confuse a computer system they use to document practice with the practice itself. The computer software program is merely an aid to support practice; it is a means to an end. When the pharmacist allows the software to define or drive what the practitioner does for a patient, the practice is certain to be ineffective and short-lived.

Documentation is the evidence of a practice.

On the other hand, it is essential to keep in mind that the patient care documentation system represents the evidence of your practice. If you do not document it, you did not do it. As with all documentation systems, considerable effort may be required to enter new patients; but

If it is not documented, it was not done!!!

in the practice of pharmaceutical care, a patient is only new once, and it is not always necessary to gather all possible patient, drug, and disease information at the very first patient encounter. The pharmaceutical care documentation system must represent a "living document" that changes, grows, and improves with your patients.

REFERENCES

1. Norman, D.D. Perceptions of the Elderly Regarding the Medicating Experience: A Discourse Analysis of the Interpretation of Medication Usage. Ph.D. thesis. Minneapolis: University of Minnesota; 1995.

2. Tomechko, M.A., Strand, L.M., Morley, P.C., Cipolle, R.J. Q and A from the Pharmaceutical Care Project in Minnesota. *Am Pharm* 1995; NS35:30–39.

RECOMMENDED READINGS

Adams, D.M. *Diagnosis: Documentation and Coding.* New York, NY: McGraw-Hill; 1997.

Dick, R.S., Steen, E.B. *The Computer-Based Patient Record.* Washington, D.C.: National Academy Press; 1991.

Proceedings of the Seventeenth Annual Symposium on Computer Applications in Medical Care. *Patient-Centered Computing.* New York: McGraw-Hill; 1994.

Slack, W.W. *Cybermedicine.* San Francisco: Jossey-Bass; 1997.

CHAPTER SIX

OUTCOMES OF PHARMACEUTICAL CARE PRACTICE

The practice of pharmaceutical care has been described and illustrated in Chapters 1 and 4. This chapter presents the practice from a slightly different perspective, that of data generated in practice by pharmaceutical care practitioners. The data presented were generated in practices which were part of the Minnesota Pharmaceutical Care Project. The project will first be described in order for the source of the data to be understood, and then the data will be presented so pharmaceutical care can be understood from a quantitative perspective.

THE MINNESOTA PHARMACEUTICAL CARE PROJECT

The concept of pharmaceutical care was converted into the practice of pharmaceutical care in an action-oriented research project called the Minnesota Pharmaceutical Care Project.[1] This project was conducted between June 1992 and November 1995 at the University of Minnesota. It was a 3-year demonstration project that required the collaboration of many aspects of the pharmacy profession. The principal investigators were from academe, while the remaining collaborators were from the Minnesota Pharmacists Association, the Minnesota State Board of Pharmacy, managed care organizations, the pharmaceutical industry, and most importantly, it included 54 pharmacists from 20 community pharmacy practice sites throughout the state of Minnesota.

In simple terms, the intent of the project was to explore the relationships between the theory and practice of pharmaceutical care. More specifically, the primary objective of the project was to determine if an innovative practice could be developed in the community practice setting. In addition, it was necessary to:

- Describe the practice in detail and with consistency so that it could be learned, practiced, and disseminated to others
- Develop a new management system to support the practice so that traditional practices could be converted to the new practice
- Develop a computerized pharmaceutical care documentation system to record patient outcomes
- Design and implement a reimbursement mechanism so the practice could survive beyond the duration of the study
- Determine the cost of providing this service and the value associated with receiving it

PROJECT METHODS

This demonstration project was conducted in a manner consistent with the qualitative methods of participatory and evaluative research. Therefore, instead of having the primary investigators identify the intervention and measure the impact, the pharmacists in the project were expected to assume the role of coresearchers. In this role they were expected to define specific interventions with direction and feedback from the primary investigators and to evaluate this impact on their own practice. Although collaborative research is much more complex to conduct, we were of the opinion that the research questions had to be answered *by pharmacists, for pharmacists, in the practice setting.* Therefore, the pharmacists selected for this project became coinvestigators and equal partners in creating the practice of pharmaceutical care.

The methods used to conduct this demonstration project are described in four major time periods. *The prestudy period* (from May 1 to October 31, 1992) involved sample site selection and preparation for the first year of the project. *The pilot-study year* (from November 1, 1992, to October 31, 1993) focused on 4 pharmacies and 10 pharmacists to determine if a new practice of pharmaceutical care could be developed. *Year 2* of the study (November 1, 1993, to October 31, 1994) was dedicated to disseminating the practice developed in year 1 to the remaining 16 pharmacies for definition, refinement, and assessment. *The final year* of the study (November 1, 1994, to October 31, 1995) was devoted to the evaluation of the data generated during the first 2 years.

The fundamental nature of this project required input and cooperation from many disciplines and areas of expertise. The broad scope of disciplines was represented in the primary investigators of the project. The project director, while a clinical pharmacist, had 10 years of management experience in businesses outside the health care industry. The medical anthropologist brought experience and expertise in qualitative methods and the cultural context of change—which is essentially what this project was all about. The clinical pharmacist brought expertise in therapeutics and practice. The principal investigator with a background in pharmacy administration was able to establish standards of practice during the project's development which kept its identity clear and the focus defined. In addition to these staff members, there was clerical support, and three practicing pharmacists functioning as support in the field. The 54 practicing pharmacists ultimately selected to participate in the project provided a wide range of practice experience. All this was required to carry the project through to completion.

The agencies financially supporting the project represented the pharmaceutical industry, third-party payers, insurers, managed care companies, regulatory agencies, and professional associations. These include: Glaxo Inc., The Merck Foundation and the Merck Company, Blue Cross/Blue Shield of Minnesota, Diversified Pharmaceutical Services (DPS), PCS Health Systems, Aetna Health Plans, and Med Centers. Each of these collaborators provided one representative at the senior management level to serve as an adviser to the project staff. In addition to those who contributed financially, this work could not have been completed without the collaborative support of the Minnesota State Board of Pharmacy, the University of Minnesota College of Pharmacy, the Minnesota Pharmacists Association, and Health Outcomes Management, Inc. The magnitude of change encompassed in the practice of pharmaceutical care is such that it demanded the development of coherent communication networks between all active participants in the change process. Multiagency discourse sustained throughout the 3-year period of the project produced essential information utilized daily to direct implementation and the practical consequences of action.

> The development of a new practice requires active participation and substantive input from all aspects of the profession.

Prestudy Period

This project was initiated following approval by the Committee on the Use of Human Subjects and Research at the University of Minnesota.

Sample-site selection was designed to achieve a representative selection of community pharmacies on the basis of geography, prescription volume, and type of ownership. The recruitment effort began with a mailing to all community pharmacies licensed in the state of Minnesota. The mailing was designed to stimulate interest in the project and it provided pharmacists with the option to receive additional information by returning a response card. A total of 229 pharmacists expressed initial interest and 100 of these, from 71 different pharmacies, accepted the invitation to attend a recruitment seminar held at the College of Pharmacy. The purpose of this seminar was to provide comprehensive information about the project and to initiate the final application process.

The final application process required the completion of written application forms by pharmacists and pharmacy managers, and consent for participation by the manager and all pharmacists practicing more than 10 hours per week in the pharmacy.

At the deadline, applications from 51 pharmacies had been received. Site visits were made to each of the pharmacies during the months of September and October. Three members of the project staff visited each site and assessed the pharmacy and its staff on the following criteria:

- The manager's, pharmacists', and technicians' level of interest in and commitment to changing their practice
- The willingness of staff (plus the needed economic resources available) to change the physical environment to accommodate patient needs
- The projected economic viability of the pharmacy for the duration of the project
- The stability of the personnel (limited retirements, changes in management) throughout the project
- The willingness of the staff pharmacists to participate as coinvestigators in a project designed to challenge every aspect of their practice for the following 3 years

Following the site visits, each pharmacy was ranked independently by three members of the project staff. The pharmacies were selected to represent the following categories:

- Urban (population of greater than 50,000) or rural (less than, or equal to, 50,000)
- Independent (less than 4 pharmacies under single ownership), chain (4 stores or more under single ownership), and clinic (if housed in the same building as a medical clinic). Hospital-operated, outpatient ambulatory pharmacies were not included in this project.
- High volume (greater than an average of 100 prescriptions filled per day) or low volume (less than or equal to an average of 100 prescriptions per day)

Attention was also directed to the approximate proportion of the final applicant pool within each category of variables described above. Twenty sites were finally selected throughout the state of Minnesota.

Pilot Study: Year 1

Of the 20 pharmacies, 4 were selected as pilot sites. These sites were selected on the basis of the staff (pharmacist and support personnel) who were willing to devote the greatest amount of time to the project and the managers' commitment to changing practice. In addition, a representative sample was maintained during the selection process. The four sites consisted of two chain pharmacies (one urban and one rural) and two independently owned pharmacies (one urban and one rural). The average volumes in these pilot sites varied from 80 to 180 prescriptions per day.

The most important selection criterion is the practice philosophy of the practitioner.

As described earlier, the purpose of the pilot year was to determine if a practice based on the pharmaceutical care philosophy could be developed and implemented in the community practice setting. To answer this question, the efforts of the pharmacists, with direction from the project staff, were devoted to the following activities:

- Educational preparation of pharmacists in the areas of philosophy, content, and the patient care process
- Development of new job descriptions and work flow processes for pharmacy staff
- Making recommendations for new physical layout and the design of patient care areas
- Development of documentation tools for pharmaceutical care practice
- The construction of a reimbursement mechanism to support the practice

An additional pilot-site year activity included the selection of 10 comparison pharmacies matched as closely as possible with the sample-site locations, practice settings, and prescription volume. These comparison sites were selected for the purpose of comparing the practice of pharmaceutical care with the articulated practices in the comparison sites. Baseline data collected included financial data, prescription volume data, workload, and workflow data.

Implementation: Year 2

The purpose of year 2 was to implement, in the remaining 16 pharmacies, the practice developed in the pilot sites during year 1. The same process described above for the first year was used during the second year. Efforts were made to improve each of the aspects developed during the first year (educational processes, job descriptions and workflow, physical layout, the documentation system, and reimbursement), with additional input from the remaining 16 pharmacies and 44 pharmacists. The improvements made during year 2 resulted in the Pharmaceutical Care Certificate Program described in Chap. 9.

Evaluation: Year 3

The third and final year of the project focused on evaluation. The qualitative data generated during the development of the practice were evaluated. This evaluation produced the Pharmaceutical Care Practice described in this text. Evaluation also produced preliminary data documenting the care pharmacists provided to patients throughout the project. These data are reported here.

RESULTS

Twenty community pharmacy sites entered the project in November 1992. The sites selected included 6 urban and 14 rural pharmacies.

Two pharmacies were considered clinic pharmacies located in a medical building. Five of these sites were chain pharmacies, while thirteen were independently owned and operated. The average prescription volumes of the project pharmacies varied from 50 to 380 prescriptions per day. On average, 55 percent of the prescriptions filled were transmitted to some third-party carrier. Fifty-four pharmacists were employed in the 20 sites (included all pharmacists working more than 10 hours per week at a site). The ages of the pharmacists varied from 25 to 73 years old. The average age was 40 years old. Twenty-five percent of the pharmacists were female. All but one of the pharmacists participating in the project possessed as a terminal degree the bachelor of science in pharmacy. The exception had a Pharm.D. degree.

Of the 20 sites, 16 remained in the project for the duration of the 3 years. The four sites that withdrew from the study did so for a number of different reasons. The first site to withdraw was a large department store chain. It withdrew from the project because the chain underwent significant corporate reorganization. Different individuals from those who originally agreed to participate in the project were assigned to the pharmacy operations and chose not to continue.

The second site, a smaller chain store, was purchased by a larger chain that already had a site in the project. Management at the larger chain chose to focus their efforts on the original site and to withdraw the newly purchased site. The third pharmacy was withdrawn because two sites from the same chain were selected for inclusion in the study. The management of the chain decided to focus its resources on one site and therefore withdrew the second from the project. The final site to withdraw from the project did so because it terminated business. We have been assured that this situation did not develop as a result of participation in the project.

The 10 comparison pharmacies identified at the beginning of the project could not be used for evaluation purposes. Insufficient documentation of patient care services existed in these pharmacies and adequate comparisons could not be made without intervening in the control pharmacies. Therefore, it was decided that the project sample sites would serve as their own controls.

This project was about change. The experience was similar to that reported in the literature; change is a long, involved, sometimes tedious, and oftentimes frustrating experience. However, the personnel involved in this project demonstrated that change in practice can occur when efforts are focused and cooperation at all levels is achieved. Together, this research team invented:

- a new professional practice (developed it, described it, and implemented it)
- a new management system to support this practice
- a new computer software documentation system to record and evaluate pharmaceutical care practice

The Minnesota Pharmaceutical Care Project implemented:
- a new professional practice
- a new practice management system
- a computerized patient care documentation system
- a reimbursement structure
- care to 9,000 patients

- a new and functional reimbursement system to reward the practitioner for this patient care practice
- care to over 9000 patients representing approximately 25,000 encounters of pharmaceutical care.

The practice created from this project, along with all of the support systems developed, will be studied, evaluated, and improved for many years to come. Although it is not the intention of this chapter to report all of the results of the study, we intend to present the most important ones, those which help to describe the practice of pharmaceutical care.

UNDERSTANDING PHARMACEUTICAL CARE PRACTICE THROUGH PATIENT CARE DATA

One of the first steps to providing pharmaceutical care is understanding patients and their drug-related needs in practice. Since few practices of this nature exist, and no comprehensive data are available, we thought it important to present the patient data generated from the Minnesota Pharmaceutical Care Project. These data will be examined three different ways. First, the entire set of patient care data derived from a 12-month period (November 1994 to October 1995) during the Minnesota Pharmaceutical Care Project will be examined. This database involves 5480 different patients who received pharmaceutical care in one of ten community pharmacies that had completely converted to the practice of pharmaceutical care and were using the same computerized documentation system. The data generated in this first group describes a community practice based on the provision of pharmaceutical care. The second subgroup is a set of patients introduced to pharmaceutical care services prior to November 1994 who continued to receive pharmaceutical care services during this same next 12-month period (November 1994 to October 1995). This subgroup of 1111 patients represents what may be termed *established patients* who used the pharmaceutical care services regularly during this 12-month data collection period. Last, a smaller subset of the second group of patients, consisting of those patients 65 years or older, will be described. The data from these patients were used to examine the cost:benefit of providing pharmaceutical care services to a group of elderly, community-based patients.

All of the patient care data described in this text were documented, collected, and initially analyzed using the Assurance Coordinated Pharmaceutical Care System developed and marketed by Health Outcomes Management, Inc., of Minneapolis, Minnesota. This patient care documentation system was developed in conjunction with the Minnesota Pharmaceutical Care Project and the staff of the Peters Institute of Pharmaceutical Care in the College of Pharmacy at the University of Minnesota. This pharmaceutical care software system uses a relational

Data are reported for three patient groups:
- 5,480 patients receiving care within a twelve month period
- 1,111 established patients receiving care throughout a twelve month period
- 249 established elderly patients (>65 years old)

database platform and is the only documentation system designed to specifically support the practice of pharmaceutical care as described in this text.

The Peters Institute of Pharmaceutical Care functioned as the primary databank for the 10 project pharmacies who contributed patient care data. All patient names and prescriber names were stripped from the data prior to combining the results from the 10 pharmacies. The Practice Management Reports and the General Analysis portions of the Assurance Coordinated Pharmaceutical Care System were used in their commercially available versions for all initial data analyses. No additional "research" subroutines were required to present the results.

GROUP 1 DATA: PATIENT DATABASE FOR ONE YEAR

During the Minnesota Pharmaceutical Care Project a total of 9399 patients received pharmaceutical care services in one of the 10 community pharmacies that contributed data through the use of the Assurance Coordinated Pharmaceutical Care System. In order to describe a pharmaceutical care practice, the data for 5480 patients receiving care for the one-year period between November 1, 1994, and October 31, 1995 were analyzed (Group 1). These 5480 different patients required 12,376 patient care encounters. This represents an average of 2.3 encounters per patient per year.

We describe the practice in terms of patients and patient encounters. Patient encounters represent the actual work that must be performed by the practitioners providing care. Initial patient encounters are documented separately from subsequent follow-up evaluations. This makes it possible for the pharmacist to compare the progress of each patient over several episodes of care and thus to document both the status of the patient at each follow-up encounter and the actual patient outcomes.

Patient Demographics

Of the 5480 patients who received pharmaceutical care during this 1-year period, 3226 (59 percent) were female. This distribution of female to male patients was remarkably consistent across the mix of 10 rural and metropolitan pharmacies in which the distribution of females ranged from 57 percent to 60 percent. The ages of the patients are displayed in Fig. 6-1.

This group of patients consisted primarily of middle-aged, employed, insured adults and their family members. Approximately 49 percent of these patients were between the ages of 30 and 65, while another 26 percent were children aged 15 or less.

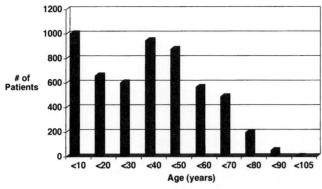

•**Figure 6-1** Ages of patients (n = 5480) who received pharmaceutical care in the Minnesota Pharmaceutical Care Project between November 1, 1994, and October 31, 1995.

Description of Drug-Related Needs

Patients seen in this generalist practice of pharmaceutical care in community pharmacies were taking an average of 2.5 different medications, as displayed in Fig. 6-2.

These included prescription and nonprescription drugs as well as physician samples and other home remedies used for self-medication. At over 60 percent of the encounters, patients were taking more than one drug, while 436 (3.5 percent) of the patient encounters involved patients taking 10 or more different medications at one time. Conversely, 2.4 percent of patients were not on any medications when they first required pharmaceutical care services. This emphasizes the importance of being proactive in identifying drug-related needs. It suggests

3.5% of patient encounters involve patients taking ≥ 10 different medications.

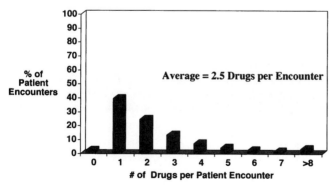

•**Figure 6-2** Number of drugs taken by patients (n = 5480) who received pharmaceutical care in the Minnesota Pharmaceutical Care Project between November 1, 1994, and October 31, 1995.

that simply reviewing a list of drugs that the patient is already taking (i.e., patient profile) is not always sufficient.

The practice of pharmaceutical care and the documentation system used to support this practice allows the pharmacist to relate each and every medication a patient is taking to its appropriate indication. This fundamental connection between drug and indication must be established and assessed by the pharmacist prior to any critique of dosage, safety, or compliance issues. The practice of pharmaceutical care requires the pharmacist to first assess the appropriateness of the indications for all medications a patient is taking; to determine if the patient has an appropriate indication for each medication, and to ascertain if each indication for drug therapy is being appropriately treated.

The amount and type of patient education is dictated by the patient's understanding of the purpose, risk, and benefits of drug therapy.

The primary source of information concerning why a patient is taking a particular medication is the patient. The patient's understanding of the indication for drug therapy (disease, illness, prevention, treat signs or symptoms, etc.) and the association of that indication with appropriate drug therapy is essential to establish as it will dictate the degree and type of patient education that will be required. Patients who have a comprehensive grasp of their illness and the risk and benefit of the drug therapy used to treat that illness require relatively little routine education. However, patients who present with little understanding of their illness and drug therapies usually require more personalized and extensive education.

In a generalist practice, "common things are common." The most frequent indications for drug therapy encountered in these 5480 patients receiving pharmaceutical care over a 1-year period are listed in order of frequency in Table 6-1.

These 12 indications represented 53 percent of all indications for drug therapy. Moreover, these are all very serious conditions. Any parent who has suffered with a young child through an episode of acute otitis media fully understands the importance of appropriate care. Similarly, the misery and suffering associated with arthritis or depression

TABLE 6-1 MOST FREQUENT INDICATIONS FOR DRUG THERAPY IN PATIENTS RECEIVING PHARMACEUTICAL CARE SERVICES DURING A SINGLE YEAR[a]	
1. Sinusitis	7. Peptic ulcer disease
2. Bronchitis	8. Estrogen replacement therapy
3. Otitis media	9. Allergic rhinitis
4. Hypertension	10. Skin infections
5. Pain	11. Depression
6. Strep throat	12. Arthritis

[a] These 12 conditions represent 53 percent of all indications for drug therapy.

TABLE 6-2 MOST FREQUENT INDICATIONS FOR DRUG THERAPY IN PATIENTS RECEIVING PHARMACEUTICAL CARE SERVICES DURING A SINGLE YEAR[a] (CONTINUED FROM TABLE 6-1)	
13. Urinary tract infection	19. Conjunctivitis
14. Common cold	20. Hypothyroidism
15. Dental infection	21. Diabetes
16. Asthma	22. Acne
17. Rash	23. Anxiety
18. Hyperlipidemia	24. Back pain

[a] The most frequent 24 conditions represent 74 percent of all indications for drug therapy.

illustrate the value of a practitioner who fully accepts the responsibility to ensure effective and safe drug therapy.

It becomes evident that pharmacists who intend to practice pharmaceutical care must be extremely familiar with the presentation, goals of therapy, treatment approaches, and outcomes associated with the most common disorders. It is important for the generalist practitioner to become effective and efficient at providing care for patients with these common conditions. These conditions present frequently, therefore efficiencies in caring for patients with common problems will allow for the extra time that will be required to provide care for patients with less common or less well understood disorders. The importance of prioritization cannot be overemphasized.

In addition to the "top 12" most commonly encountered disorders, Table 6-2 lists the next most frequent indications for drug therapy encountered in a generalist community-based pharmaceutical care practice.

This second list expands the first and includes a large portion of the disorders encountered in a generalist practice. When combined with the first list, these 24 indications for drug therapy represent a cumulative 74 percent of all of the indications seen by the generalist. These data have strong implications for programs designed to prepare pharmacists to provide pharmaceutical care and for professional education programs in pharmacy. A strong case can be made that colleges of pharmacy should make absolutely certain that students receive instruction and experience with patients who suffer from these most common disorders.

The patients' most common needs define and prioritize the practitioner's learning agenda.

Since the late 1990s, there has been a growing discussion of the attributes and potential liabilities of disease state management programs. These programs vary, but they essentially begin with a disease in which pharmaceutical industry representatives have an interest, and pharmacists are encouraged to "manage" the care of patients with the particular disease. Protocols are often preestablished and promoted as a

Asthma, hyperlipidemia, and diabetes represent the 16th, 18th, and 21st most common indications for drug therapy.

guide for the practitioner. How the particular disease is chosen often seems less than rational. The most popular disease state management programs available have chosen asthma, hyperlipidemia, or diabetes. These represent the 16th, 18th, and 21st most common indications for drug therapy in a generalist's practice. Certainly, patients with any one of these disorders would benefit from pharmaceutical care services. However, these three conditions combined represent only 7 percent of all of the indications for drug therapy and only about 11 percent of patients encountered in community pharmacies, as listed in Table 6-3 below.

New patients with these selected "targeted" disorders present themselves so infrequently to a community pharmacy that it would be extremely difficult to build a new practice, or maintain a viable existing generalist practice based on a disease state management approach. During the 1 year of pharmaceutical care services provided for the 5480 patient in the Minnesota Pharmaceutical Care Project, the average pharmacy encountered a new patient with hyperlipidemia only once every 2 weeks.

New patients with selected diseases (such as asthma, hyperlipidemia, and diabetes) are encountered so infrequently as to make the building of a viable practice on this basis impractical.

Patients with sinusitis, bronchitis, and otitis media present three times more frequently than patients treated with disease state management protocols.

Let us take this discussion a bit further. Imagine for a moment that a pharmacist who wants to begin to provide pharmaceutical care services decides to follow the industry's lead and begins to "practice" with patients who have hyperlipidemia. The pharmacist fully intends to expand to asthma patients, then to diabetic patients. Then what? How will the next patient population be chosen. Who will decide?

Logically, practitioners who want to expand their practices to as many new patients as possible would choose to provide care for patients with the most commonly encountered disorders (sinusitis, bronchitis, otitis media). This patient group would represent three times more new patients than the asthma-hyperlipidemia-diabetes disease state management group. In addition, this most commonly encountered group of patients would also include 28 percent of the asthma-hyperlipidemia-diabetes disease state management patients, because so many patients present with multiple medical conditions (comorbidities).

Asthma, hyperlipidemia, and diabetes represent only 7% of all indications for drug therapy.

TABLE 6-3 DISEASE STATE MANAGEMENT IN PATIENTS RECEIVING PHARMACEUTICAL CARE SERVICES FOR 1 YEAR[a]

DISEASE STATE	NUMBER OF PATIENTS	PERCENT OF PATIENTS
Asthma	$n = 236$	4.3
Hyperlipidemia	$n = 231$	4.2
Diabetes	$n = 207$	3.8

[a] These three conditions combined represent only 7 percent of all indications for drug therapy.

A group of researchers and pharmacy practitioners in Florida developed a Therapeutic Outcomes Monitoring (TOM) program using asthma as a prototype disease. They set out to determine whether community pharmacists could provide care using such a disease-state oriented program and assess the performance of the Therapeutic Outcomes Monitoring program. After considerable protocol preparation, training, and field testing, they found that virtually all patients who received care responded positively to the Therapeutic Outcomes Monitoring services. However, enrollment of patients was difficult and the lack of documentation of care was a major problem. Although this initial Therapeutic Outcomes Monitoring project was considered to be a technical success, this disease-state approach was not successful from a patient enrollment or marketing perspective.[2]

If the pharmacist wanted to be certain that he or she was going to have the greatest impact on patient care, he or she might chose to expand practice to include disorders that are known to have significant risk factors leading to hospitalization, injury, and death. In this case, expanding practice to include patients with hypertension, osteoporosis, and depression could certainly have a major impact on the health and well-being of the people in the community. Again, by expanding practice to include patients with hypertension, osteoporosis, and/or depression, 22 percent of the patients in a generalist's practice would receive pharmaceutical care, and approximately 40 percent of all drug therapy problems could be identified and resolved. Thus, it becomes somewhat obvious that a rational approach to drug therapy is not only essential on a patient-by-patient basis but it is also required in order to establish and maintain a viable practice.

We compared the most common indications for patients of different age groups within the sample of 5480 patients. We chose to look at two different groups, the youngest (21 years old and younger), and the oldest (65 years old and older). As expected, the most commonly encountered indications for drug therapy vary among these groups. Table 6-4 lists in order the most frequent indications for drug therapy in

TABLE 6-4 THE MOST FREQUENT INDICATIONS FOR DRUG THERAPY IN PATIENTS ≥ 65 YEARS OLD[a]

1. Hypertension	6. Diabetes
2. Upper respiratory infections	7. Estrogen replacement therapy
3. Peptic ulcer disease	8. Pain
4. Arthritis	9. Hypothyroidism
5. Hyperlipidemia	10. Angina pectoris

[a] These 10 conditions represent 52 percent of all indications for drug therapy in patients ≥ 65 years old.

TABLE 6-5 FREQUENT INDICATIONS FOR DRUG THERAPY IN PATIENTS ≥ 65 YEARS OLD[a] (CONTINUED FROM TABLE 6-4)	
11. Anxiety	17. Asthma/chronic obstructive
12. Cardiac dysthythmias	pulmonary disease
13. Urinary tract	18. Allergic rhinitis
infection	19. Insomnia
14. Depression	20. Rash
15. Glaucoma	21. Prostatitis
16. Skin infection	22. Congestive heart failure

[a] The 22 most common conditions represent 75 percent of all indications for drug therapy in patients ≥ 65 years old.

patients who were 65 years of age or older when they received pharmaceutical care.

Again, a small number of disorders (10) represents a large portion of the medical indications for drug therapy (52 percent). As would be expected, this older group presents with more cardiovascular risk factors—such as hypertension, hyperlipidemia, diabetes, and angina pectoris. The next 12 most frequently encountered indications for drug therapy in patients of this age group are listed in Table 6-5.

In contrast to the elderly, Table 6-6 lists in order the 12 most frequently encountered indications for drug therapy in patients 21 years old or younger when they received pharmaceutical care from their community pharmacist.

The list in Table 6-6 represents an interesting array of mostly eye, ear, nose, and throat (EENT) and dermatological disorders. While these disorders appear commonly among the young, they are not commonly featured in the core curricula of many colleges of pharmacy. Many pharmacists who begin to develop pharmaceutical care practices find that they must learn or "relearn" much of the practical information about these common disorders in order to care for their younger patients.

TABLE 6-6 MOST FREQUENT INDICATIONS FOR DRUG THERAPY IN PATIENTS ≤ 21 YEARS OLD	
1. Otitis media	7. The common cold
2. Strep throat	8. Skin infection
3. Bronchitis	9. Allergic rhinitis
4. Sinusitis	10. Pain
5. Conjunctivitis	11. Acne
6. Asthma	12. Rash

Drug Therapy Problems

A primary responsibility of practitioners providing pharmaceutical care is to identify, resolve, and prevent drug therapy problems. Drug therapy problems, identified in individual patients, must be resolved because, left unresolved, drug therapy problems prevent the patient from realizing the full benefits of drug therapy. Therefore, it is helpful to understand the distribution and frequency of drug therapy problems. Drug therapy problems have not been routinely identified, so we are describing for the first time the distribution of drug therapy problems in the community-based, noninstitutionalized population.

During the 12,376 patient encounters, the pharmacists identified a total of 7223 drug therapy problems. These 7223 drug therapy problems included patient encounters involving multiple drug therapy problems and patients who had the same type of drug therapy problem recur at multiple encounters. To eliminate any confusion, only the 4228 unique types of drug therapy problems are summarized below. However, it should be understood that this figure is a very conservative estimate of the drug therapy problems in the ambulatory population.

Throughout the year, these 5480 patients had 4228 unique types of drug therapy problems that the pharmacist determined were significant (important or dangerous) enough to require a specific intervention to resolve. Table 6-7 lists the distribution of the unique types of drug therapy problems that were identified and resolved by the pharmacists.

43% of patients have active drug therapy problems.

It is interesting that approximately the same proportion of drug therapy problems was associated with each of the primary drug-related needs of patients. These include appropriate indication, effectiveness,

TABLE 6-7 Drug therapy problems (DTPs) in patients who received pharmaceutical care services during a 1-year period ($n = 5480$ patients)

	Number of DTPs	Percent
Indication		
Need additional drug therapy	991	23
Unnecessary drug therapy	288	7
Effectiveness		
Wrong drug	672	16
Dosage too low	610	15
Safety		
Adverse drug reaction	899	21
Dosage too high	246	6
Compliance		
Inappropriate compliance	522	12
Total	4228	100

Approximately 30% of the drug therapy problems involve inappropriate indications, 30% involve ineffective medications, 30% involve unsafe therapy, and 10% involve compliance problems.

These data indicate that 2 out of 5 patients in a community, who are fully insured in a managed care system including a pharmacy benefit plan, experience drug therapy problems a practitioner can identify and resolve.

Patient compliance is much higher when a therapeutic relationship is established.

and safety. Thirty percent of drug therapy problems was associated with "appropriate indication," 31 percent with "effectiveness," and 27 percent with "safety." If no practitioner is providing pharmaceutical care, it would appear that the natural or actual distribution of drug therapy problems would be spread "evenly" throughout indication, effectiveness, and safety issues.

It is important to understand that these drug therapy problems were identified in patients who were not institutionalized (hospital or nursing home), living in the community, and fully insured, including managed care services and a pharmacy benefits plan. These data suggest that the practice of pharmaceutical care does represent a valuable approach to drug therapy and that there is no other health care professional who presently assumes complete responsibility for a patient's drug therapy being appropriate, effective, safe, and convenient.

In addition to the drug therapy problems associated with indication, effectiveness, and safety, an additional 12 percent of drug therapy problems was associated with compliance. At first glance these data are not consistent with numerous other reports of compliance problems occurring in 30 to 50 percent of patients. The difference is that in pharmaceutical care, appropriateness of the indication for drug therapy is established first, then the effectiveness of drug therapy is assessed. Next, the safety of the patient's drug therapy is assessed, and only after this orderly, structured assessment is complete is the patient's drug-taking behavior assessed for compliance problems.

If no practitioner accepts the responsibility to provide pharmaceutical care based on this approach, then all drug therapy problems might be "clumped" into the category of patient noncompliance. This yields inflated noncompliance figures, and results in expensive and time-consuming interventions to improve compliance. These are often ineffective as they do not address the patient's real drug therapy problems. This is most likely the reason why attempts to improve patient compliance have yielded only minimal and short-lived results. Why, for example, would any well-meaning practitioner want to improve compliance in patients who are taking unnecessary medications or who are engaged in inappropriate (wrong) drug therapy? Why would patients increase their use of a medication causing them an adverse reaction? Why would patients increase use of a medication that is not meeting their expectations and not providing any noticeable benefit? Only after all of the drug therapy problems associated with indication, effectiveness, and safety are identified and resolved can compliance behavior be assessed and modified as necessary. To do otherwise is to engage in irresponsible "blaming of the victim."

Twenty-three percent of the drug therapy problems identified and resolved by pharmacists occurred because patients needed additional drug therapy. Certainly, encouraging a visit to the community pharmacist for appropriate drug therapy or a referral for a medical condition or illness represents the most cost-effective approach an organized health care system can provide its patients.

These data call into question the common practice of simply relying on a pharmacy "profile" (list of drugs the patient has already purchased) to provide complete care for the patient. The most common type of drug therapy problem was the need for additional drug therapy to treat conditions that were not previously being treated. These drug therapy problems are overlooked when the pharmacist focuses on a prescription or drug order. Therefore, a proactive approach by the pharmacist is needed.

The data in Table 6-7 also indicate that 7 percent of the drug therapy problems were identified in patients who were taking drugs that were not necessary. An additional 16 percent of drug therapy problems were found in patients who were taking the wrong drug product. This 23 percent of drug therapy problems, or almost one out of every four, required the pharmacist to work with the patient and/or the prescriber to discontinue drug therapy. In some of these cases, a different drug was substituted. On the other hand, 15 percent of drug therapy problems occurred in patients who were taking a dosage of medication that the pharmacist determined was too low and therefore not effective. Ineffective therapy can be very expensive and inconvenient to the patient. The pharmacist must make certain that the drug is effective yet not dosed so high that it introduces the next set of problems—those of safety.

One out of four drug therapy problems involves patients taking unnecessary medications or the wrong drug.

Drug therapy problems associated with safety issues accounted for 27 percent of all drug therapy problems identified and documented. In general, problems of safe drug therapy fall into two related but distinctly separate categories. Approximately 21 percent of drug therapy problems occurred in patients who experienced an adverse drug reaction, and the pharmacist intervened on the patient's behalf by discontinuing the offending agent and, when necessary, substituting drug therapy that was considered safer for that patient. An additional 6 percent of drug therapy problems was the result of taking a dosage of the medication that was too high. In these cases, the pharmacist intervened on behalf of the patient to reduce the dosage of the drug rather than to substitute another drug product.

The 4228 drug therapy problems were identified and documented in 2343 different patients. Therefore 43 percent of the patient population experienced at least one drug therapy problem during the year, while 3137 patients did not have a drug therapy problem during that same time period. In a generalist's practice, therefore, approximately 4 out of every 10 patient encounters involve a patient experiencing a drug therapy problem that can be identified by a pharmacist and resolved, thus allowing the patient to experience the full, safe benefit of the prescribed and/or recommended drug therapy. Some patients experienced several drug therapy problems. Figure 6-3 indicates the number of patients who had up to five or more drug therapy problems during the year.

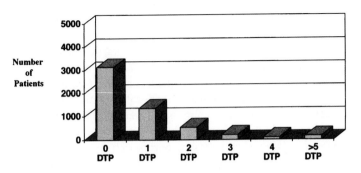

•Figure 6-3 The number of patients who had drug therapy problems among those patients (*n* = 5480) who received pharmaceutical care services in the Minnesota Pharmaceutical Care Project between November 1, 1994, and October 31, 1995.

18% of patients have more than one drug therapy problem.

Note that 25 percent of patients had a single drug therapy problem, while 18 percent had multiple drug therapy problems throughout the year. Figure 6-3 represents the typical distribution of patients with drug therapy problems encountered in a generalist community-based practice.

Predicting Drug Therapy Problems

Given the high incidence and broad distribution of drug therapy problems, many have asked: "How can we know which patients are going to have drug therapy problems and who will not?" This question is asked by those who intend to provide care only to those individuals with "significant" need. Our data suggest that those who have drug therapy problems and those who do not cannot be differentiated by some easily identifiable demographic variable. Instead, the most effective way a pharmacist can tell who has a drug therapy problem is to complete an assessment. Determining the pharmaceutical care needs of patients is similar to determining other health care needs, such as dental care, where the most effective method to determine if and how much dental care a patient actually needs is for the dentist to look in the patient's mouth and conduct an assessment of the patient's dental care needs. It is also essential to keep in mind that in addition to identifying and resolving drug therapy problems, the other significant responsibilities in pharmaceutical care are to prevent drug therapy problems and to meet therapeutic goals.

The philosophy of pharmaceutical care directs that each patient who needs care should receive it. Therefore, even patients who do not have a drug therapy problem may require pharmaceutical care in order to prevent drug therapy problems and to ensure that their therapeutic goals for each medical condition are in fact being met. It serves no one's purpose, other than perhaps the accountant's, to deny patients access to pharmaceutical care at least until after an assessment of the patient's drug therapy is made. An examination of the data will provide evidence to support this.

In order to examine the predictability of drug therapy problems and who might need pharmaceutical care, we have examined several variables and their relationship to the presence or absence of drug therapy problems. Figure 6-4 shows the relationship between the average number of drug therapy problems and the number of active medications a patient was taking.

Clearly, on average, the more medications a patient needs, the greater the risk of experiencing a drug therapy problem. However, one must keep in mind that the majority of patients do not have a drug therapy problem at any given time. For example, of the 542 patient encounters involving patients who were taking four or more medications, 141 experienced drug therapy problems (35 percent) and 401 did not (65 percent). Similarly, of the 425 patient encounters involving patients on five or six active medications, 49 percent had drug therapy problems and 51 percent did not. Thus, it would seem that a much more effective method of determining who needs pharmaceutical care is for the pharmacist to perform a structured assessment of the patient's drug-related needs rather than simply counting the number of prescriptions the patient has purchased.

Figure 6-5 describes the relationship between the number of medical problems per patient encounter and the average number of drug therapy problems.

In general, patients who have multiple medical problems also experience more drug therapy problems. However, of the 3623 patient encounters involving patients with multiple medical problems, 1821

> The more medications a patient needs, the higher the risk to experience a drug therapy problem.

> Patients who have more medical problems also experience more drug therapy problems.

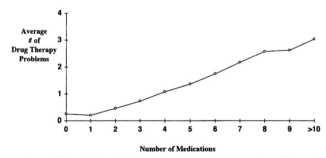

•**Figure 6-4** The relationship between the average number of drug therapy problems and the number of medications a patient was taking among those patients (*n* = 5480) who received pharmaceutical care in the Minnesota Pharmaceutical Care Project between November 1, 1994, and October 31, 1995. There were 12,367 patient encounters.

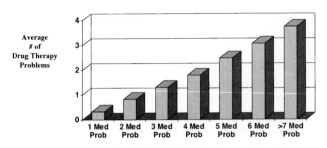

Number of Medical Problems per Patient Encounter

•**Figure 6-5**   The relationship between the number of medical problems (Med Prob) per patient encounter and the average number of drug therapy problems among those patients ($n = 5480$) who received pharmaceutical care in the Minnesota Pharmaceutical Care Project between November 1, 1994, and October 31, 1995.

Age, gender, type and number of medical conditions, or number of active medications are not reliable predictors of which individual patient will have drug therapy problems.

(50 percent) had no drug therapy problems identified when the pharmacist assessed their drug-related needs.

As described earlier, the age and gender distribution of patients who have drug therapy problems and the patients who did not have drug therapy problems are very similar. Also, the list of the most frequent medical conditions seen in patients who did not have a drug therapy problem identified at their first encounter is almost identical to the list of medical conditions most frequently encountered in the general patient population (see Table 6-1). In patients without a drug therapy problem, the most frequent medical indications for drug therapy included hypertension, bronchitis, sinusitis, allergic rhinitis, otitis media, streptococcal sore throat, pain management, depression, estrogen replacement therapy, and skin infections.

In summary, individual characteristics such as age, gender, type or number of medical conditions, and number of active medications are not reliable predictors of which *individual* patients will have drug therapy problems. Rather, it is only through a structured assessment of the patient's drug-related needs that the pharmacist and the patient can work together to determine the complexity of the patient's drug-related needs and identify those drug therapy problems needing resolution and those that must be prevented.

Complexity of the Patient

A method to describe and compare patients' pharmaceutical care needs is to use a resource-based relative value scale as a description of the complexity of the care each patient requires. The resource-based relative value scale is described in Chap. 8. The variables to describe a patient's complexity include the number of medical problems that require drug therapy, the number of drug therapy problems, and the number of active medications the patient is taking. Patients with no active drug therapy problems and only one or two active medications, taken to treat a single medical condition, are characterized as requiring the lowest level (level 1) of resources to meet their pharmaceutical care needs. Similarly, as the complexity of a patient's needs increases through the identification of drug therapy problems requiring resolution along with additional medical problems requiring drug therapies, the level of expertise and necessary resources increase up to the highest or fifth level. The fifth level on the pharmaceutical care resource based relative value scale represents a very complex patient requiring a comprehensive assessment and care plan because these patients have four or more medical problems requiring eight or more active medications and at least four drug therapy problems needing resolution. Figure 6-6 represents the distribution of patient complexity for patients encountered in a generalist community-based pharmaceutical care practice.

As in any generalist professional practice (general medical practice, pediatrics, law, dentistry, physical therapy, nursing, chiropractic), the majority of the patients' needs are of the lower complexity, level 1 or level 2 variety. Although patients with complex needs do, in fact, present themselves to generalist practitioners, it is the unusual patient whose medical conditions and drug therapies are such that he or she is at immediate risk of serious morbidity or mortality or has a high probability of severe prolonged impairment without appropriate and immediate interventions to comprehensively manage all drug therapies (level 5). Of the over 23,000 patient encounters documented in the 3-year Minnesota Pharmaceutical Care Project, approximately 1 percent of patient encounters involved patients requiring the very highest level of resources and pharmaceutical care services.

The most effective method in determining if a patient has a drug therapy problem is to complete an assessment.

The major variables determining patient complexity are as follows:
• the number of active medical problems,
• the number of drug therapy problems, and
• the number of active medications.

A generalist practice consists mainly of patients of low complexity (1–2 active medications treating 1–2 medical problems and experiencing 1–2 drug therapy problems).

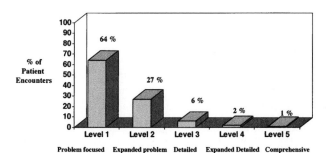

•**Figure 6-6**   The distribution of patient complexity—using a resource-based relative value scale—among patients who received pharmaceutical care in the Minnesota Pharmaceutical Care Project between November 1, 1994, and October 31, 1995.

Figure 6-6 can also be used to describe the workload distribution for practitioners who provide pharmaceutical care services. As the great majority of patient encounters (91 percent) involve patients with level 1 or 2 pharmaceutical care needs, it behooves the practitioner to develop the appropriate skills to identify patient needs and provide care for these patients as effectively and efficiently as possible.

Ineffective care wastes time and requires additional resources to correct inappropriate drug therapies, treatment failures, toxicities, and compliance failures. Inefficiencies in identifying a patient's drug-related needs and problems will cost the practitioner in terms of time, patient convenience, and loyalty. In effect, this could radically alter any positive therapeutic relationship. Pharmaceutical care practitioners must develop and maintain their practice skills at a level that allows them to provide care expeditiously, so as to leave time for the care of the fewer, but substantially more complex patients who are at immediate risk of experiencing drug-related morbidity and/or mortality.

A generalist practitioner also encounters a small number of complex patients who are at immediate risk of experiencing drug-related morbidity and mortality.

GROUP 2 DATA: SUBSET OF ESTABLISHED PATIENTS

As we have emphasized throughout this text, pharmaceutical care practice is based on a rational approach to drug therapy, requiring the practitioner to assume responsibility for the actual outcomes of each patient's drug therapy. Therefore, each patient's therapy must be evaluated at appropriate follow-up intervals to determine the actual outcomes (positive or negative) of the pharmaceutical care provided. In order to evaluate patient outcomes from pharmaceutical care, we examined the follow-up status of 1111 patients who had received care for an entire 12-month period. Each of these patients had at least one encounter with the pharmaceutical care practitioner prior to the beginning of the year and each also received pharmaceutical care at a minimum rate of two encounters during the year. This group might be described as comprising established patients. Figure 6-7 describes the distribution of the actual documented patient status and outcomes for these established patients. The terms used to describe patient outcomes and status are defined in Chap. 4.

Evaluating patient outcomes is most meaningful when compared to preestablished goals of therapy.

The patient's problems were resolved and drug therapies discontinued in 10 percent of the situations (see Fig. 6-7). This represents a relatively small number of patients due to the nature of a generalist's community-based practice in which many or most medical conditions are chronic disorders and therapeutic goals often involve trying to improve or stabilize the patient's condition. Patient outcomes were improved or stable in 37 percent of the cases, while only 8 percent of patients' conditions were worse at follow-up evaluation. It is important to note that even through the best efforts of experienced pharmaceutical care practitioners, prescribers, and their well-intentioned patients, not all drug therapy results in successful patient outcomes. Despite these efforts,

Most patient medical conditions are either chronic or recurring, therefore the goals of therapy involve stabilizing or improving the patient's condition, not curing or resolving them.

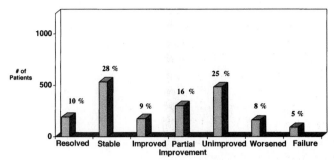

•**Figure 6-7** The distribution of actual documented patient outcomes for 1111 patients who received pharmaceutical care in the Minnesota Pharmaceutical Care Project and who had at least two follow-up evaluations from November 1, 1994, to October 31, 1995.

8 percent of patients conditions were worse at their follow-up evaluation and 5 percent were considered treatment failures. In practice, these patients required continued care and reassessment to determine how best to meet their drug-related needs. These data support the notion that if one accepts responsibility for patient drug therapy outcomes, one must be prepared to manage both successes and failures.

In order to quantitate the impact of pharmaceutical care in this community-based patient population, we compared actual patient outcomes according to their earliest and latest (most recent) follow-up evaluation. There were 1111 different patients who had at least two follow-up evaluation visits, at which time the pharmacist documented the status of the patient and progress toward meeting therapeutic goals.

Figure 6-8 separates the earliest evaluation documented for each patient from the latest outcome evaluation for these 1111 established patients. Figure 6-8 also demonstrates a "shift to the left," representing an important and substantial improvement in the actual patient out-

> A practitioner who accepts responsibility for actual patient outcomes has to be ready to manage both treatment successes and treatment failures.

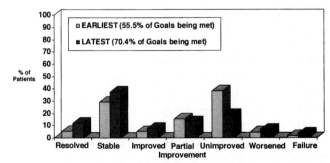

•**Figure 6-8** The earliest evaluation documented for each patient versus the latest outcome evaluation for 1111 patients who received pharmaceutical care in the Minnesota Pharmaceutical Care Project from November 1, 1994, to October 31, 1995.

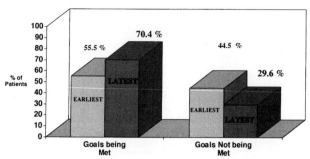

•**Figure 6-9**   A comparison of those patients whose therapeutic goals were met versus those whose goals were not met among 1111 patients who received pharmaceutical care in the Minnesota Pharmaceutical Care Project from November 1, 1994, to October 31, 1995.

Pharmaceutical care improves patient outcomes.

Pharmaceutical care increases the number of patients meeting therapeutic goals by 15% within the first year.

comes at repeat follow-up evaluations associated with the provision of pharmaceutical care. Most of the shift comes from the improvement in patients where status was unimproved or worse and the practitioner identified a drug therapy problem, intervened, and altered the patient's care plan to better meet their need.

The impact of pharmaceutical care can be evaluated by looking at those patients who had therapeutic goals met and those whose goals were not met (Fig. 6-9). To clarify the examination of the influence of pharmaceutical care on patient outcomes, all patients whose status was partially improved, improved, stable, or resolved were grouped into a "goals being met" category, and those whose status at follow-up was unimproved, worse, or considered a treatment failure were grouped in the "goals not being met" category. During this 12-month period, which is a relatively short period to observe substantial changes in many chronic medical conditions, there was a significant improvement in the outcomes of patients receiving pharmaceutical care. At the earliest evaluation, only 55.5 percent of patients' drug therapies were meeting the desired therapeutic goals, whereas 70.4 percent of these same patients had their therapeutic goals met at the later follow-up outcome evaluation. The results are statistically significant using chi square analysis ($X^2 = 34.39$, $p<.001$), indicating that there is an association between the pharmaceutical care provided for the patients and therapeutic goals they were able to achieve.

Examination of the earliest and latest follow-up evaluations of these 1111 established patients also indicates that the level of patient complexity was substantially reduced during the 1-year period. During the earliest follow-up, 1002 patients required either level 1 or level 2 services. As described in Fig. 6-10, the remaining 109 patients were more complex and required levels 3, 4, or 5 pharmaceutical care services. However, the later follow-up data indicate a clear improvement in that

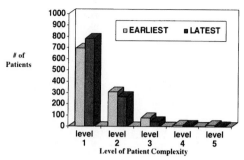

•**Figure 6-10** A comparison of the levels of patient complexity among 1111 patients who received pharmaceutical care in the Minnesota Pharmaceutical Care Project and who had at least two follow-up evaluations from November 1, 1994, to October 31 1995.

only 64 patients required the more complex levels 3, 4 or 5 pharmaceutical care. These data support the conclusion that a practitioner who practices pharmaceutical care can measurably improve the effectiveness, safety, and outcomes of drug therapy for patients. In addition to improved therapeutic outcomes, these patients' drug-related needs became less complex, on average, due to the resolution of drug therapy problems combined with positive progress in treating and managing diseases through the use of appropriate individualized drug therapy.

Patients' drug-related needs become less complex due to the resolution of drug therapy problems.

The Economic Impact of Pharmaceutical Care

The data generated for Group One were used to describe the economic impact of pharmaceutical care. Based on the resource-based relative value scale described in Chap. 8, the average charge for pharmaceutical care for all patients ($n = 5480$) was $12.14 per patient encounter (1994 U.S. dollars). Just as patients improved their health status throughout the year, the cost of those services for the group of "established" patients ($n = 1111$) declined from an average of $13.57 at their earliest encounter to $11.85 at their latest pharmaceutical care encounter.

Over this 1-year period, their drug therapy problems were identified and resolved, they were more able to meet their therapeutic goals, their therapies became less complex, and the resources required to provide pharmaceutical care decreased, thus reducing direct costs. It is also clear from these data that to maintain a viable practice, practitioners must continually add new patients not only to replace patients who leave, move, or expire but also to replace the revenue associated with the decline in per patient revenue due to improved health and positive outcomes.

It is instructive to examine the cost of care associated with certain individual patient characteristics. As with virtually all forms of health

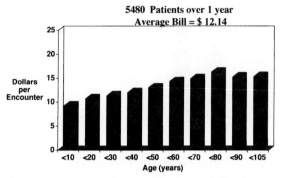

•**Figure 6-11** Average patient cost for pharmaceutical care services by decade of life among 5480 patients who received pharmaceutical care in the Minnesota Pharmaceutical Care Project between November 1, 1994, and October 31, 1995. The average charge was $12.14 per encounter.

care services, from the earliest years through the eighth decade of life, the cost of pharmaceutical care increases. Figure 6-11 represents the average patient charge for pharmaceutical care by decade of life.

Although the average charges for the older patients were generally higher than those for the younger groups, almost half (47 percent) of the revenue from these community-based practices was generated through caring for patients ages 31 to 60. Also, 62 percent of all patient care revenues was generated by caring for the drug-related needs of female patients. These types of demographic influences on practice revenue are important to take into account when beginning a new practice or when exploring the most effective approaches to expanding a pharmaceutical care practice (see Chap. 7).

Additional validation of the data generated through the provision and documentation of pharmaceutical care to a community-based population can be found in the observation of the trend that patients who were smokers required more costly pharmaceutical care (an average of $13.80 per patient encounter) than those adults who did not smoke ($12.34). The Health Outcomes Management, Inc., pharmaceutical care software allows the practitioner to maintain separate and unique data for each patient concerning the use of nicotine, alcohol, and caffeine. This is very useful in the analysis of these common patient risk factors that are not contained in most traditional prescription dispensing records.

Table 6-8 illustrates the increasing cost of providing pharmaceutical care for adult patients who use alcohol.

In the 709 patients with a documented alcohol history, the average pharmaceutical care bill increased by as much as 22 percent per encounter for patients who had six or more drinks each week compared to adults who did not use alcohol. Caffeine use had a similar effect on pharmaceutical care needs and costs (Table 6-9). Patients who did not

TABLE 6-8 ALCOHOL USE AND THE COST OF PHARMACEUTICAL CARE

	NUMBER OF PATIENTS	COST OF CARE
Nondrinkers	$n = 432$	$12.45
Drinkers		
< 2 drinks/week	$n = 208$	$13.12
2–6 drinks/week	$n = 52$	$13.61
> 6 drinks/week	$n = 17$	$15.12

use any caffeine required $1.81 less in pharmaceutical care services per encounter than those who used two or more cans or cups of caffeinated beverages daily.

Nicotine, alcohol, and caffeine are potent drugs known to influence the health and drug-related needs of individuals who expose themselves to these substances on a regular basis. This constitutes important patient-drug information that must be incorporated into the pharmacist's comprehensive assessment of the patient's drug-related needs.

GROUP 3 DATA: THE VALUE OF PHARMACEUTICAL CARE IN AN ELDERLY POPULATION

In October 1995, Jeffery Johnson and Lyle Bootman at the University of Arizona published an important set of data which described the expense burden to the U.S. health care industry caused by drug-related morbidity and mortality.[3] They projected that $76 billion was spent each year to cover the direct costs of drug-related morbidity and mortality. This amount of money is almost unimaginable and brings to mind an observation by the great physicist and teacher Richard P. Feynman[4] when he said "There are 1×10^{11} stars in the galaxy. That used to be a huge number. But it's only a hundred billion. It's less than the national debt. We used to call them astronomical numbers. Now we should call them economical numbers."

The figure of $76 billion is astounding and represents almost $300 per year for every man, woman, and child in the United States to pay for the lack of positive outcomes of drug therapy. The majority of these costs, over 60 percent, were considered to be avoidable through the provision of pharmaceutical care. The $76 billion in health care costs con-

TABLE 6-9 CAFFEINE USE AND THE COST OF PHARMACEUTICAL CARE

	NUMBER OF PATIENTS	COST OF CARE
No caffeine use	$n = 232$	$11.95
Caffeine use		
1–2 cans/cups/day	$n = 185$	$12.54
> 2 cans/cups/day	$n = 121$	$13.76

sisted of $48 billion for hospitalizations required to diagnose and treat drug therapy problems, $14 billion in additional nursing home expenses associated with long-term care costs for patients experiencing drug-related morbidity and mortality, $8 billion in added physician and urgent center visits to treat drug-related events, $5 billion in emergency room visits to treat drug therapy problems, and $2 billion in additional drug costs to treat and prevent morbidity and mortality from drug therapy problems[3].

We used these estimates of direct costs associated with drug-related morbidity and mortality to describe the patient benefits and costs associated with the delivery of pharmaceutical care. Cost:benefit calculations can be quite complex and involved. Therefore we took care in designing and calculating these figures by engaging the collaborative effort of Professor Steve Schondelmeyer, who holds the Century Mortar Club Chair in Pharmacoeconomics and is the Director of the Pharmacy Research in Management and Economics (PRIME) Institute at the College of Pharmacy, University of Minnesota. National estimates of direct cost data reported by Johnson and Bootman and expenditure estimates for pharmaceutical care provided for elderly patients in the Minnesota Pharmaceutical Care Project were used to determine the economic impact of pharmaceutical care. These data indicate that there is an extremely high potential for positive economic rewards when pharmaceutical care is provided to patients.

The following describes the cost:benefit analysis for pharmaceutical care. Johnson and Bootman's research data indicate that in 1992 dollars, $76,557,711,000 were required to pay for the expenses of 221,166,506 patient encounters associated with drug-related morbidity and mortality. Using the consumer price index data, this represents approximately $88 billion in terms of 1997 dollars. Of these costs, Johnson and Bootman indicate that 10 percent are caused by idiosyncratic drug therapy problems and are therefore unavoidable. The share of drug-related costs associated with the care of the elderly ($\geq$ 65 years old) was projected to be 34 percent of the total drug-related costs. These data include only noninstitutionalized elderly taking one or more prescription medication in a year and who received pharmaceutical care during that year. This represents approximately $27 billion in costs associated with drug-related morbidity and mortality. These cost estimates were further reduced to account for Johnson and Bootman's assumption that only about 80 percent of direct costs of drug-related morbidity and mortality are preventable. Therefore, the total direct health care costs associated with drug-related morbidity and mortality in Americans of age 65 or above was $21 billion. This amount was used to estimate the possible savings to be realized by the provision of pharmaceutical care to this Medicare-eligible population.

Data from the Minnesota Pharmaceutical Care Project were then used to estimate direct costs of providing pharmaceutical care for noninstitutionalized elderly receiving at least one prescription within a year. Of the 9399 patients whose care was documented during this project, 1747 received pharmaceutical care services prior to November 1994 and also continued to receive services throughout the following 12 months. This population of "established" patients was used for the cost:benefit analysis because their cost data represent the cost of providing care to a given population for an entire year. Of these 1747 established patients, 249 were 65 years old or older. These 249 patients who received pharmaceutical care represent 39.4 percent of the total number of patients aged $\geq$ 65 who were eligible to have received pharmaceutical care at some time during that year. Of these patients, 147 were receiving drug therapy for at least one of the following conditions targeted by Medicare legislation: asthma, chronic obstructive pulmonary disease, congestive heart failure, depression, hyperlipidemia, diabetes, or hypertension. These disease states were chosen based on proposed legislation that would phase in payment for pharmaceutical care for Medicare-eligible patients in the United States beginning with patients with these targeted medical conditions.[5]

The portion of eligible patients $\geq$ 65 years old receiving pharmaceutical care was 39.4 percent. Therefore, the possible savings were reduced from $21 billion to $8.5 billion (Table 6-10).

These costs are further reduced by a factor of 0.746 due to the fact that 74.6 percent of drug therapy problems identified in the elderly during the Minnesota Pharmaceutical Care Project were documented in patients with one or more of the targeted-medical conditions (Table 6-11).[5]

Last, our cost:benefit analysis estimated that health care costs would be decreased only if the patient's outcome at the follow-up evaluation was documented to be positive (i.e., patient's problem resolved, stabilized, improved, or partially improved). This occurred in 69 percent of the elderly patients in the Minnesota Pharmaceutical Care Project. Therefore, the direct cost of drug-related morbidity and mortality that could be avoided by providing pharmaceutical care to nonhospitalized elderly Americans taking at least one prescription drug is estimated at $4,400,000,000. This is described in Table 6-12.

There is a high cost, to both the patient and the payer, for not providing pharmaceutical care.

TABLE 6-10 COST:BENEFIT RATIO OF PHARMACEUTICAL CARE IN PATIENTS $\geq$ 65 YEARS OLD
Percent of eligible patients using pharmaceutical care services: 39.4% = $8,500,000,000

Sources: From the Minnesota Pharmaceutical Care Project, Peters Institute of Pharmaceutical Care, College of Pharmacy, University of Minnesota, Minneapolis; and Johnson and Bootman.[3] With permission.

TABLE 6-11 COST:BENEFIT RATIO OF PHARMACEUTICAL CARE IN PATIENTS ≥ 65 YEARS OLD WITH TARGET CONDITIONS[a]

Percent of drug therapy problems experienced by the
elderly with ≥ 1 of the targeted conditions
74.6% = $6,300,000,000

[a]Asthma, chronic obstructive pulmonary disease, congestive heart failure, depression, hyperlipidemia, diabetes, hypertension.
Source: Minnesota Pharmaceutical Care Project, Peters Institute of Pharmaceutical Care, College of Pharmacy, University of Minnesota, Minneapolis; and Johnson and Bootman.[3] With permission.

TABLE 6-12 COST:BENEFIT RATIO PHARMACEUTICAL CARE IN PATIENTS ≥ 65 YEARS OLD WITH TARGET CONDITIONS

69% of drug therapy problems resolved, stabilized,
improved, or partially improved
$4,400,000,000

Source: Minnesota Pharmaceutical Care Project, Peters Institute of Pharmaceutical Care, College of Pharmacy, University of Minnesota, Minneapolis; and Johnson and Bootman.[3] With permission.

TABLE 6-13 COST:BENEFIT RATIO PHARMACEUTICAL CARE IN PATIENTS ≥ 65 YEARS OLD

Costs to provide pharmaceutical care to
elderly with one or more of the targeted conditions
$382,448,205

Source: Minnesota Pharmaceutical Care Project, Peters Institute of Pharmaceutical Care, College of Pharmacy, University of Minnesota, Minneapolis; and Johnson and Bootman.[3] With permission.

Based on the resource-based relative value scale of reimbursement developed in the Minnesota Pharmaceutical Care Project, the direct costs of providing pharmaceutical care on a nationwide basis to this same group of elderly patients was $382,448,205 (Table 6-13).

This represents a cost:benefit ratio of 11.4:1. It indicates a remarkably valuable investment for any health care system responsible for the care of elderly patients. These data indicate that there is an estimated 11-fold benefit for every investment in the provision of pharmaceutical care for patients ≥ 65 years old (Table 6-14).

In summary, practices are established, expanded, and improved based primarily on the results of the patient care provided. Therefore, it

Table 6-14 Cost:benefit ratio pharmaceutical care in patients ≥ 65 years old with target conditions
Benefit:cost ratio with estimated savings
11.4 : 1

For every dollar invested in providing pharmaceutical care, the health care system has the potential to benefit by $11.00.

is important to be able to describe your practice, not only in words, as we do in Chaps. 1 and 4, but with empirical data including patient outcomes. This chapter described the practice of pharmaceutical care using empirical data from over 5000 patients receiving pharmaceutical care during a 1-year period. The practitioner must have access to essential patient data, use those data to care for individual patients, and critically review outcome data from groups of patients to constantly improve the value of the entire practice.

Pharmaceutical care is a good investment.[6] These cost:benefit data add validity to the idea that medications, while the most commonly used therapy, are one of the least expensive forms of treatment available. In general, medications are potent and can result in great good along with great harm. The patient care data resulting from the Minnesota Pharmaceutical Care Project indicate that the provision of pharmaceutical care not only improves actual patient outcomes, but is a logical and powerful economic investment.

Pharmaceutical care optimizes commonly available, inexpensive, yet effective therapies resulting in positive outcomes for patients and payers.

References

1. Tomechko, M.A., Strand, L.M., Morley, P.C., Cipolle, R.J. Q and A from the pharmaceutical care project in Minnesota. *Am Pharm* 1995; NS35:30–39.
2. Grainger-Rousseau, T.J., Miralles, M.A., Hepler, C.D. Therapeutic Outcomes Monitoring: Application of Pharmaceutical Care Guidelines to Community Pharmacy. *JAPhA* 1997; NS37:647–61.
3. Johnson, J.A., Bootman, J.L. Drug-related morbidity and mortality: A cost-of-illness model. *Arch Intern Med* 1995; 155:1949–1956.
4. Feynman, R.P. *Six Easy Pieces*. Reading, MA: Addison-Wesley; 1994.
5. HR 3757 IH, 104th Congress, second session, July 8, 1996, by Mr. Pallone.
6. Johnson, J.A., Bootman, J.L. Drug-related morbidity and mortality and the economic impact of pharmaceutical care. *Am J Health Syst Pharm* 1997; 54: 554–558.

Recommended readings

Benson, D.S. *Measuring Outcomes in Ambulatory Care*. Chicago: American Hospital Publishing; 1992.
Cutler, P. *Problem Solving in Clinical Medicine: From Data to Diagnosis*, 2d ed. Baltimore: Williams & Wilkins; 1985.
Levin, H.M. *Cost-Effectiveness: A Primer*. Beverly Hills, CA: Sage Publications; 1983.
Miller, M.C., Knapp, R.G. *Evaluating Quality of Care*. Germantown, MD: Aspen; 1979.
Mishan, E.J. *Cost-Benefit Analysis*. New York: Praeger; 1976.

CHAPTER SEVEN

BUILDING A PRACTICE UTILIZING THE PRACTICE MANAGEMENT SYSTEM

UNDERSTANDING THE PRACTICE MANAGEMENT SYSTEM

The key to a successful practice is to add new patients continually so the practice can become financially viable and survive over the long term. Providing care to many patients, on a repeat basis, requires an efficient and effective organization. To accomplish this, a practice management system that facilitates the work that must be done—in this case, to provide pharmaceutical care, must be developed and implemented.

Just as it is necessary to have an orderly, systematic approach to managing a *patient*, it is also necessary to have an orderly, systematic approach to managing a *practice* when providing pharmaceutical care. This requires a practice management system that supports the practice—a system that enables practitioners to provide pharmaceutical care.

A practice management system includes all the support required to provide the service to patients in an effective and efficient manner. Most frequently, the practice management system includes the following:

- A clear statement of the mission for the practice (a clear description of the service provided). This mission then defines an appropriate environment and culture in which the service is provided.

- All the resources required to deliver the service (including physical, financial, and human resources)

- The means by which the service can be evaluated. The evaluation processes must measure the practitioner's ability to manage the patient, and the ability of the manager to manage the practice. This requires an effective documentation system.

- The means to reward the practitioner and financially support the longevity of the practice (reimbursement mechanisms). The ability to attract

> The key to a financially viable, successful practice is to add new patients continually, one patient at a time.

> A practice management system is a new concept in pharmacy.

237

payment reflects the value of the service to the patient in the short term and to society in the long term.

The decision maker in a practice management system is referred to by many names, including *manager, boss, office manager, business manager,* and *president* as well as others, some much less flattering. For the purpose of our discussion, we will refer to the individual who is responsible for making the management decisions, as the *practice manager.* This individual may be a practitioner, a businessperson, or a practitioner with business expertise. Regardless of the background or the specific position of the individual, we will refer to the decision maker as the practice manager.

> The practice management system must provide all of the support a practitioner requires in order to provide pharmaceutical care to a large number of patients.

THE PRACTICE MANAGEMENT SYSTEM AS A COMPONENT OF PHARMACEUTICAL CARE

It is necessary to place the practice management system in the context of practice. Figure 7-1 indicates that the practice management system has as its foundation the same philosophy of practice, as does the patient care process.

We can also see from the figure that the patient care process and the practice management system directly impact each other on a constant basis. This is expected since the patient care process represents the work that must be accomplished, and the practice management system facilitates or inhibits that work. As the patient care process changes, the practice management system must be transformed within the parameters prescribed by the philosophy of practice.

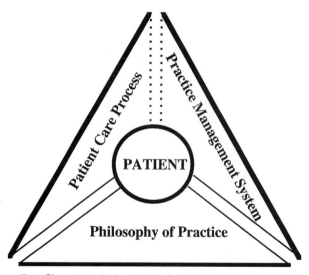

•**Figure 7-1** Pharmaceutical care practice

	PHILOSOPHY OF PRACTICE	PATIENT-CARE PROCESS	PRACTICE MANAGEMENT SYSTEM
TABLE 7-1 PRACTICE COMPONENTS AND THEIR CHARACTERISTICS			
Purpose	Prescriptive	Descriptive	Predictive
Those influenced	All practitioners, all patients	Individual practitioner, individual patient	A group of practitioners, a group of patients
Relevant time frame	Continuous	Present	Future

The philosophy of practice is different in that it is a constant; it does not change on a day-to-day basis but only changes or evolves over time. In fact, it only changes as a result of the entire profession critically examining its beliefs and behavior, agreeing on particular changes, and redefining its collective purpose. This may take years.

The philosophy of practice and the patient care process both have their unique characteristics as components of a professional practice, as does the practice management system. Table 7-1 compares the characteristics of the three components. The philosophy of practice and the patient care process have already been discussed.

The practice management system must serve a "predictive" purpose. The long-term success or failure of a practice is determined by the success or failure of the practice management system supporting it. The decisions made by the practice manager will impact all those involved in the practice. All of the practitioners, patients, and staff will, at one time or another, be affected by management decisions. However, this impact will only be realized in terms of future events. The practitioners, patients, and staff affect decisions on a day-to-day basis, whereas the practice manager affects decisions in the long term. This is the nature of the practice management system.

The long-term success of a patient care service is dependent on the support the practitioner receives from the practice management system.

We will describe each element of the practice management system by applying these concepts to the task at hand: building a pharmaceutical care practice.

BUILDING A SUCCESSFUL PRACTICE

Building a successful pharmaceutical care practice is not a simple task. There are few established, so this is largely unchartered territory without significant experience on which to rely. In addition, the magnitude of the change from a dispensing mission to a patient care mission is so great that, to our knowledge, few practitioners have accomplished it

Changing from dispensing pharmacy to pharmaceutical care requires a revolutionary change at the personal level.

fully. Other practitioners such as physicians, dentists, and nurses have made substantial improvements in their practices, but none have completely changed their focus from a product to patient care. A change of this scope requires an evolutionary change on the professional level, but on the individual practitioner level, it requires a personal, revolutionary change. Only if you are prepared for this will you find the energy required to build a practice. However, it can be done, it has been done, and—with the guidance that follows—it will be significantly easier than it appears at first glance.

We will describe, one step at a time, what it takes to build a successful practice of pharmaceutical care. Although it is not our intention to provide a course in management at this point, we will discuss the principal steps involved. We have depended upon those who have already built practices to provide the framework for this process,[1-3] into which we have liberally integrated our experience with building almost fifty such practices to date.

There are five major steps to building a practice:

Building a successful practice requires:
- preparation
- putting the patient first
- attending to the staff
- installing the physical and technical resources
- obtaining payment.

1. Preparing to build a practice
2. Focusing on the patient
3. Focusing on the staff
4. Creating an appropriate practice
5. Accomplishing reimbursement

The material presented here will be applicable for building a practice in any community ambulatory practice setting. We have three specific settings in mind where we believe the principles presented are immediately applicable. First, the professional pharmacy that has a small "front end," containing only nonprescription medications and medically related materials. Examples of these pharmacies include the national and international franchises of Medicap and the Medicine Shoppe. In this case, we assume that the entire business will be converted to pharmaceutical care services with *dispensing as a support function*.

The second scenario in which this material is applicable is the clinic-based pharmacy, which resembles the professional pharmacy described above. This pharmacy is often in the same building as a hospital, physician's office, or managed care group practice. The "front end" is usually limited to prescription and nonprescription drug products and other medically-related materials. Or it is possible that the clinic-based pharmacy may offer no products for sale. It may consist of the pharmacist's office next to the physician's office. The material presented here is also applicable to this practice situation.

The third scenario for the use of this material is the commercial pharmacy. We define the commercial pharmacy loosely as a pharmacy in which the prescription business is only a part of the total business transactions. This pharmacy might have a number of other departments including nonprescription drugs, durable medical equipment, greeting cards, foods, beauty aids, photography, video rental, and lottery ticket sales. Most independent pharmacies and all of the chains (except the professional chains described above) would be considered, by this definition, to be commercial pharmacies. The material presented here is applicable to a commercial pharmacy *only* if dedicated space is identified and treated as a separate, independent, identifiable pharmaceutical care service. This physical space, usually from 200 to 500 square feet, along with a dedicated pharmacist practitioner and appropriate support staff, must be regarded as independent from the remainder of the operation, since the "rules" for the patient care service are completely different from the "rules" required to manage retail, product-oriented pharmacy.

There are five fundamental steps to building a new pharmaceutical care practice. Perhaps the most important aspect of using this building process appropriately is that each step be completed in succession. For this process to be useful, it is necessary to start at the first step and complete each one before progressing on to the next. This appears to be elementary, however, it is necessary to emphasize since it is usual and customary for pharmacists to attempt to build a practice by focusing on changing the physical environment. This happens to be part of step 4 in the process. Or, pharmacists want to begin with reimbursement since they are focused on financial need. This is step 5 in the process! Starting anywhere other than step 1 will lead to a short-lived, failed experiment.

It is also necessary to complete all five steps. Skipping a step will halt the building process. Since everyone makes changes at a different rate, the time frame required to complete each step will vary with individuals. It is the order and the completeness as opposed to the time frame that we wish to emphasize. Let us begin the process of building a successful, sustainable pharmaceutical care practice.

PREPARING TO BUILD A PRACTICE

Getting started means the pharmacist must understand clearly, and define explicitly, the service that will be offered to patients. This is the most important step and impacts all subsequent decisions. It seems simple enough, but to succeed many pharmacists must change the way they think about their business enterprise.

Instead of thinking about a commercial, product-focused business, we must now come to understand a service enterprise. Delivery of products and the delivery of services, in this case, pharmaceutical care, are two distinct and different enterprises. Adding a pharmaceutical care

One must thoroughly understand pharmaceutical care before building a practice.

To begin, the practitioner must "internalize" the service to be offered to patients.

service to an existing product-focused business requires a new understanding of business, different expectations of your personnel, and different management strategies in order to ensure success. To many experienced pharmacists, it requires leaving behind much of what is understood about pharmacy as a dispensing profession. This new orientation is critical to starting in the "new direction," but it is also quite difficult given the traditional paradigms of pharmacy. Table 7-2 helps to focus attention on the differences between dispensing products and providing pharmaceutical care.

Practice management requires that the terminology be used specifically and consistently. It includes *practice*, *service*, *care*, *patients*, and *consumers*, all which make up the core of the new business. We will use these terms repeatedly, so we must have a common understanding of their meaning.

Dispensing products and providing pharmaceutical care are two different enterprises and require different management systems.

TABLE 7-2 DIFFERENCES BETWEEN DISPENSING PRODUCTS AND PROVIDING PHARMACEUTICAL CARE	
DISPENSING PHARMACY	PHARMACEUTICAL CARE
Product business.	Service (people) business.
Objective is to bring product to the customer.	Objective is to bring the pharmacist to the patient.
Decisions focus on the business.	Decisions focus on the patient.
Inventory generates revenue.	Patient care generates revenue.
Available service supports the product.	Available product supports the service.
Success measured as number of prescriptions.	Success is measured as patient outcomes.
Space is organized to display and sell products.	Space is organized to meet patient's needs.
Records are kept primarily to meet legal requirements concerning the drug product.	Documentation supports patient care.
Schedule for refill determined by customer supply of drug product.	Schedule for follow-up determined determined by risk and benefit of drug therapies and needs of the patient.
Business is passively sought through the generation of prescriptions.	Business is actively sought through the recruitment of patients.

Practice

Although the term *practice* has traditionally been used in pharmacy to denote a "place of practice" or a "practice setting" and *only* that, in a health care professional practice the term means something quite other than the physical environment in which one works. (See Chap. 1 for a detailed discussion of a practice.) For our present purposes, a practice comprises a set of knowledge, skills, and attitudes applied for the purpose of solving a specific set of problems and thereby improving the well-being of another human being. Practice requires an assessment care plan, and follow-up evaluation for each patient receiving care. A practice is what occurs between the practitioner and the patient. In pharmaceutical care, practice involves identifying, resolving, and preventing drug therapy problems that interfere with appropriate, effective, safe, and convenient drug therapy taken by patients. As a pharmaceutical care practice is built, the practitioner applies unique knowledge, skills, and attitudes to the care of each patient, one person at a time.

> Practice comprises a set of knowledge, skills, and attitudes applied for the purpose of solving a specific set of problems and thereby improving the well-being of another human being.

Service

Service aspects of health care cover three basic areas: the interpersonal interactions between practice personnel and the patient (consumers), the systems (including policies, procedures, and processes) in which all must function, and the consumers' impressions based on interactions with the practice (appearance of the physical environment, etc.). Whenever *service* is referred to, it will mean the aspects of care that lead to a high level of consumer (patient) satisfaction (reactions to specific episodes of service) and positive consumer attitudes of service quality (long-term attitudes about the nature of service provided by the practice).[1] *Quality service* will be used to refer to both aspects of care.

> Services are aspects of care that lead to a high level of consumer (patient) satisfaction and positive attitudes about quality.

Care

Care is the modus operandi of the practitioner in health care. It is the manner in which practice is executed. It is how the practitioner fulfills his or her responsibilities. It is the attitude, the value system, the philosophy of practice of the practitioner. Care encompasses both the technical and the nontechnical aspects of practice. Recall that to care for another person requires that you take the time to determine the needs of that individual, are willing to gather the resources necessary to meet that individual's needs, and are willing to stay in contact to make certain that all that you did for the other person was helpful and did not cause any new problems. All this is done with compassion and sensitivity toward the individual.

> Care is a manner in which practice is executed.

Patient

The patient is the recipient of care and the focus of pharmaceutical care practice.

The term *patient* is used to describe the recipient of care and the focus of pharmaceutical care practice. Although this term has traditionally been used to describe someone with a disease or illness who is receiving treatment, we will use it to refer to individuals who interact directly with the practitioner and who are experiencing the practice on a patient-specific level. When we refer to this person at the management level, we will use the term *consumer* to suggest a different type of accountability at the level of *delivering* the service.

Consumer

The term "consumer" represents the rights and voice of the patient.

Although we chose not to use this term to describe the recipient of care and the focus of pharmaceutical care practice on a patient-specific clinical basis, we recognize that as a practice is developed, it is essential to be sensitive to consumer culture. Unless we respond to the patient "as consumer" we will not attend, in enough detail and with enough care, to the voice of the consumer or to the demands of the payer. Thus, we use the term *consumer* to reflect the rights and the voice of the patient.

We recognize that there are different types of consumers of our services. They may be thought of as primary consumers (patients), secondary consumers (payers, insurers, etc.), and tertiary consumers (hospitals, referrals, etc.). We will focus on the primary or individual consumer.

As was mentioned earlier, to succeed at pharmaceutical care, the practitioner must introduce a new service to the patient. The service is the aspect of the practice which the patient experiences and remembers at each encounter, so it is very important to "get it right." Because pharmacy as a profession has been product-focused for so long, we will briefly explain why service is so important to building a pharmaceutical care practice.

The pharmacist will have to change the expectations the patient has of the pharmacist. Keep in mind, the expectations patients have today are the direct result of what has been done to or for them in the past. The expectations patients develop in the future will be a direct result of what is done for them today. The fastest way to change patient expectations is to provide services that patients want and need. The pharmacist has to establish that he or she has something to offer of value beyond the product. The quickest way to do this is to provide a valuable service.

The fastest way to change patient expectations is to provide services that patients want and need.

Although this sounds uncomplicated and often is, it can be confusing because, in the case of a professional practice generally and drug therapy specifically, the patient may require help in identifying his or her drug-related needs. Often, the pharmacist is able to best determine what service is needed, while the patient is best at helping to determine how the service should be delivered. Both are essential for quality service.

Pharmacists must fight the temptation to use what has been learned from experiences in the dispensing (product) business to predict what will happen in a pharmaceutical care (service) practice. There are many myths and assumptions associated with the dispensing enterprise which will not apply to the new pharmaceutical care practice. These include the ideas that

- Patients will not wait.
- Patients will not pay.
- Patients will not understand.
- Patients do not care to know.
- Patients will not tell the pharmacist about their health care needs.
- Physicians will not like it.
- Pharmacists are too busy.
- Pharmacists' liability will increase.
- Pharmacists do not have the ability to provide care.

Do not use assumptions of the dispensing paradigm to form a plan to conceptualize and implement a new pharmaceutical care practice. As mentioned earlier, dispensing and pharmaceutical care are different enterprises, and in our experience, any extrapolated "old paradigm" assumptions will be of little value. Therefore, we must learn from those who have built successful service businesses. Following are basic lessons learned by other service providers that can serve as a foundation for building a new practice.[1] A quality service can accomplish the following:

- Attract new patients
- Increase patient loyalty and the retention of existing patients
- Increase the retention of service-oriented personnel
- Decrease liability
- Increase a practice's attractiveness for group or network affiliation

And, because the quality of the care provided will ultimately determine if a patient returns or not, we include here the clinical rationale for providing pharmaceutical care.[1] A quality service will

- Lead to improved identification, resolution, and prevention of drug therapy problems
- Improve compliance with treatment regimens
- Improve patient outcomes
- Increase the opportunity for continuity of care

With these basic concepts as the foundation and the starting point, we must create a mission for the organization, the practice—a description of the service to be offered—that is clearly stated and able to be

Assumptions from the dispensing paradigm do not form an appropriate foundation for pharmaceutical care.

communicated explicitly. We suggest the following:

> The mission of this organization (or the service to be provided) is to meet the individual and collective drug-related needs of our patients in a compassionate, caring, and professional manner and to execute the services our patients need as effectively, comprehensively, and efficiently as possible.

FOCUSING ON THE PATIENT

Practitioners build practices. They will either make it happen, or be the rate-limiting step. The manager, the physical plant, the pharmaceutical industry, computer systems, and third-party payers do not build practices. They can facilitate or make it difficult for practitioners to build successful practices. Building a practice means that the practitioner has to place the patients' interests first. It means the answer is always "Yes, I can help." The most important concept to communicate to the new pharmaceutical care practitioner is the following, which is adopted from Silker's description of a successful dental practice:[2]

Practitioners build practices in conjunction with their patients.

> Strive to discover your patients' priorities and value systems and integrate their desires with your broad knowledge of drug therapy to develop a care plan that is in your patients' best interest and your practice will flourish.

Creating a financially viable service means giving people what they need, the way they want it. It is important to let patients know that meeting their needs and desires is central to the service. This is so important that it may be appropriate to prominently display a sign with the following message:

> Our goal is to provide the very best pharmaceutical care, support, information, and quality products you need for a healthy life.

However, before posting this signage, it is important to know patients' drug-related needs and provide the service that will meet these needs. This seems obvious and simple. Neither is the case.

No practitioner in the present health care system has systematically assessed for patients' drug-related needs; therefore little or no data exist on what ambulatory patients need and want as it relates to their drug therapy. In addition to this lack of data, pharmacists are not taught, nor are they accustomed, to critically assess a patient's drug-related needs. Therefore it may feel uncomfortable or even risky for the pharmacist to initiate a pharmaceutical care practice.

Two major goals must be met to build a practice:
1) change the expectations patients have of the pharmacist's services, and
2) introduce a new health care service.

There are two concepts to understand. First, pharmacists must change the expectations patients have of them. Second, practitioners have to introduce a completely new health care service to their patients. It is fairly clear that one can change the patient's expectations of the pharmacist only by acting differently. *Talking about changing patient perceptions, promising to change your practice, planning to change, and wishing change would occur will not be successful.* It is necessary to act differently. Changes in a patient's expectations require that the pharmacist behaves in a manner consistent with pharmaceutical care. The answer is the same for the second issue. The only way to introduce a completely new health care service is to provide it, to show patients, how they can benefit, and how to use the new service.

To maintain a therapeutic relationship it is necessary to find out what the patient thinks of the services provided. This cannot be done immediately. The service must be provided first and the practitioner must learn how to be efficient and effective at its delivery. For the first 6 to 9 months of the new service, engaging in a process of inquiry is essential. This means asking patients for their opinions about the new service provided. In addition, listen, empathize, and respond to patient's opinions. This is especially important when a new service is first introduced.

> The most useful data for building a practice come from patient feedback.

During the discovery process of what really matters to patients it is essential to gather data and information to address the following questions:

- What is important to patients about the non-clinical aspects of their experiences with pharmaceutical care?
- How is the practice performing in these important areas?

Methods to obtain this vital information include patient interviews, surveys, focus groups, suggestion boxes, consumer advisory boards, formal exit interviews, and even less formal walk around discussions with staff and patients.[1] The important message is that patients are asked what they want, and they understand that their suggestions will be acted upon in a timely manner.

FOCUSING ON THE STAFF

The ultimate success of any practice will depend on the quality of the service delivered. Service is provided by people. Nothing will have greater impact on that service than the people who provide it. The commitment, cooperation, and participation of all practice personnel is essential for success. By practice personnel, we are referring to the practitioner (pharmacist) who provides the care, the support staff (clerks, technicians, secretaries, etc.) who support the practitioner and make things happen on a day-to-day basis, and the practice manager who makes things happen on a long-term basis. Depending on the size of the practice as well as the specific nature of the practice, the number and specific type of personnel may vary. However, the three categories of personnel mentioned above will fulfill the majority of responsibilities involved in building a pharmaceutical care practice.

> If staff are to help care for patients, then care for the staff.

Many different factors concerning the practice personnel can influence the success of a practice, but none so much as communication.

Both the willingness and the ability to communicate with each other and with patients will be the best predictors of whether a practice will succeed. Care means communication. Quality care means quality communication.

A number of different sources present tips to communicate well.[1-3] All of these references are useful, but we would like to emphasize a few suggestions which are most relevant to building a pharmaceutical care practice, where not only the service is new, but the vocabulary to describe it is new. These suggestions apply to both staff and patients:

- Make the technical content of explanations appropriate.
- Determine that the intended message is being understood.
- Do not be afraid of words that show caring and emotion.
- Ask open-ended questions.
- Answer questions completely.
- Use the skills of empathy, listening, and managing conflict.

These ideas appear too simple to be helpful. However, we have found that if these behaviors are stated explicitly and expected by all practice staff, they can have a significant impact on the success of a practice.

It takes all practice personnel to provide a quality service. A good place to begin is to make certain all personnel first understand the mission of the organization and the service they are expected to deliver. Second, each person must understand his or her own role and the role of all others making up the practice. The primary roles of the pharmacist practitioner, support staff, and the manager are described below.

It takes all practice personnel, working in concert, to provide a quality service.

The Role of the Pharmacist

The pharmacist practitioner is responsible for the day-to-day, moment-to-moment, decision making concerning direct patient care and all that is associated with this responsibility. No other staff is allowed to interfere with the completion of these responsibilities.

The Role of the Support Staff—Technicians, Clerks

The support staff are responsible for facilitating the patient care process, including patient flow, work flow, and meeting any other needs the patient might have, such as questions concerning hours of operation, access to services, eligibility for services, costs, billing procedures, scheduling, and other general information. The staff support the practitioner providing direct patient care.

The Role of the Practice Manager

Practice managers are responsible for obtaining resources needed by practitioners and staff to do their work. They must establish a management plan for the practice on a long-term basis, develop policies and standardize procedures that facilitate the patient care process, and at the same time not interfere with direct patient care. If the practice manager is successful, he or she will be "invisible" to the patient (and the staff).

Creating an Appropriate Practice

The patient and his or her drug-related needs "drives" the practice. How effectively this happens depends on the ability of the practitioner to create the "right" patient experience.

Creating the right experience for the patient will be difficult if the pharmacist focuses on him or herself first. Even more menacing is to begin by focusing on the physical plant. There is a natural tendency to do this since it is tangible and much easier to address than attitude, culture, or communication. An exercise which may help to ensure that the right experience is created for the patient, first, is to visit a different pharmacy and while approaching the patient care area, ask the following questions:

> Obtaining and using resources appropriately is all about creating the right experience for the patient.

- When a patient enters the pharmacy, is it clean, neat, professional, quiet?
- Does the patient know where to go to receive pharmaceutical care from the pharmacist?
- Is the space identified clearly so the patient is not immediately confused?
- Is the person meeting/greeting the patient pleasant and focused on the patient first?
- Is there appropriate space for the patient (and his or her children) to wait to see the pharmacist and to receive the service?
- Is there private/semiprivate space available for the patient to discuss his or her care with the pharmacist?
- Does the patient always come first?
- Does the flow of the work focus on the patient and his or her needs?
- When the telephone rings, is it answered professionally to reinforce that the patient comes first?
- When the pharmacist is interrupted, is it done professionally and with the respect of the patient foremost?
- Does the patient have access to what he or she needs while in the pharmacy?
- Can patients sit comfortably?
- Are there educational materials available?
- Are there facilities for handicapped patients?
- Is the lighting sufficient?
- Are there interruptive noises in the pharmacy from paging systems, computer printers, modems, or radios?

Now with these answers in mind, the pharmacist must return to explore his or her own pharmacy and ask the same questions.

Another dimension of professionalism can be added by visiting other practitioner officers, for example that of a dentist, chiropractor, physician, or veterinarian. Their experiences can add to basic knowledge about how to handle patient problems, how to bill patients, how to attract new patients, and how to manage the challenges of starting a new practice.

Each aspect of the patient's experience requires consideration, down to the smallest detail. For example, does your name tag encourage patients to relate to you in a personal, informal manner, or is it intimidating? Can it be read from a distance? Pharmacists, managers, and support staff are often too close to the day-to-day operations to see clutter, mess, poor signage, inventory not put away, messy notes hanging on walls and counters, or notices to staff attached to doors, desks, and shelves. Therefore, it is necessary to ask patients what *they* see, what *they* hear, and what *they* experience. Such feedback is very important. Consumers constantly transform a practice, so practitioners must constantly adapt in order to provide the quality service that will contribute to the development of a successful practice.

> Each aspect of the patient experience must be critically examined, down to the smallest detail.

Physical or Technical Resources

The physical resources that must be considered are physical plant including space, furniture, telephones, computers, software programs, medical equipment, reference material, and any photocopy or fax machines needed. The physical plant must meet all of the expectations suggested above for the "right" patient experience.

In order to effectively plan workable physical space to provide pharmaceutical care, it is useful to consider how to deal with several minimum requirements. These include the following:

1. A semiprivate, quiet area for patient and pharmacist to meet. Keep in mind that for busy practices, each pharmacist providing pharmaceutical care will need a semiprivate area to practice. Providing some fully private space to meet with patients with very special needs is also important. However most patients prefer a comfortable, open, yet semiprivate area. Some patients prefer to remain standing if the interaction with the pharmacist is only going to require a few minutes, but some patients need to sit or prefer to sit while meeting with the pharmacist.

2. A neat, clean surface in the patient-pharmacist meeting area. Be mindful to avoid leaving clutter, stacks of paper or office supplies in the semiprivate patient care area. These will be distracting to patients and will diminish the patient's confidence that the pharmacist's full attention is on the patient. A clock is useful to help both patients and pharmacists keep track of time spent in consultation. Also, having paper and pen available for patient use is helpful and often reassuring, helping patients to feel that you really want them to understand, remember, and participate.

3. A desk and work space for the pharmacist. This space will be necessary to research patient questions, access drug information, complete documentation and other patient records, and consult current reference materials.

4. Computer system for patient care documentation with full printing capabilities. This system should also provide CD-ROM capabilities for drug information as well as medical information software and should offer internet access to medical, drug and other health related information.

5. Consideration should be given to the space provided for patients when they are waiting to meet with the pharmacist. This space can be useful to display samples of health-related information available from your service, educational videotapes, samples of self-care diagnostic procedures, products, and references concerning herbals, nutritional, and other therapeutic approaches to patient needs.

The major criteria to be considered in designing a physical plant in any particular setting is whether patients feel comfortable and whether pharmaceutical care can be provided in this setting. If these two objectives can be accomplished, then appropriate physical space is designed.

> The major criteria to be considered in designing the physical space are whether patients feel comfortable and whether pharmaceutical care can be provided.

Get Started

Discussions, planning, and worrying do not take care of patients. There is only one way to change a practice paradigm, and that is to actually begin to take care of patients' drug-related needs, and stick with it. Every pharmacy practitioner who has successfully changed his or her practice can point to a day of change—that is, the day on which he or she actually started providing pharmaceutical care and accepted the responsibility for patient outcomes.

> Designate the first day, and get started!

Choose a day. Let all the staff know that it will be an important day. This first day will serve not only as the beginning for accounting and management purposes, but everyone involved will constantly use the first day as a comparison of future developments and improvements.

Begin by providing pharmaceutical care for a minimum of two new patients each day. This is a minimal level of patient care. Two new patients a day will provide the direct patient experience necessary for professional and economic growth. As in all new endeavors, practice requires doing something over and over in order to gain mastery. It is important to remain committed to providing care for at least two new patients every day. During this early stage of development, it is often tempting to "skip" a few patients or a few days because "things are hectic." Such temptations must be resisted at all times. Continuity of care begins with a fundamental understanding of sustained effort.

> Building a practice requires that a minimum of two new patients be cared for each day.

After much consternation about how to initiate a practice and with which type of patient to begin, many pharmacists start where they are most comfortable—patients with whom they are most familiar. However, it must be emphasized that if the patients are frequent visitors to the pharmacy, then they may be complex patients with many medical conditions and a large number of drug-related needs. This is not always the easiest place to start. Usually the best rule is simply to start with the next patient.

Two new patients each day represent a rapidly growing workload due to the follow-up evaluations required for every patient. Some patients will require numerous follow-up evaluations even for acute problems, and those with chronic disorders (the majority of patients) will require constant, repeated follow-up evaluations on a long-term basis. This has a direct impact on practice workload. For example, on the tenth day of a new practice period, care has been provided for at least 18 patients accumulated from the previous 9 days. Some, for instance 3, of these "established" 18 patients may need their follow-up evaluations at once, so you will be providing direct care for 5 patients on day 10 (2 new patients and 3 established patients). It is important to keep good, clear, and concise documentation, as the work of a practice can grow exponentially.

Establish a charge for the service from the beginning.

Let patients know how much they will be charged for this new service. There are several ways to accomplish this: first, by charging them directly the same way other general practitioners have done for decades. Without a charge, services are always undervalued. The practitioner should present new patients with an invoice for the service. This can also include drug product charges. Some practitioners feel they should not require reimbursement until they have developed their new skills, so they display the value (intended charge, for example $20) on the invoice and "zero it out," indicating that it will usually cost $20, but this time there will be no charge. By displaying the usual and customary fee, you are changing patients' expectations of payment. People pay for services they consider valuable and important.

Find out from the staff how well the practice is progressing.

After 2 weeks of active practice, it is important to meet with all of the staff, discuss how they think the new service is being accepted by patients, and solicit suggestions. Review patient care documentation to see that it is complete and concise. If the practice has multiple pharmacists, discuss the problems and successes of each individual. Collaboration with staff is important and group meetings can lead to the exchange of important information. As areas of improvement are identified, staff activities can be directed to better support the provision of pharmaceutical care. This process is repeated at week 4 and week 6.

After six weeks of building a practice two patients at a time, a summary of data should be presented to all staff. This can easily be accomplished through a pharmaceutical care computer documentation system. It will help everyone to understand the number of patients receiving care, the age distribution, the most common indications for drug therapy, and the number and types of drug therapy problems identified and resolved. Additionally, a summary of the number of drug therapy regimens that have been changed as well as the number and costs of unnecessary clinic visits, nursing home admissions, or hospitalizations that have been prevented should be presented. These data, although very preliminary, provide the essential feedback for evaluating progress and making changes where necessary.

Financial Considerations

As with all professional services, it is the responsibility of the practitioner to understand the financial implications of the services provided to patients. In the case of pharmaceutical care services, pharmacists have a strong tendency to quickly try to compare and contrast financial estimates from their dispensing, product-oriented activities with financial projections for a pharmaceutical care service. This is often done prematurely and leads to false conclusions. As stated earlier, pharmaceutical care and the dispensing of pharmaceutical products are two very different activities. This means that data used to describe the financial position of a product type of business are often quite different from the data required to describe the financial status of a service.

> Data which best describe a patient care practice are different from the data used to describe dispensing practices.

There are important reasons why premature financial comparisons of existing dispensing activities and planned patient care services are often erroneous. Many privately owned and operated pharmacies do not perform the financial analyses for their dispensing operations—analyses that would be necessary to use as a base to make accurate projections for pharmaceutical care services. In the case of many corporately owned and operated pharmacies, these types of financial analyses may be performed but are seldom accessible to the practitioner at the local practice site. As an example, almost every pharmacy uses the number of prescriptions or orders filled per day (new and refill) as a measure of the work performed that day. In this case the prescription is the unit of measure, and it is also the unit of measure for most financial determinations. In the case of pharmaceutical care, the patient is the fundamental unit of measure, and thus the number of patients (new and established) seen by the pharmacist is most useful for financial analysis of pharmaceutical care services. Additionally, because much of primary care is actually delivered and paid for on the basis of a family unit (child of parent or parents), it is also helpful to determine service activity based on the family unit in the pharmaceutical care practice.

Time is another unit used in many pharmacy financial analyses. However, pharmacist time spent filling and dispensing prescriptions might vary considerably if technicians or technology perform some or all of the prescription processing. Pharmacist time in the patient care service operations is primarily face-to-face time with patients. Because different methods as well as different data sources must be used for sound financial analyses, many comparisons yield meaningless conclusions. Therefore, rather than compare traditional dispensing financial data with pharmaceutical care service data, we will focus on the major financial consideration associated with the provision of pharmaceutical care.

We will focus on two categories of information required to make this activity financially feasible: the investment required to deliver phar-

> Learn about both the costs and the benefits of providing pharmaceutical care.

maceutical care and the potential return on investment generated from the service. Because everyone will be starting from a very different place in terms of personnel, we will discuss the new costs to be invested and which may be assigned to the service. It is important to understand that when implementing pharmaceutical care within an existing pharmacy operation, some of the required investment is new due to the implementation of pharmaceutical care. Also, some of the costs associated with this service are presently being incurred, and whether these preexisting costs are to be assigned to the service and deducted from the dispensing operations for accounting purposes is a local management decision. Although a level of financial sophistication that can accurately distinguish these costs and properly apply them to various portions of the operations of the total pharmacy "business" is ideal, it is seldom actually accomplished.

The following sections address the three most fundamental questions asked by pharmacists when planning, designing, implementing, and evaluating pharmaceutical care services:

- What do I have to invest to get started?
- What will it cost once pharmaceutical care is up and running?
- What return on investment should I expect for providing pharmaceutical care?

In order to address these essential questions in a complete manner, one must examine new investment requirements and new returns possible from pharmaceutical care by considering both tangible and intangible costs and benefits.

What Do I Have to Invest to Get Started?

It is often tempting to discuss the readily apparent tangible investments required to begin providing pharmaceutical care, but in practice, it is more useful to begin by recognizing and planning for the intangible investments. These can include substantial personal energies and commitments to change paradigms, prejudices, and priorities. Redirecting oneself from a business dedicated to product dispensing to patient-centered, need-focused activities can require substantial investments in personal time, thought, reflection, honesty, critical analysis, and humility. Although these personal investments are difficult to quantify, they are real and must be recognized, evaluated, and supported throughout the initial implementation process.

A substantial investment in leadership must also be available during the initial implementation phase of pharmaceutical care. New ideas, a clear vision of the practice and the service, plus the ability to communicate this new vision to others is essential in the implementation of pharmaceutical care. In the provision of a new patient care service, the initial leadership must emanate from the practitioner providing care. Waiting for a governmental agency or regulating body to grant their approval or waiting for a professional association or educational institution to take the lead in patient care activities will not be effective.

Enthusiasm is another essential ingredient required to successfully begin offering pharmaceutical care. Again, initial enthusiasm to help patients identify and meet their drug-related needs must come from the individual practitioners. This enthusiasm will be apparent to patients, their families, colleagues, and other health care providers as well as pharmacy support personnel.

> Enthusiasm is an essential ingredient.

A new learning curve will probably be necessary for both the pharmacist and support personnel. This learning curve applies not only to the provision of patient care but to understanding and participating in a new service operation within the pharmacy. This requires a new and different management method. The new management learning curve includes the ability to support patient care service and use outcome data from the documentation system to critically evaluate the new service. This learning curve must be steep, as it is important to provide practitioners, who are just beginning to provide pharmaceutical care, with timely feedback on how well or poorly their patients are progressing as a result of the services provided.

> Be prepared to accept a new learning curve.

In addition to the time and monetary investment associated with educational programs that prepare practitioners to provide pharmaceutical care, practitioners must be willing to invest the time and energy required to progress up the patient care learning curve. As with all new patient care services, practitioners and patients both must learn how best to communicate, trust, and work together to ensure that all drug-related needs are being met and that each medication is appropriately indicated, effective, as safe as possible, and can be taken appropriately by the patient.

Time and personal energy are two common investments that cut across all the intangible investments required to ensure the successful implementation of pharmaceutical care. The time and energy required may be even greater for the first few practitioners who decide to offer pharmaceutical care in a given community. This is often the case because there are still numerous unknowns when trying something innovative in a new setting. Once these first pioneers have invested sufficient time and energy and discovered the most effective methods to deliver pharmaceutical care, practitioners who follow can learn from these experiences and can begin more efficiently.

In addition to the intangible investments, there are several tangible investments that must be made. The first to be considered is personnel. Pharmacists, technicians, clerks, and other support personnel must be available to support the initiation of pharmaceutical care. In the case of personnel, how the pharmacist's time is accounted for will depend on whether additional personnel time is required or if time dedicated to the provision of pharmaceutical care is reassigned from dispensing activities to patient care activities. In our experience, the majority of pharmacies have sufficient pharmacist personnel to provide pharmaceutical care once the dispensing operation is transformed into an efficient technician-driven system. Having a technician-driven dispensing system with pharmacist support only for legally required checking of filled prescriptions is essential to provide pharmaceutical care and will make most existing dispensing systems more efficient. If the costs associated with pharmacist's time dedicated to providing pharmaceutical care have been transferred from the dispensing operation, this reduction makes the prescription processing operation less costly. If the prescription dispensing system is made efficient through the appropriate use of support personnel and technology, it is very unusual for the hiring of additional pharmacists to be required in order to provide pharmaceutical services.

Time and personal energy will have to be invested.

In addition to investing time in patient care activities, pharmacists must also plan to invest time to establish new professional relationships with community physicians, nurses, dentists, and other health care providers who will need to be aware of the new service in order to refer patients. Describing pharmaceutical care services to health care administrators in a particular geographic area will also require an initial investment of time. Local businesses and other employers should be contacted to inform them, their employees, and their families of the availability and benefits of the new pharmaceutical care services.

The amount of time given to direct face-to-face patient care by the pharmacist during the early stages of the new service will depend to a great extent on the goals and objectives set forth in the initial planning stages. Obviously, if the initial objective is to provide pharmaceutical care services for all patients who present to the pharmacy between 9 A.M. and 6 P.M. every day, it will require a much greater initial investment of pharmacist time than it will if the initial objective is to provide pharmaceutical care services for two new patients each day. It is important to understand the balance in the investment of pharmacist time required during the initial offering of pharmaceutical care services. It is essential that when first offering pharmaceutical services, the pharmacist be provided sufficient opportunities to practice and improve patient care skills.

Practice requires practice.

The practice learning curve requires seeing and caring for a sufficient number of patients to become proficient. "Practice requires practice" should be the pharmaceutical care practitioner's mantra. Limiting the scope of pharmaceutical care services too severely in the beginning can paradoxically slow or even prevent the service from becoming a success. Starting too slowly in order to minimize pharmacist time investment will end in frustration and failure because the pharmacist will not make adequate progress on the patient care learning curve and patients will not be satisfied with the new service. Fewer than two new patient encounters per day do not provide sufficient practice opportunities for pharmacists and will represent a poor initial investment. This critical balance in the initial investment of pharmacist time to patient care must be considered when deciding whether to use potential payment from a third-party plan, or a disease state management protocol, as a place to begin offering pharmaceutical care services. If that third-party plan or disease state management protocol cannot provide sufficient patient-pharmacist encounters to ensure a minimum of two new patients each day, then it will not represent an effective place to begin. Data from the Minnesota Pharmaceutical Care Project indicate that a pharmacy must fill at least 600 prescriptions every 3 months from a given third party plan or from a selected disease-state protocol to generate enough patients to ensure two new patients each day requiring pharmaceutical care.

It is essential to invest sufficient technician time in the initial provision of pharmaceutical care services. As described earlier, the dispensing operations need to become technician-driven and the patient care services require new and sometimes extensive documentation. The pharmaceutical care documentation requirements can also be supported by appropriately trained technical support personnel.

Other initial tangible investments that must be considered include computer hardware to support required patient care documentation as well as drug and medical information programs available through CD-ROM technology. Pharmaceutical care software license and support fees also need to be considered when initiating pharmaceutical care. Additional telephone lines may be required to support patient follow-up evaluations, a computer modem, internet access, or fax machines. Other initial tangible investment that may not already be available in the existing pharmacy operation include current reference texts, signage to direct patient flow, a desk for pharmacist working space, and chairs for patients and pharmacists to use during consultations. Table 7-3 lists the reference texts found to be useful for practitioners.

Many pharmacists will incur educational costs to improve their patient care knowledge and skills. Technician training in prescription processing and/or patient care documentation may also require initial economic and time investment. Other initial investments that may need to be considered include the costs of marketing the new services to patients, health care providers, and payers.

In summary, there are numerous tangible and intangible initial investment considerations required to offer pharmaceutical care. In a typical pharmacy, objectives should be established to complete the initial start-up phase within a maximum of 6 months. If a longer time period is allowed, enthusiasm and energy will wane and the service is

The maximum time for the start-up phase is 6 months.

at risk of never becoming operative. The exact cost of the start-up investments is very much dependent on the capabilities of the personnel, facilities, and resources available within the existing pharmacy operations.

What Will It Cost Once Pharmaceutical Care Is Established?

Following the initial start-up time, there will be both tangible and intangible investment costs. These are required to maintain, expand, and continually improve the service. Again, it will be necessary to maintain a degree of enthusiasm for the provision of pharmaceutical care. As with generalist practices in other health care professions, repetitiveness and constantly encountering similar patient problems, medical conditions, and drug therapy problems can diminish the practitioner's enthusiasm

TABLE 7-3 REFERENCE LIST FOR PHARMACEUTICAL CARE	
REFERENCE	AUTHORS AND/OR PUBLISHER
Drug Facts and Comparisons	Facts and Comparisons
Griffith's 5 Minute Clinical Consult	Williams & Wilkins
Handbook of Nonprescription Drugs	American Pharmaceutical Association
Physicians' Desk Reference	Medical Economics Company
Goodman & Gilman's The Pharmacological Basis of Therapeutics	McGraw-Hill
Harrison's Principles of Internal Medicine	McGraw-Hill
Pharmacotherapy: A Pathophysiological Approach	Appleton & Lange
AHFS Drug Information	American Society of Health-System Pharmacists
Drug Information for the Health Care Professional Vol 1 A and B, Advice for the Patient Vol II, USPDI	Rand McNally
Geriatric Dosage Handbook	American Pharmaceutical Association
Pediatric Dosage Handbook	American Pharmaceutical Association

for practice. Therefore, it is important to be willing to direct energy and time to constantly improving patient care skills as well as keeping current in the areas of drug, therapeutics, and other health related knowledge and services. To continue to offer the highest quality patient care service possible, each practitioner must demonstrate the leadership required to be willing to identify weaknesses in the present services and experiment with methods to improve effectiveness, efficiency, or scope of the pharmaceutical care being offered to patients.

It is important to be able to sustain a financially viable practice or patients will not be able to benefit from the pharmaceutical care they need. Financial plans that recognize the tangible investment costs required to maintain a viable practice are essential to ensure that patients can receive the care they need on a long-term basis. Personnel costs are among the high-priority investment costs. Adequate pharmacist, technician, and other support personnel need to be in place in order to provide services. The numbers and actual costs of personnel will depend on the scope of the services provided, the number of patients receiving care, and the complexity of the patient drug-related needs met by the service. Over time, it is important to plan for potential personnel replacement as pharmacists and technicians move to other practices or retire.

In order to maintain a viable pharmaceutical care practice, several tangible investment costs must be considered in the financial analysis of the service. These include depreciation of the hardware required for the patient care documentation system, ongoing software license and support fees, office supplies, phone line charges, internet access fees, updating of electronic and text references, and ongoing marketing investments to expand the service to new patients.

It is essential to recognize the investment costs required to expand care to new patients. Bringing new patients into a practice is essential not only for growth but simply to maintain a constant flow of patient encounters. Without adding new patients, the practice will become smaller and smaller because existing patients improve and no longer require pharmaceutical care, move from the community, receive care from another health care institution (hospital, long-term-care facility), or expire.

It is essential to continually attract new patients into a practice.

Finally, if costs such as rent, utilities, security, and other overhead expenditures dedicated to the provision of pharmaceutical care are separately allocated to the investment costs of the practice, then they must be accounted for in the financial consideration of the long-term viability of pharmaceutical care.

What Return on Investment Should I Expect for Providing Pharmaceutical Care?

In order to examine the entire scope of financial considerations, it is important to address the question of what return on investment one can

The rewards realized from pharmaceutical care are both tangible and intangible.

expect from the service. Like the investment costs associated with establishing and maintaining a viable practice, the return or reward side of the equation must recognize both intangible and tangible dividends.

In almost all cases, pharmacists' career satisfaction immediately improves once they actively and directly become involved in patient care. Taking care of patients and experiencing with them improved outcomes, enhanced health status, and increased loyalty are important positive rewards realized from the provision of pharmaceutical care. Many of the pharmacist's activities associated with the provision of pharmaceutical care are clinically engaging in the broadest sense. Practitioners enjoy a noticeable improvement in career satisfaction and feel that they are contributing in a meaningful way to their patients' quality of life.

Professional recognition from peers, colleagues, physicians, nurses, and other health care providers is also enhanced through the practice of pharmaceutical care. Physicians recognize the improvement in patient care as well as patient understanding of their drug therapies. This leads to a new, more professionally satisfying relationship between prescribers and pharmacists. When both consider their primary responsibility to be the improvement of the patient's health, teamwork and collaboration logically follow. Rather than the numerous phone calls and questions concerning refill authorizations, product availability, generic substitutions, and formulary regulations required in the dispensing operation, pharmaceutical care requires a very different interaction between prescribers, pharmacists, and other health care professionals. The patient's needs become the nucleus of all questions, comments, and inquiries for those actually providing care.

Practitioners providing services to patients discover that physician and nurse colleagues will refer patients to them in order to be confident that all of the patient's drug-related needs are being met and that drug therapy problems are being identified and resolved or prevented.

Support personnel within the pharmacy also become more confident and comfortable as their roles and responsibilities are clearly defined within both the dispensing operations and the pharmaceutical care. Initially, when they are reassigned to support the prescription processing and filling operations, it is not uncommon for some pharmacy technicians and clerks who have been responsible for much of the consumer contact in the product dispensing operation to miss this patient contact. Also, some support staff may see their new assignments as being the responsibility of the higher-paid pharmacist and feel they are being given too much responsibility within the dispensing operation. During this transition period, there may be some turnover among the support staff. It is important to recognize this potential and deal with it immediately, as it is vital that both the technician-driven dispensing operations and the practice are run efficiently.

Financial considerations resulting from the implementation of pharmaceutical care include monetary rewards. Many pharmacies realize an increase in drug product sales as a direct result of the new practice. This increase in sales includes not only prescription drug products but can extend to nonprescription drug products, home diagnostic kits, durable medical supplies, as well as health and beauty products. Pharmacies prepared to offer both product and advice on the proper use of health food items, vitamin supplements, natural products, and alternative medicine remedies can also account for enhanced sales following the implementation of patient-centered pharmaceutical care.

Direct reimbursement for pharmaceutical care services is another tangible return on the investment dedicated to these services. Patients who pay for their prescription and nonprescription products can be directly charged or billed for the pharmaceutical care they receive. During the early stages of implementing the new service, many practitioners are hesitant to ask for payment for the service. However, it is essential that a business plan be in place to charge patients for the service. All other health care services need to be paid for and so does pharmaceutical care. There are several professional and practical issues that need consideration when charging private-pay patients for pharmaceutical care.

Owing to the rapid spread of managed care organizations, pharmacy benefit management firms, health maintenance organizations, and insurance companies throughout the health care industry, there is a tendency for pharmacists to hope and wait for a third-party payer to offer to reimburse them for providing pharmaceutical care. This strategy, as we have noted earlier, has not proven to be effective. One reason is that as with all health care services that are presently recognized and reimbursed, pharmaceutical care must first be provided and patients must find it valuable before a third-party carrier is likely to offer it as a benefit to their clients. For a pharmacist to take the position of "I will only provide pharmaceutical care after the third parties offer to pay me to do so" will result in no new service offerings and cause a stalemate that will endure longer than the pharmacist's anticipated professional life span. The service must be provided and validated before reimbursement can be expected.

For example, in just a few short years, the practice of chiropractic has evolved from a profession fighting for its very existence to a recognized health care service reimbursed by many of the major payers.[3] Much of their success is due to chiropractors' dedication to providing a service that is valued and paid for by multitudes of patients.

Requests for third-party payers to reimburse pharmacists providing pharmaceutical care have been met with success by individual pharmacists and by groups or networks of practitioners. Individual pharmacists or pharmacies can easily make the new services available to local businesses as a benefit to their employees. There are several forms of "cafeteria" insurance plans offered in which the employee has a fixed amount of money to spend on health care–related items and services. From these funds, the employee can decide to purchase needed eyeglasses, pay for needed dental services, or pay for needed pharmaceutical care. Most such plans require the patient to pay for the service and then to submit a receipt for reimbursement by the employer. Pharmaceutical care documentation systems should have the capacity to print individual patient invoices to assist patients in obtaining reimbursement from employers and insurance carriers.

Individual pharmacists are at a great disadvantage when dealing with large third-party payers because the practitioner can offer services to only a small portion of the carrier's clients. The impact a single practitioner can demonstrate is minimal compared to the thousands, tens of thousands, or even millions of patients represented by the third-party carrier. Therefore many individuals and groups of practitioners have formed organizations or networks to offer greater access for patients. Large networks of pharmacists providing consistent pharmaceutical care using the same computerized documentation system are more likely to provide payers with improved patient care results and evidence of the value of the service.

As with most other health care services paid for by third-party payers, documentation of pharmaceutical care must be complete and accurate, and billing must be easily administered through a computerized patient care documentation system that can be audited. Payment in the form of fee for service is no longer considered a workable approach by many payers. Rather, a billing system based on patient needs, patient complexity, and the risk the patient is experiencing is more compatible to the reimbursement systems presently directed to other health care services. Attempts to request payment for each and every pharmacist intervention or activity are viewed as a request for fee for services (i.e., the more individual interventions the pharmacist does, the higher the bill will be). Very few if any other health care providers receive reimbursement based solely on a payment-by-the-hour basis. To request third-party payers to reimburse on a per hour basis will likely be unsuccessful; it is seen as paying for inefficiency (i.e., the longer it takes, the more you make).

Reimbursement for pharmaceutical care can be realized if the rules are followed.

During the Minnesota Pharmaceutical Care Project,[4] the resource based relative value system for reimbursement had five levels of payment ranging from $7.45 for the most straightforward patient encounters to $55.89 for the level 5 encounters, involving the most complex patients with four or more drug therapy problems, four or more active medical problems, and eight or more medications. Figure 6-6 describes the portion of patient encounters at each level of reimbursement. The amount charged at these levels is described in Table 8-2. The average charges for pharmaceutical care ranged from $11.30 to $16.00 for various patient populations. Using a figure of $15 as an average charge per patient encounter, one can estimate the potential new revenue that can be generated. Four examples of the potential new revenue from a single practitioner providing pharmaceutical care are presented below. Each example illustrates a different set of assumptions about the patient population and practitioner commitment.

Example 1:

- The practitioner dedicates 6 hours a day, 5 days a week, 50 weeks a year to providing pharmaceutical care.
- The practitioner provides care for 5 patients each hour.
- The average patient encounter is billed at $15.

In this example the pharmacist would provide care during approximately 7500 patient encounters throughout the year and generate $112,500 in potential gross billings for the service.

Example 2:

- The practitioner spends an average of 8 minutes of face-to-face time with each patient.
- The practitioner spends 7 hours per day, 5 days per week, 48 weeks per year providing direct patient care.
- The average charge per encounter is $10.

In this example the pharmacist would provide care during 12,600 patient encounters throughout the year and generate $126,000 in potential gross billings for the service.

Example 3:

- The practitioner spends an average of 20 minutes of face-to-face time with each patient.
- The practitioner spends 4 hours per day, 5 days per week, 48 weeks per year providing direct patient care.
- The average charge per encounter is $20.

The amount of revenue generated is determined by the number and complexity of patients cared for by the pharmacist.

In this example the pharmacist would provide care during 2880 patient encounters throughout the year and generate $57,600 in potential gross billings for the service.

Example 4:

- The practitioner provides care for a population of 1000 patients.
- The average patient requires 2.5 pharmaceutical care encounters each year.

- The distribution of patient complexity and charges for the service, based on the resource based relative value scale, is distributed as in Fig. 6-6 (i.e., 64 percent of encounters are level 1 and billed at $7.45; 27 percent are level 2 and billed at $18.63; 6 percent are level 3 and billed at $33.53; 2 percent are at level 4 and billed at $46.85; and 1 percent are level 5 and billed at $55.89 per encounter.)

In this example the pharmacist would provide care during 2500 patient encounters throughout the year and generate $33,264.50 in potential gross billings for the service.

In summary, to determine the amount of revenue necessary to make the investment in a new pharmaceutical care practice feasible, it is necessary to consider the costs of providing care to a patient on an individual basis. It is also necessary to consider practice patterns, potential patient populations to be served, and the potential for reimbursement from private-pay, as well as third-party payers.

ACCOMPLISHING REIMBURSEMENT

Now is finally the appropriate time to discuss reimbursement. Although we are sensitive to the need for financial support of the practice in order to sustain long term, it is also important to realize that if all the previous steps are not completed before the reimbursement discussion is initiated, important information, decisions, and priorities will be missed, and reimbursement will never be achieved.

Reimbursement will be realized only after the service is provided, and quality can be demonstrated.

To review, before reimbursement can be realized, the following must be accomplished:

1. The service to be offered must be clearly understood.
2. Patients must be placed first and the right experience created for them.
3. The staff must be prepared to provide the service.
4. The practice must be prepared with the appropriate personnel, physical requirements, and financial support.
5. The service must be provided. Quality must be demonstrated. Now, reimbursement can be sought.

Chapter 8 will describe pharmacists' previous experience with reimbursement and alternative approaches to payment for pharmaceutical care.

REFERENCES

1. Bradford, V. *The Total Service Medical Practice.* The Healthcare Financial Management Association. Chicago, Irwin; 1997.
2. Silker, E.L., Riewer, D.M. *Dentistry: Building Your Million Dollar Solo Practice.* Lakeshore, MN: Silk Pages Publishing; 1995.
3. Koch, W.H. *Chiropractic: The Superior Alternative.* Machias, ME: Bayeux Arts; 1995.
4. Tomechko, M.A., Strand, L.M., Morley, P.C., Cipolle, R.J. Q and A from the Pharmaceutical Care Project in Minnesota. *Am Pharm.* 1995; NS35: 30–39.

RECOMMENDED READINGS

Bennis, W., Parikh, J., Lersem, R. *Beyond Leadership: Balancing Economics, Ethics and Ecology*. Oxford, England: Blackwell; 1994.

Caroselli, M., Edison, L. *Quality Care: Prescriptions for Injecting Quality into Healthcare Systems*. Boca Raton, FL: St. Lucie Press; 1997.

Nadler, D.A., Shaw, R., Walton, A.E. *Discontinuous Change: Leading Organizational Transformation*, San Francisco: Jossey-Bass; 1995.

CHAPTER EIGHT

A REIMBURSEMENT SYSTEM FOR PHARMACEUTICAL CARE

Reimbursement for pharmaceutical care means payment for what the pharmacist knows and applies for the benefit of the patient. As we critically examined the alternative methods to accomplish this, we became aware of pharmacy's efforts to obtain reimbursement for what have traditionally been identified as cognitive services.

Pharmacists have sought payment for cognitive services, those services that go beyond the dispensing of the medication, for decades. However, in spite of these persistent and varied efforts, the literature fails to document widespread, long-term, direct reimbursement for activities referred to as cognitive or clinical pharmacy services. Although there are examples of an individual or a small group of practitioners succeeding in their efforts to obtain compensation, their impact has not been long-lasting or broad-based. Nor is there significant discourse within the profession on how best to manage reimbursement for these services.

Reimbursement is important for the long term health of a practice, therefore, we did not want to perpetuate pharmacy's declining economic experience. We have found that a number of factors may have contributed to pharmacy's failure to receive payment for patient care. These include the following:

1. the lack of a clear definition of the service for which payment is sought
2. the lack of a consensus about the value of the different services
3. the lack of the pharmacist's willingness to provide the services on a consistent basis
4. the lack of separation of payment for product and services
5. the lack of a documentation system recording the impact of the service on patient outcomes

Each of these factors is discussed below. Following the discussion we propose a list of lessons to be learned from this experience. Finally

> Payment for pharmaceutical care is based on what practitioners do with what they know for the direct benefit of the patient.

> Payers in the health care system only pay for services actually delivered.

we discuss how we used this experience to take a different approach to obtain reimbursement for pharmaceutical care using the Resource-Based Relative Value Scale.

REIMBURSEMENT FOR PHARMACY SERVICES

It is difficult to determine when the concept of cognitive services first appeared in the pharmacy literature. No single meaning for the concept has emerged, and many synonymous referents are used throughout the literature. The Cognitive Services Working Group of the American Pharmaceutical Association's (APhA's) Academy of Pharmacy Practice and Management (Clinical/Pharmacotherapeutic Section) defines it as "those services provided by a pharmacist to or for a patient or health care professional that are either judgmental or educational in nature rather than technical or informational. Examples of such services are patient education programs, drug level monitoring, hypertension monitoring, diabetes counseling, and home visits for medication consultation."[1]

Martin includes the concept of technical information in her explanation when she states that cognitive services are "those services that provide counseling, education, or technical information."[2] Other terms appearing throughout the pharmacy literature to mean conceptually the same thing as cognitive services include *professional services*, *value-added services*, *clinical pharmacy services*, *consulting services*, and *patient-oriented* (or *patient-focused*) *services*. Although many definitions exist for each of these and each has a slightly different emphasis (or breadth or scope), it may be useful to compare a few. Gagnon defines value-added services as those activities, benefits, or satisfactions delivered alone or in conjunction with a product.[3] Shepard includes drug utilization evaluation and review, delivery service, written patient information, private consultation rooms, drive-up windows, courteous service, and convenient business hours in his conceptualization of value-added services.[4] Rupp describes value-added services more narrowly than did either Gagnon or Shepard when he states that value-added services are "extra-distributive, professional, cognitive services that add or create value for the patient. We're not talking about auxiliary services such as having delivery services available. Value-added services include things like drug screening, drug therapy monitoring activities, patient medication profile monitoring activities, counseling activities, and a certain amount of triage and referral activities."[5]

Clinical pharmacy, another synonym for cognitive services in the hospital setting, has been defined by the American College of Clinical Pharmacy as "a health science specialty which embodies the application, by pharmacists, of the scientific principles of pharmacology, toxicology, pharmacokinetics and therapeutics to the care of patients."[6] In the Office of the Inspector General's Report on the Clinical Role of the

Payment requires a clear definition and understanding of the service you are willing to deliver on a consistent basis.

Community Pharmacy, clinical pharmacy services are defined more broadly as "functions performed by the pharmacist on behalf of the patient to identify, resolve and prevent drug-related problems."[7]

The most contemporary term to be used synonymously with *cognitive services* is *pharmaceutical care*. However, when this occurs, "pharmaceutical care" is being used differently than originally intended by those first defining it for contemporary use[8] and differently than in the manner described here. Strand and colleagues indicate that cognitive services are the tools a pharmacist uses as interventions to prevent or solve a patient's drug-therapy problems when completing the patient care process.[9-11] Therefore, most of pharmaceutical care practice is omitted when the term *cognitive services* is synonymously used with it. Great caution should be taken to use words as originally intended.

Cognitive services and pharmaceutical care are not synonymous.

Although specific definitions for each of these terms are somewhat different, it is important to note that throughout the literature and in practice, these terms are often used interchangeably. Perhaps this has contributed to the confusion and lack of recognition and payment for the services.

We can integrate all of this information and settle on a definition for cognitive services to be used here as *the use of specialized knowledge by the pharmacist for the patient or health care professionals for the purpose of promoting effective and safe drug therapy.* Pharmacists have included many different activities in this broad definition. Take, for example, the following: patient counseling and education, medication profile monitoring, drug utilization evaluation, medication compliance monitoring, formulary development and enforcement, prescribing error detection and intervention, and blood level testing, most of which focus on the drug and not the patient.

Although cognitive services have been delivered for many years and are presently being provided by pharmacists practicing in all types of pharmacy practice settings (e.g., hospitals, long-term-care facilities, home health care agencies, ambulatory care clinics, emergency centers), this manuscript will describe and discuss those available to ambulatory patients in community pharmacy settings, since this is the primary context under discussion for pharmaceutical care. *Community pharmacy* refers to walk-in pharmacies in noninstitutionalized settings and includes chain drugstores, independent pharmacies, and apothecaries.[7] Only when concepts developed in other practice settings are relevant to what occurs or should occur in the community pharmacy setting will that information be included in this discussion.

Pharmacy has undergone significant change over the past thirty years. Hepler, in what we consider a landmark paper, identifies three major periods in twentieth-century pharmacy: traditional, transitional, and patient care.[12] During the first stage, pharmacists procured, prepared, and evaluated drug products. Both medicines (product) and advice (cognitive services) were provided to "customers," and drugs were frequently provided without a prescription. This stage closed as pharmaceuticals were increasingly being manufactured by industry and therapeutic choice became the responsibility of the physician.

During the transitional stage, pharmacy experienced a period of professional flux. Indeed, in the mid-1960s clinical pharmacy practice was born, and rapid expansion of function and role occurred. Perhaps because clinical pharmacy was formalized by those practicing in the hospital pharmacy setting, the pharmacist's functions (consistent with clinical pharmacy practice) were described to reflect those performed in the hospital.[13-14] Although most could have been easily translated into community practice functions, community pharmacy continued, in the main, to function as dispenser of prefabricated drugs and intensified a long-lasting focus on product rather than cognitive service as their essential raison d'être. It is instructive to note that the American Pharmaceutical Association's Code of Ethics from 1922 to 1969 prohibited the pharmacist from discussing "therapeutic effects or composition of a prescription with a patient." Also, in 1951 the Durham-Humphrey amendment to the Food, Drug and Cosmetic Act introduced prescription-only status for most effective therapeutic agents, thereby effectively restricting the pharmacist to a dispensing role.

In 1969 Francke called for a separation of pharmacies and drugstores while at the same time deploring the mercantile nature of the latter.[15] Few community pharmacists took this admonition seriously. One important exception was Eugene White in Virginia, a pharmacist who rejected the commercialism of mainstream pharmacy and instead opened an office providing therapeutic services. His views were, and continue to be, radical. He asserted, as far back as 1954, that pharmacists "should work intimately with physicians and prescribe drugs based on physicians' diagnoses."[16]

Clinical pharmacy in its nascent form appeared to emphasize "patient-oriented practice," but many conceptualizations placed drugs at the forefront and the patient receded once again to the background. A widespread misunderstanding of Brodie's exhortation to emphasize responsibility for "drug-use control" served to legitimize and encourage a preoccupation with product, not patient.[17,18] However, it was during this transitional period that innovative services such as clinical pharmacokinetics developed, thereby moving the pharmacist closer to the bedside. But, the highly technical nature of this new clinical science furthered the focus on the drug and its delivery rather than on the patient and his or her specific drug-therapy problems.[8]

Although the "clinical role" as it unfolded in the sixties has continued to develop and mature, it has done so with limited economic reward. Smith correctly observes that a problem faced by clinical pharmacists is that of being directly compensated for the less tangible cognitive dimensions of their services.[19] Smith notes that the only two clinical services that routinely receive direct payment are (1) pharmacokinetic dosing with consultation and (2) general consultation to extended-care facilities. In the case of community practice, no cognitive services are routinely reimbursed, and these services continue to be subordinated to the more measurable act of dispensing pharmaceuticals with a tangible value.

A REVIEW OF SERVICES

The term *cognitive services* has been shown to include many different activities performed by the pharmacist. Therefore, it is important that a conceptual framework be used to compare and contrast cognitive services with pharmaceutical care to arrive at a reimbursement approach which will function effectively.

We have organized pharmacists' cognitive services into three different categories of activities or responsibilities. The first category consists of those services which benefit the general good of society by promoting health and disease prevention. The second category consists of services that benefit an organization, an institution, or other health care professional. The third category of services include those which benefit a specific patient by addressing a specific issue, problem, or need. Table 8-1 places the cognitive services to be discussed within this conceptual framework.

The literature describing the delivery of cognitive services in the institutional setting, the long-term setting, and the ambulatory (clinic)

TABLE 8-1 CONCEPTUAL FRAMEWORK FOR PHARMACISTS' COGNITIVE SERVICES

SERVICES THAT BENEFIT SOCIETY	SERVICES THAT BENEFIT AN ORGANIZATION	SERVICES THAT BENEFIT AN INDIVIDUAL
Drug information (general)	Formulary development and enforcement	Triage, referral
Drug abuse prevention		Patient medication profile monitoring
Health education	Drug utilization evaluation (retrospective, concurrent)	
Screening programs (disease prevention)	Counterdetailing	Prescribing error detection and intervenion
		Blood-level testing
		Drug therapy monitoring
		Patient-specific counseling and education
		Medication compliance monitoring
		Nonprescription product counseling

setting is extensive. In addition, over 300 articles provide evidence of the positive impact clinical pharmacy services have in the institutional setting on patient outcome, the cost of drug therapy, and the prescribing patterns of physicians.[20] However, it should be noted that clinical pharmacy services are provided to relatively few patients in hospitals and are not routinely reimbursed.[21–25] The literature that focuses on the delivery of cognitive services in community pharmacy practice looks quite different, both in terms of the number of citations describing the services and the number of articles reporting the impact of service provision. The review presented here will be limited to the literature reporting community pharmacy practice examples and reimbursement.

Services that Benefit Society

The prevention of illness and the promotion of health are obviously primary missions of all health professionals, and pharmacists are no exception. McKenney and colleagues provide a very useful organization for pharmacist activities in community preventive health care.[26] They also describe the extent of pharmacist involvement in the delivery of these services. They observe that although "pharmacist involvement in such activities may be sporadic, seldom advertised beyond the target community, and rarely documented in the professional literature, it is difficult to find a pharmacist who has not participated in such an activity at one time or another."[26]

More recently, pharmacists have demonstrated an active involvement in designing and implementing immunization delivery programs.[27–32] The specific pharmacists' activities vary with each practice site. Grabenstein describes roles that are common to most pharmacists involved in immunization programs: teaching and providing patient counseling, screening patients, maintaining patient immunization profiles as well as general drug profiles, sending reminder letters concerning booster doses, identifying vaccine-drug interactions, promoting National Adult Immunization Awareness Week and World Health Day, distributing self-assessment tests, encouraging legislators and other health policy makers to provide reimbursement for immunization by Medicare and Medicaid and by other third-party payers, developing contingency plans for influenza outbreaks and providing resource materials for all who are interested in acquiring additional knowledge and information.[33]

Some of the more contemporary services offered by pharmacists in the area of health promotion and disease prevention include serum cholesterol monitoring,[34–35] blood glucose monitoring, provision of information on home diagnostic products, involvement in smoking cessation programs,[36–38] and drug therapy monitoring.[39–41]

It is interesting to note that a consumer survey in rural and urban Pennsylvania counties identified pharmacists as providing less health information than any other health care professional.[42] The following explanations were offered: (1) pharmacists are not recognized by the public as primary sources of health information, (2) the information pharmacists provide is not the kind of information the public wants, or (3) pharmacists do not accept that it is their role to provide health information beyond prescription counseling. All three possibilities suggest additional attention be paid to this category of cognitive services. However, it is important to consider that health promotion and prevention services do not represent a "unique" contribution by the pharmacist. This is important when seeking reimbursement in this cost-conscious environment.

Services that Benefit an Organization

The development and maintenance of drug formularies is a service provided by many pharmacists working in institutional settings. Evidence that documents drug cost savings with the use of drug formularies is quite convincing. In spite of this, discussion of formulary use in the community practice setting is limited to third-party payers, both private and governmental. It is unfortunate, however, that most have been developed and maintained without direct involvement of the community pharmacist. Although past activity in this area has been minimal, formulary development and maintenance provides an opportunity for community pharmacists to have an impact on both the quality and cost of drug therapy.

Drug use evaluation, a method discussed in great detail, is becoming more important to community pharmacists because of recent legislation mandating this activity. The Medicaid drug rebate law, passed as part of the 1990 Omnibus Budget Reconciliation Act, seeks to ensure that Medicaid recipients receive high quality pharmaceutical services at reasonable costs and recognizes the role pharmacists play in providing drug therapy.[43] One of many stipulations of the law establishes a national drug use review (DUR) system requiring pharmacists to counsel patients. The Medicaid drug rebate law represents the largest organized effort at community pharmacy–based drug use review (or evaluation). The recent work completed by pharmacists at the Iowa Pharmacists Association, in conjunction with the American Pharmaceutical Association, will provide guidance as the specific rules and regulations are established for the Medicaid drug rebate law.[44] As these services become less the responsibility of the practitioner and more the responsibility of managed care organizations, individual practitioners lose the ability to obtain reimbursement.

Services that Benefit the Patient

Patient-specific education is clearly the most common cognitive service described in the pharmacy literature. It is difficult to examine this literature critically for three reasons. First, many different terms are used to refer to this category of pharmacist activity. Hence, we find *patient information, patient education, patient counseling,* and *medication counseling,* to name but a few. Second, descriptions of what the pharmacist actually does when he or she provides patient education or information are usually vague or absent completely. Finally, there is evidence that pharmacists do not provide patient education routinely or systematically. Instead, it appears that pharmacists often provide the counseling services that are of interest, familiar, and/or are convenient to the pharmacist.

> Cognitive services, that are defined by the practitioner for the practitioner's benefit and are delivered on the practitioner's schedule, are generally neither highly valued nor reimbursed.

A representative list of patient education programs available from the community pharmacist is broad in scope. Such a list might include programs about the following: epilepsy management,[45] asthma management,[46] diabetes,[47] adverse drug reactions, possible interactions,[48] the care and prevention of painful stings,[49] cancer chemotherapy,[50] and geriatric education.[51–52] Although many types of patient education programs are offered by pharmacists, not many are recognized or reimbursed by third parties. White suggests that "the quality and effectiveness of patient education programs must be proven before pharmacists will be reimbursed for these services."[53] Programs which have received third-party recognition include a hemophilia training program, task-oriented programs such as home hyperalimentation, and home use of intravenous antibiotic therapy for cystic fibrosis patients,[54] and selected disease-state monitoring programs.

There is limited evidence that pharmacists' provision of patient education has a sustained positive impact on the patient. McKenney has demonstrated that good patient education can benefit hypertensive patients.[55] Fifty randomly assigned patients were provided with blood pressure monitoring, health education, reinforcement, and prompting as they returned to their community pharmacy for prescription refills. The number of patients with blood pressure control increased from 20 to 79 percent in the study group, and compliance rose from 25 to 70 percent in these patients.

There is significantly more literature available describing the development of patient education programs than there is reporting the successful delivery of such a program in the community pharmacy setting.[56–58] Perhaps this reflects the pharmacist's dilemma of whether to provide drug-specific and disease-specific information to selected patients or whether all patients deserve to receive the necessary information about all of their drugs for all of their diseases. In fact, there appears to be no consensus among pharmacists as to what cognitive services patients deserve or need or what can ethically be expected from the pharmacist. This is certainly an issue that requires further debate and study and contributes to the reimbursement dilemma.

Rupp and colleagues studied the pharmacist's role of identifying and correcting prescribing errors. In a study of nine community pharmacies in Indiana, it was found that 2.6 percent (153) of new prescriptions dispensed by pharmacists over a 2-week period required intervention to correct or resolve a prescribing error.[59] In 38 of these, experts agreed that the documented error may have resulted in patient harm if pharmacist intervention had not occurred. The cost of the pharmacist's time to conduct an intervention was estimated to be $1.75, while the value of pharmacist intervention, as determined by the cost of medical care avoided, was estimated to be $7.15. This represents the first estimate of the value that cognitive services add to the patient's prescription.

A corollary to the above study was conducted in pharmacies throughout five states.[60] Of the 33,011 new prescriptions dispensed at the participating pharmacies during the 5-day collection period, 623 (1.89 percent) were found to be associated with one or more prescribing-related problems. The mean value that pharmacists added to each new prescription by screening for prescribing problems was $2.32. However, the pharmacists were not directly reimbursed for these services. Additional studies will be needed to standardize the service provided and to create an average value for providing the service.

A drug monitoring service for geriatric patients is described by Stanaszek and Baker.[61] Many issues associated with drug taking by the elderly are discussed. In addition, steps involved in monitoring a new prescription are described. Although a number of very useful concepts are presented, the authors also demonstrate the difficulty pharmacists have in knowing where specific tasks begin and end. These include determining the nature of the knowledge and information required by a patient undergoing counseling for a new drug, drug utilization review, provision of patient education programs, efforts to increase compliance with medication regimens, and monitoring for adverse effects, drug interactions, and onset of symptoms, as well as participation in screening programs and chronic disease management. The reader is led to believe all of these services are important but is given little direction as to how each is actually provided. This perplexity exists throughout the cognitive service literature.

Blood level testing is a relatively new cognitive service offered in the community practice setting. Potassium and cholesterol levels have both been measured in this setting.[62,63] It is almost certain that a number of additional blood tests will be soon available in the community practice setting, since methods for easy measurement are currently under study for theophylline, hepatitis A viral antibodies, ferritin levels, total bilirubin, and serum and plasma creatinine. Although there are "cognitive" elements associated with blood level testing, it remains to be determined whether pharmacists will develop laboratories or patient-oriented reasons or purely for the commercial advantage.

A large number of different patient-specific services has been offered by pharmacists, however, none of them have been offered or reimbursed consistently or systematically. Pharmaceutical care addresses a number of these issues.

THE VALUE OF COGNITIVE SERVICES

The value of a service is judged by the recipient and not by the provider of the service.

It is frequently argued that reimbursement depends on first demonstrating the value of the service. The following studies describe the value a patient places on cognitive services, both quantitatively (with payment) and qualitatively by describing their support for the service.

As early as 1973 we find evidence that consumers expect and want professional attention and services.[64] But, in general, they are unaware of the specific services community pharmacists can perform. Monsanto and Mason[65] report that the majority of consumers in their study appeared to be aware of nondispensing services, but the majority had only used advice on nonprescription drugs and advice on minor health problems. They also found that the percentage of consumers willing to use nondispensing services was higher than the percentage of consumers who had used them in the past. It is interesting to note that consumers in this study demonstrated a growing interest in receiving advice on diagnostic test kits and information on poison prevention.

Gagnon conducted a consumer perception study in which he distributed a nine-page self-administered pretested questionnaire to determine consumer receptivity toward various services that can be offered in the community pharmacy.[66] A total of 934 questionnaires were analyzed. Gagnon found that the needs of consumers are focused in three areas: (1) personalized professional contact with the pharmacist, (2) access to the pharmacist when the consumer needs him or her, and (3) financial services (receipts, invoices, and drug expenditure records). Other findings from the study indicate that the importance of pharmacists' services decreases with age and with more years of education. The recommendations made by Gagnon emphasize the need for pharmacists to understand what the patient wants and needs.

A one-year study was undertaken to identify patient-oriented nondistributive services provided in a community pharmacy setting and to evaluate consumer satisfaction with those services.[67] Direct or personal services provided by the pharmacist ranked highest (checking with physician, checking for interactions, and medication counseling). Sixty-one percent of the respondents reported that a pharmacist's consultation had saved a physician office visit. Pharmacy location and pharmacist consultation ranked higher than the financial considerations of prescription price or availability of charge accounts.

Hirsch and colleagues conducted a study of patients, physicians, and third-party prescription plan administrators in order to identify those pharmacy services they believe are important and valuable, and to determine whether third-party plan administrators would reimburse pharmacists for such services.[68] Focus groups of patients and physicians indicated that both wanted personalized services related to medications. Physicians believe that pharmacists are talking to patients about their medications, while patients report that they want more drug information, but pharmacists are not always providing it for them. The third-party plan administrators (a sample of 41 administrators was included in the mail survey) indicated that they believe pharmacy services are important to consumers. One-third of the third-party plan administrators said their companies would consider implementing a structural pharmacist incentive plan to improve enrolee satisfaction.

Consumers' Willingness to Pay

Eighteen patients were evaluated in a pilot study focusing on a theophylline consultation service established in a community pharmacy.[69] Each patient indicated a willingness to pay approximately $25 for the performance of a serum theophylline level and a consultation. Patient acceptance of and satisfaction with the service was high.

Another pilot program supported by a college of pharmacy was initiated in two community pharmacies in Florida.[70] Patients were charged $35 for laboratory values and assessment of cardiovascular risk factors. Appropriate referrals were made to a physician for patients identified to be at significant risk. A pharmacist provided patient education regarding diet and other methods available for controlling cholesterol for a separate $10 fee. The program attracted four to six patients per week.

Schondelmeyer and Trinca[71] used one pilot and four primary study sites to determine consumer demand for a pharmacist-conducted prescription counseling service. Demand was evaluated both in terms of whether the patient chose to receive the service and at which pricing level the patient chose to receive it. The counseling service differed from the activities engaged in by many pharmacists in two ways. First, the counseling service was formally planned and delivered in a uniform method. Second, it was delivered as a personalized health care service to meet each consumer's individual needs. Of a total sample of 218 subjects, 88.1 percent used the service when there was no charge, 24.7 percent at a $1 charge, 36.3 percent were willing to and did pay $2 for the counseling service, and 16.7 percent used the service when charged $3. Also of interest was the finding that pharmacists substantially overestimated the role of cost as a reason for consumers refusing the counseling service. A larger number of patients than expected did not want information about their medication.

A number of surveys assessing the consumer's willingness to pay for clinical services have been completed.[72,73] One survey of consumer attitudes toward paying for a community pharmacy–based medication reminder system provides initial trends which need further study.[74] The researchers found a trend suggesting that individuals who experience more benefits of a service would be more likely to pay for it. The survey also suggested that although the percentages of males and females willing to pay were similar, females appeared to be willing to pay a greater amount for the services. Although patients covered by third-party prescription benefits tended to be more likely to pay for the service than private-pay patients, private-pay patients appeared willing to pay more for it. Perhaps the most important observation from this study is that willing-to-pay patients rated the importance of the service significantly higher than not-willing-to-pay patients.

Einarson and colleagues conducted two studies to evaluate patient attitudes about drug monitoring services. The first, a pilot study, evaluated 27 patients who paid $10 to have a serum cholesterol determined.[63] All subjects stated, on a pretest questionnaire, that they were strongly in favor of such a service, that they would use it, and that they would pay an average of $11.60 for the test. On the posttest questionnaire, patients expressed strong satisfaction with various aspects of the service, and the amount that they were willing to pay increased significantly to $14.35.

The second study by Einarson and colleagues evaluated the feasibility of a community pharmacy–based blood level testing service with the use of a questionnaire.[62] A majority of subjects ($n = 443$) reported that they would use such a pharmacy-based service and would pay an average of $11.54 for it. A total of 186 patients was tested for potassium or cholesterol levels during the 5-week study. Following the use of the service, patients expressed satisfaction and reported a willingness to pay an average of $14.47 when offered in the future. A financial analysis showed that the blood level testing service would be financially feasible if 18 blood level tests were performed each day at a charge of $10 or eight tests at $15.

A Value-Added Pharmacy Services (VAPS) program, sponsored by Marion Merrell Dow, Inc., reported that patients expressed significant satisfaction with the services provided.[75] This in-pharmacy service campaign provided written patient information, verbal patient counseling, labeling to promote refill compliance, poison antidote charts and emergency prescription beepers, and more comfortable waiting/counseling areas. A comparison between 19 experimental VAPS pharmacies and 16 control pharmacies before, during, and at the conclusion of the program was conducted by researchers at the University of Texas, the University of Maryland, and the University of North Carolina. Patients who visited the VAPS pharmacies reported an increase in overall service delivery of 19 percent, compared with a 4 percent increase in control stores. Of the services provided, patients indicated the greatest interest in information services, particularly written information and verbal counseling. Ninety-two percent of all patients rated written and verbal information as "useful" or "extremely useful." In a qualitative analysis, patients also said they prefer services that enhance convenience, such as longer hours and faster service.

When the preceding literature is combined with the benefit of clinical pharmacy services, it is fair to conclude that significant evidence exists to support the value of cognitive services. Why, then, is reimbursement not forthcoming based on all this evidence? This evidence is necessary, but it has not proven to be sufficient for reimbursement. Four explanations are possible: (1) the cognitive services have not been clearly defined, (2) the services are not provided consistently or systematically, (3) there is a lack of an organized effort on the part of the profession to seek a standardized approach to reimbursement, and (4) reimbursement decisions often are based not on cost-effective or clinical evidence but in political, emotional, financial, or purely marketing considerations.

PHARMACISTS' WILLINGNESS TO PROVIDE SERVICES

A major contributing factor to the reimbursement challenge is whether the pharmacist is willing and able to provide cognitive services. Berardo and colleagues directly observed pharmacists to determine how often patients are counseled when they receive a prescription.[76] They found that pharmacists counsel patients about prescription medications from 0 to 48 percent of the time. They also determined that the counseling itself consumes, on average, 36 seconds (varies from 3 to 146 seconds). The type of information provided most often consisted of how to take the medication, information on side effects, dosage amount, and number of doses per day. Also of interest was the "busyness" index calculated from the number of prescriptions waiting to be filled, the number of new prescriptions brought in, the number of incoming and outgoing phone calls, and the number of other encounters the pharmacist had with patients, clerks, and interns. The index was then correlated with the percent of prescriptions dispensed during each half hour, which included patient consultations. It was found that there was no significant relationship between busyness of the pharmacist at any particular time and the amount of patient consultation he or she conducted. These data do not support the commonly expressed concern that pharmacists are too busy to counsel patients.

Mason and Svarstad completed a study involving 40 pharmacists randomly selected from independently-owned, rural, community pharmacies in Wisconsin.[77] The investigators used a "shopping technique" and demonstrated that pharmacists did little patient interviewing to detect or prevent medication usage problems but did prepare profiles for more than three-fourths of the encounters. Verbal instruction was provided in 70 percent of all encounters. It is particularly significant that this study demonstrated a link between pharmacists' attitudes toward medication counseling and their behaviors on all five counseling dimensions studied. The authors emphasize that more counseling by pharmacists is not always better and significantly more research is needed to determine relationships between attitudes and practice.

The lack of payment for the delivery of cognitive services is the most frequent explanation provided by pharmacists when asked why more cognitive services are not provided to patients. Many policy makers agree with these pharmacists. For example, the report published by the Office of the Inspector General identified the product-based reimbursement structure in community pharmacies as the first barrier in the provision of clinical pharmacy services. The report states that "the drug distribution system has always operated in a competitive environment, over the past decade competition has increased dramatically with the burgeoning growth of mail service pharmacies and discount chains. Consequently, the economics of practice tend to keep prices down and to compensate with higher volume. The result typically is a focus on product and price rather than provision of clinical services for which there is no economic incentive."[7]

A high level of agreement exists concerning the need to redesign economic incentives and develop systems to obtain reimbursement for cognitive services. There also appears to be sufficient literature to explain how to obtain reimbursement for these services in the community practice settings.[78–80] However, a paucity of literature exists when one looks for examples of successful community pharmacies achieving reimbursement for one or all of the cognitive services described earlier.[81] It is interesting to note that once again, institutional pharmacists, long-term-care pharmacists, and, most recently, home health care pharmacists have all been significantly more successful at establishing successful reimbursement models than those in community practice.

PAYMENT FOR COGNITIVE SERVICES

Pharmacy's first attempt to obtain reimbursement for professional activities occurred in the 1950s.[82] Although not all calculations of dispensing fees contained a "professional" component, the professional fee was a mechanism to argue for the "cognitive" or "service" component provided by the pharmacist for the patient's benefit. Although the "professional fee movement" was successful to the extent that most reimbursement formulas today contain some type of a professional fee, it was largely unsuccessful in that a number of the fees were so limited as to include only basic remuneration for (1) the cost of the ingredient and the container, (2) the cost incurred in the actual dispensing of the prescription, and (3) the profit necessary to sustain the business and to permit its growth. There is little or no room left for the costs associated with the provision of cognitive services to the patient. Moreover, there is a problem associated with increasing professional fees, or adding an additional counseling fee (or clinical service fee) to the price of the prescription. This problem, as succinctly stated in the Office of the Inspector General's Report, is that "as long as the overall reimbursement scheme is directly tied to the volume of transactions, there will be a strong incentive to increase the number of sales rather than expand services."[7]

The addition of a fee to the price of a medication is not the only mechanism for reimbursement. An additional method is to charge a monthly or yearly fee for the cognitive services provided. This method permits the service to be provided in the case of a prescription drug product, a nonprescription drug product, or no product involvement. Also, the service includes a medication history that is used to rule out therapeutic duplications, drug interactions, and adverse drug reactions. The history is made available to the patient's physician or to the hospital pharmacist should the patient need hospitalization. This method of reimbursement has been successfully implemented in Pharma-Card, an independent community practice in Valparaiso, Indiana.[83] The technique used by Richard Brychell, owner and operator of the practice, is to charge an annual professional fee based on the number of services used by a particular family and based on the amount of money saved for the family.

Another mechanism that can be used for reimbursement is to charge separately for each service provided. A few examples are reported in the literature. A pharmacist in Blacksburg, South Carolina, provides cholesterol screening and counseling in his pharmacy.[84] A fee of $7 is charged each time the service is provided. Two additional for-fee consulting services have been described.[85] One is based on a self-care concept in which the pharmacist charges $3 for an on-demand service taking about 3 min. The other program is structured to be initiated on physician referral for a comprehensive clinical evaluation of the patient's therapeutic regimen. The pharmacist reports all recommendations directly to the physician, for which the patient pays the pharmacist approximately $50. While both of these innovative pharmacists report that their efforts are rewarding, utilization of the service is disappointing. They conclude that success of these programs depends on the public's education and third-party realization of the cost-effectiveness and value of the pharmacist's services.

UNRESOLVED ISSUES

There is a growing consensus that "service" will be the "competitive edge" for business in the 1990s and beyond.[86,87] Shepard not only discusses why pharmacists must provide "value-added services" to survive financially but explains how the community pharmacist can differentiate cognitive services from the product to meet patients' needs.[88] Many pharmacists perceive cognitive services to be the potential "savior" of community pharmacy business. This is increasingly the case, since competition based on the retail price of the prescription product has become meaningless in view of the current levels of reimbursement by government and third-party payers. If pharmacists choose to use cognitive services as their "competitive edge" in the future, then the tools described by Shephard and Gagnon can help to conceptualize and market these services.[3]

Pharmacists have been providing important cognitive services for patients for many years. As has been described, patient profile monitoring, drug utilization review, drug-use evaluation, drug interaction evaluations, individualized dosing, blood level testing, and monitoring of specific drug therapy were all introduced as services provided by pharmacy personnel. In spite of these many services being "available" from the pharmacist, many questions concerning the delivery of these services continue to be asked. Consider the following:

- If these services are being provided and are of value to the patient, then why is the pharmacist not being paid, by the patient and/or by the third-party payer, for their delivery?
- If these services are being provided and are of value to the patient, why are patients not demanding the services?
- Why are patients, physicians, nurses, and administrators relatively unaware of the services provided by the pharmacist?
- Why are pharmacists unable to convince decision makers that their services are necessary and that pharmacy personnel are cost-effective?
- If these services are being provided and are of value to the patient, then why are pharmacists experiencing difficulty differentiating their job responsibilities from those of the technician?
- If these services are being provided and are of value to the patient, then why are 3 to 20 percent of hospitalizations due to drug-related morbitity?
- Why is drug-related morbidity and mortality costing this country over $78 billion a year, and why are drug-related incidents, half of which are preventable, responsible for thousands of deaths every year?

Although specific answers are difficult to find in the literature, a number of factors may be contributing to the aforementioned issues. For example, many cognitive services are presently provided by the pharmacist without any written evidence. We identified, at the time of writing, only two systems of documentation of cognitive services reported in the literature.[79,83] This lack of documentation precludes reimbursement for any particular service.

A service that is not documented is "invisible" to payers.

Second, it is not customary for the pharmacist to provide a *consistent* set of services to each patient, so it is difficult for the patient to identify a specific service from one visit to the next. Nowhere in the literature is there a stated set of minimum cognitive services required for a patient. Even the Standards of Practice created by the American Pharmaceutical Association in 1978 reflect a descriptive set of standards created by surveying present practice.[89] Therefore, instead of stating the practices required to achieve a certain outcome, the standards describe what was presently being offered by pharmacists. This has created a situation whereby a pharmacist may provide medication profile monitoring but not prescription-related problem resolution. Or, the pharmacist may provide patient counseling but not medication compliance monitoring. This type of inconsistent delivery of service, with more emphasis placed on the pharmacist's desire and ability to deliver a particular service than on what the patient needs, has contributed significantly to the questions concerning value.

Third, since the services are provided sporadically, at a time deemed convenient for the pharmacist and not necessarily when the patient demonstrates a need, it is difficult for a decision maker (i.e., administrator and payers) to place importance on the service in question, therefore making it difficult to justify the assignment of personnel, resources, and payment to the tasks.

The review of cognitive services undertaken above presents a picture of some disarray. First, there is no single, consensual agreement within the profession as to what the term *cognitive services* means. The list of services described by this term is lengthy, and descriptions of the services tend to be vague and inconsistent. Services are delivered sporadically and are evaluated inconsistently. With the exception of one study,[60] no research has been directed toward measuring the impact of cognitive services on patient outcomes.

Pharmaceutical care addresses the issues discussed above. First, the service for which payment is sought is explicitly defined (see the patient care process in Chap. 4). Second, there is only one practice and the value of it is described in Chap. 6. We have found no disagreement about the value of identifying drug therapy problems and resolving them. Third, documentation will verify whether or not the pharmacist has provided the service (Chap. 5). Separation of drug product and the patient care service is complete from a reimbursement perspective. Now consider how a reimbursement approach was selected for pharmaceutical care.

REIMBURSEMENT FOR PHARMACEUTICAL CARE

The issue of reimbursement becomes much simpler once patient care is separated from the drug product. It is then possible to examine how other health care providers are paid for patient care services. However, it is helpful to first establish the objectives of an "optimal" reimbursement mechanism. The objectives of a reimbursement system for pharmaceutical care are that it will:

- Reimburse the practitioner for *all* the work performed, regardless of whether or not a prescription is involved

The issue of reimbursement becomes much clearer once patient care is separated from payment for drug product.

- Be based on patient need and not practitioner services, since all other health care practitioners are moving to this method of payment
- Allow for payment in community, hospital, long-term care, or wherever pharmaceutical care is provided
- Be consistent with the practice so the philosophy of practice and the reimbursement system do not interfere with each other
- Be consistent with the method used to reimburse other health care practitioners for patient care

With this as a conceptual framework, all available reimbursement approaches that could meet these objectives were considered. Three candidates were identified: the fee-for-service system, the capitation method, and the resource based relative value scale approach. We will discuss each and explain why the resource based relative value scale approach was selected for pharmaceutical care practice.

FEE FOR SERVICE

The fee-for-service system is a traditional, well-established approach that has been in use for many years. A practitioner is paid based on the number and type of services provided and documented. Each time a service is provided, a charge is generated. The decision to provide a service is based on decisions made by the practitioner for a specific patient. Payment has traditionally been made with the expectation that a service will be performed only if it is necessary and appropriate and therefore justified.

This approach has a number of limitations associated with its use. First, every effort is currently being made to eliminate this system of payment, since it has proven to be very expensive and encourages practitioners to provide more services than necessary in order to receive higher levels of payment. It seemed somewhat shortsighted to select a reimbursement system that has gone out of favor and would appear to have a short life. It appeared difficult to obtain reimbursement for a new pharmaceutical service using an archaic payment system.

Another limitation of the fee-for-service system is that it does not meet a number of the objectives outlined above. For example, if all the work of the pharmacist is to be reimbursed, then each and every activity of the pharmacist has to be argued as a reimbursable service. This appears to be a tremendous task, especially in the political-economic environment of cost cutting and service minimization. Nor does fee-for-service focus on what the patient needs; instead, the focus is on what the practitioner does. We know that this is not the direction in which the health care system is moving, so a system that promotes practitioner-driven reimbursement has little chance of surviving in the long term.

It is less clear whether the fee-for-service system can accommodate the practitioner in all practice settings. Because practitioner-driven activities are quite dependent on practice setting, especially in the traditional sense of pharmacy, it is likely that this would require approval of activities performed at one practice setting at a time.

The philosophy of pharmaceutical care centers on the patient and his or her drug-related needs, not the practitioner. This is inconsistent with the fee-for-service approach. Caring requires that the practitioner brings whatever resources are necessary to meet a patient's needs, regardless of whether they are on the reimbursement list of services or not. And pharmaceutical care involves a list of new practitioner activities such as identifying drug therapy problems, preventing drug therapy problems, and follow-up evaluation. Each activity would have to be negotiated on its own merit. This is a difficult challenge for a completely new service.

The fee-for-service approach is being used less and less by other health care providers as a system for reimbursement. Whether it be managed care organizations or the federal government, the majority of decision makers in the health care industry today are trying to minimize the services paid by fee for service. Pharmacists have had a long history of unsuccessfully negotiating this form of reimbursement for its services. Therefore, this does not appear to be a viable alternative for pharmaceutical care.

THE CAPITATION METHOD

Capitation payment is an increasingly popular approach with which to purchase health care services. This payment method awards the provider a fixed amount of reimbursement for a predetermined level of services paid out on a per patient basis for a fixed period of time. For example, a dentist may be paid $10 per month per patient for all dental care. Usually, the capitation payment method has significant financial risk built into the contract for both the provider and the purchaser. For example, the dentist would be paid the fixed amount for all patients, whether they used few services or many services. The risk to the provider is that too many patients would request more services than the $10 per month would reimburse and money would be lost. The risk to the payer is that very few patients would request minimal services, so that the payer would be purchasing services not received. The specific risk assumed by each is negotiated annually on a contract-specific basis.

Capitation is a risky business.

This payment method appears to meet many of the objectives outlined above. All of the practitioner's activities associated with providing care are reimbursed by the payer. In addition, payment focuses on the patient and not on the practitioner's activities. Therefore, the philosophy of pharmaceutical care would appear to be accommodated by this payment system. The practice setting has little to do with a per-patient method of reimbursement, and more and more practitioners are being paid through a capitation method. So why not select the capitation method of payment for pharmaceutical care?

Although pharmacists will likely be paid on a capitation basis in the future, there is presently too much risk associated with this method. A successful capitation system requires that the practitioner be familiar with all costs associated with providing the service, the usage rates for the service, the variability in usage rates, and the impact the service is able to have on the patient. Ultimately, data generated in pharmaceutical care practice and gathered from the documentation system will provide the information necessary to design a successful capitation system for pharmaceutical care. However, in the meantime, a more suitable system is required.

Data and experience in providing pharmaceutical care are necessary to negotiate capitation contracts.

THE RESOURCE-BASED RELATIVE VALUE SCALE SYSTEM

The method of payment based on the resource-based relative value scale (RBRVS) became widely known and used in January of 1992 when it was adopted as the new Medicare physician payment system.[92] The federal government now uses this system to pay for a broad range of health-care services.

The basic principles underlying the RBRVS are not new, however. Physicians and insurers have been using this system since the first relative value scale was developed by the California Medical Association in 1956. In an RBRVS, services are ranked according to the relative costs of the resources required to provide them. For example, if service A consumed twice as many resources (time, overhead expense, difficulty) as service B, then service A would have a relative value of twice as much as service B. The relative value scale then must be multiplied by a dollar conversion factor to become a payment schedule.

The data which led to OBRA 89, the federal legislation which enacted the Medicare physician payment reform provisions, were generated in a national study which began in 1985 at Harvard University.[90] The study funded the development of RBRVS for almost thirty physician specialties. The American Medical Association (AMA) was intimately involved in this study, under subcontract from Harvard, to facilitate general medicine's acceptance of the system. The AMA eventually accepted the results of the study and supported the development of a national system of payment for physician services based on a RBRVS system. This system comprises three components: (1) the relative physician work involved in providing a service, (2) the practice expenses, and (3) practice liability insurance costs. There are other factors that were built into the provision. For example, a 5-year transition period was accepted (beginning in 1992), geographic differences were taken into account in calculating practice expenses, specialty differentials in payment for the same service were eliminated, and a process for determining the annual update in the conversion factor was defined. Suffice it to say that a tremendous amount of time, energy, research, and discussion went into the development of this system for physician payment.[92] This system has been broadly applied to include payment for nonphysician practitioners' services, including the following:

> Payment for the majority of patient care services today is established from a resource based relative value system.

- Physical and occupational therapists
- Physician assistants
- Nurse practitioners and clinical nurse specialists in certain settings
- Certified registered nurse anesthetists
- Nurse midwives
- Clinical psychologists
- Clinical social workers

This payment reform is very comprehensive. It standardizes payment levels and policies across nearly 230 different carrier areas. Further details about the development of this system and its ultimate application in payment reform can be found in the literature.[91,93]

RBRVS Applied to Pharmaceutical Care

This system was deemed to work for all these patient care providers, so should it not work for pharmacists? To answer this question, all of the parameters of the RBRVS system were applied to pharmaceutical care practice. This resulted in the Pharmaceutical Care Reimbursement Grid (Table 8-2) developed as part of the Minnesota Pharmaceutical Care Project described in Chap. 6.

This Pharmaceutical Care Reimbursement Grid was adapted from the original physician care model.[90] The following discussion describes the grid variables, the level of reimbursement calculations, and a discussion of its use in pharmaceutical care practice.

Payment Level Calculation

Across the top of the Pharmaceutical Care Reimbursement Grid is displayed the "Level" of payment. There are five distinct levels relating patient needs and resources required. Payment by the resource based relative value scale is calculated at one of these five levels. The level of payment in this system is based on patient need and patient need is placed into one of these five categories. The payment level, or level of patient need, is calculated to be at the lowest level where all the following qualifying criteria are met: (1) the number of medical conditions for which the patient is currently being treated, (2) the number of drug therapy problems the patient has at present, and (3) the number

> Payment is based on the level of patient need.

			LEVEL 3 (1.8)	LEVEL 4 (2.5)	
KEY COMPONENTS	LEVEL 1[a] (0.4)[b] D99201[c]	LEVEL 2 (1.0) D99202	D99203	D99204	LEVEL 5 (3.0) D99205
Workup of drug-related needs	*Problem-focused* 1–2 active medications	*Expanded problem-focused* (additional history required) 1–2 active medications	*Detailed* 3–4 active medications	*Expanded detailed* (additional history required) 5–8 active medications	*Comprehensive* >8 active medications
Pharmacists's assessment of drug therapy	*Problem-focused* 0 drug therapy problems	*Expanded Problem-focused* (additional patient information required) 1–2 drug therapy problems	*Detailed* 2–3 drug therapy problems	*Expanded detailed* (additional patient information required) 3 drug therapy problems	*Comprehensive* ≥4 drug therapy problems
Care planning and follow-up evaluation	*Straightforward* 1 medical problem	*Straightforward* 1–2 medical problems	*Low complexity* 2–3 medical problems	*Moderate complexity* 3 medical problems	*High complexity* ≥4 medical problems
Contributory Factors					
Nature of presenting drug-therapy problem (risk)	*Minimal* Self-limited	*Low* Transient in nature, good prognosis with appropriate drug therapy	*Moderate* Risk of morbidity is moderate, prognosis is uncertain	*Moderate to High* increased probability of prolonged impairment without appropriate drug therapy	*High* Risk of morbidity is high. High probability of severe prolonged impairment
Counseling and/or coordination of care	Counseling and/or coordination of care with other providers or agencies are provided consistent with the nature of the problem(s) and the patient's and/or family's needs				
Time guidelines (face-to-face time)	5 min	10 min	20 min	30 min	≥45 min
Reimbursement amount	$7.45	$18.63	$33.53	$46.58	$55.89

TABLE 8-2 PHARMACEUTICAL CARE REIMBURSEMENT GRID

[a]Service level.
[b]Resource-based relative value unit.
[c]Billing code.

of medications the patient is currently taking. The levels of need vary from the simplest, most straightforward "problem-focused" at level 1 to the most complex "comprehensive" needs of patients at level 5. The quantitative criteria are displayed on the grid. For example, a patient is placed at level 3 when the patient has 3 to 4 active medications, 2 or 3 drug therapy problems, and 2-3 medical conditions. Note that the patient is placed at the lowest level where *all three criteria* are met. A number of variables go into the calculation of the level of patient need, and therefore the level of payment. Some of these variables contribute directly and are called *key components*, and others contribute indirectly and are called *contributory factors*. These factors are presented down the left hand side of the grid in Table 8-2. Let us discuss how these variables integrate to create the level of patient need.

Although a different "intensity" of work is provided by the practitioner at each of the five reimbursement levels, the nature of the work is the same at *all* levels. The first three of the components that define the intensity of the work are the *key components* in determining the level of reimbursement, where the final two are considered to be *contributory factors*. The work includes the following:

- The extent of the workup of patient's drug-related needs
- The complexity of the assessment and identification of drug therapy problems
- The nature of the risks reflected in care planning and follow-up evaluation
- The amount of counseling and/or care coordination needed
- The amount of face-to-face time spent with the patient

We will discuss each of the components of the work in detail. This work and the relative resources required to do the work create the five levels of care.

Determining the Extent of the Workup of Drug Therapy

The resource-based relative value scale recognizes five different levels of workup. The major criterion determining the different levels is the number of active medications the patient is presently taking. This affects the amount of information necessary to provide pharmaceutical care and the amount of integration required. The most straightforward workup is called a *problem-focused workup* and involves patients taking one to two medications. The next level is an *expanded problem-focused workup* and is appropriate for patients requiring one to two medications but in whom more extensive medication history is required and documented. With three or four active medications, the practitioner must conduct a *detailed workup*, with five to eight, *an expanded detailed workup*. Finally, when a patient requires more than eight medications, which, for example, is frequently the case with an elderly patient, a *comprehensive workup* of drug therapy is required.

Level of patient need is determined by the number of:
- active medications
- drug therapy problems
- medical conditions

The basic elements of pharmaceutical care are required at all five levels of patient need.

Determining the Complexity of the Assessment Process

The complexity of the assessment process follows the same descriptive categories as presented above for the levels of workup. However, the variable of interest is the number of active drug therapy problems identified. Table 8-2 makes the following distinctions:

- The first (and lowest level of reimbursement) reflects patients with no active drug therapy problems at this time.
- Level 2 reflects one or two active drug therapy problems.
- Level 3 reflects two or three drug therapy problems.
- The fourth level is for those patients with three active drug therapy problems.
- The highest level of reimbursement encompasses all patient encounters for which four or more drug therapy problems are identified.

Each drug therapy problem requires a sophisticated decision-making process for its identification and its resolution.

Determining the Nature of the Risks Reflected in Care Planning and Follow-up Evaluation

The level of risk associated with the patient is determined by the number of active medical conditions, since this variable represents major risks to a patient. Clearly, number and type of medications as well as number and type of drug therapy problems also represent risk, but these contribute in their own way to the level of reimbursement. Therefore the risks of the medical condition will impact the nature and scope of the care plan and follow-up evaluation required.

Each medical condition will require the practitioner to establish therapeutic goals, appropriately intervene to establish an appropriate plan to accomplish these therapeutic goals. In addition, it will be necessary to monitor the progress of the patient through a follow-up evaluation. The level of effort required will be the direct result of the number of active medical conditions.

Determining the Amount of Counseling and/or Care Coordination Needed

Counseling is defined as a discussion with a patient and/or family concerning one or more of the following areas:

- Risks and benefits of treatment options
- Instructions for management (treatment) and/or follow-up
- Importance of compliance with chosen treatment options
- Risk reduction interventions
- Patient and family education

No specific criteria have been designated on the reimbursement grid for this variable since it is assumed that the appropriate level of counseling for each level of workup, assessment, care planning, and follow-up evaluation will take place.

Coordination of care with other providers or agencies is provided consistent with the nature of the problems with the patient's and/or family's needs. No specific criteria have been designated for this variable, since it is assumed that whatever care coordination is required, will take place.

Determining the Amount of Face-to-Face Time Spent with the Patient

The amount of time listed on the reimbursement grid, at each level of payment, are guidelines, representing a range of times which may be higher or lower depending on actual practice circumstances. It is also important to note that the specific times refer only to "face-to-face" time. Face-to-face time is defined as that time the practitioner spends with the patient and/or family. This includes the time in which the practitioner performs such tasks as completing a workup of drug therapy, making an assessment, preparing a care plan, and counseling the patient.

The only practitioner time recognized in this payment system is the time spent face-to-face with the patient.

Practitioners will also spend time doing work before and after the "face-to-face" time with the patient, performing such tasks as reviewing records, tests, arranging for follow-up services and communicating further with other professionals and the patient through written reports and telephone contact. This is all non-face-to-face time and is not included in the time component for the visit codes.

Refer back to Table 8-2 which describes the criteria at each of the different levels of payment.

Other Grid Notation

Across the top of the Pharmaceutical Care Reimbursement Grid in Table 8-2 you will see two other numbers in the "Level" of payment box. The number in parenthesis, the resource based relative value unit referred to as "b" on the grid (e.g., in level 1 the number is 0.4), represents the relative number of resources required to provide care at this particular level of payment (patient need). Level 1 requires 40 percent of the resources required at level 2. Level 5 requires 300 percent more resources than does providing care at level 2. These relative values were calculated based on "best estimates" from the first pharmaceutical care practices put in place.[95] Validation from additional pharmaceutical care practices will be necessary, as it becomes available.

The last number in the "Level" of payment box in Table 8-2, referred to as "c" on the grid, represents the CPT (current procedural terminology) billing code, which we created in a format consistent with the other systems in place.[94] This number was assigned for use during the Minnesota Pharmaceutical Care Project.

Calculating the Reimbursement Amount

The original reimbursement amount was calculated based on the variables described above and reflects the expected resources required to provide care at each level. Therefore the calculation of costs includes tangible and intangible costs of delivering the service, and a reasonable financial return. These costs, multiplied by the relative value for each level of care, create the reimbursement amount at each level. Remember, these figures were calculated based on a limited number of pharmacies in 1993 dollar figures. Therefore, recalculation in today's dollar terms and validation from additional pharmaceutical care practices will be necessary, once they become available. As part of the Minnesota Pharmaceutical Care Project,[92] pharmacists at ten different community pharmacy practices received reimbursement for their services from three different third-party payers. The payment system was successfully implemented and in 1994, the average payment for pharmaceutical care patient encounters was $12.14.

Meeting the Reimbursement Objectives

It should be apparent how the RBRVS meets all of the reimbursement criteria we established for the optimal approach. Certainly it allows payment for all components of pharmaceutical care, since payment is based on patient need. Second, the patient is the focus of the payment system. This approach is completely consistent with the philosophy and practice of pharmaceutical care, as can be seen by our ability to adapt each aspect of the medical care RBRVS to the practice and vocabulary of pharmaceutical care. Finally, we are using the same system as other health care providers and can therefore document the impact of pharmaceutical care on managing health care expenditures. The resource based relative value scale meets all the reimbursement objectives of pharmaceutical care practice.

> In a generalist practice, the amount of payment negotiated at levels 1 and 2 will have the greatest economic impact on the financial viability of the practice.

REFERENCES

1. Working Group Bibliography. Payment for cognitive services: The future of the profession. *Am Pharm* 1989; NS29(12):34–38.
2. Martin, S. Traditional values, innovative practices: Pharmacists who provide cognitive services. *Am Pharm* 1990; NS30(4):22–27.
3. Gagnon, J.P. Defining and marketing value-added pharmacy services in a community pharmacy. *Pharm Times* 1989; August:61–62, 66–67.
4. Shepherd, M.D. Pharmaceutical care: Adding value to the future. *Am Pharm*, 1991; NS31(4):55–59.
5. Value-added services help pharmacists help patients.

Day summary. APhA Annual Meeting, New Orleans, LA, 1991.

6. Kelly, K. The American College of Clinical Pharmacy. *Drug Intell Clin Pharm* 1979; 13:564.

7. Report on the clinical role of the community pharmacist (draft). U.S. Department of Health and Human Services, Office of the Inspector General, January 1990.

8. Hepler, C.D., Strand, L.M. Opportunities and responsibilities in pharmaceutical care. *Am J Hosp Pharm* 1990; 47:533–543.

9. Strand, L.M., Morley, P.C., Cipolle, R.J., et al. Drug-related problems: Their structure and function. *DICP Ann Pharmacother* 1990; 24:1093–1097.

10. Strand, L.M., Cipolle, R.J., Morley, P.C. Documenting the clinical pharmacist's activities: Back to basics. *Drug Intell Clin Pharm* 1988; 22:63–67.

11. Strand, L.M., Cipolle, R.J., Morley, P.C. *Pharmaceutical Care: An Introduction*. Current Concepts. Kalamazoo, MI: The Upjohn Company; 1992.

12. Hepler, C.D. The third wave in pharmaceutical education: The clinical movement. *Am J Pharm Educ* 1987; 51:369–385.

13. Report of the Task Force on the Pharmacist's Clinical Role. *J Am Pharm Assoc* 1971; NS11:482–484.

14. Francke, D.E. Relationship between clinical pharmacology and clinical pharmacy. *J Clin Pharm* 1972; 12:384–392.

15. Francke, D.E. Let's separate pharmacies and drugstores. *Am J Pharm* 1969; 141:161–176.

16. McLeod, D.C. Philosophy of pharmacy practice, in McLeod, D.C., Miller W.A., eds. *The Practice of Pharmacy*. Cincinnati, OH: Harvey Whitney Books; 1981, p. 7.

17. Brodie, D.C. Drug use control: Keystone to pharmaceutical service. *Drug Intell Clin Pharm* 1967; 1:63–65.

18. McGhan, W.G., Brodie, D.C., Lindon, J. The theoretical base of pharmacy. *Am J Hosp Pharm* 1991; 48:536–540.

19. Smith, H.A. *Principles and Methods of Pharmacy Management*, 3d ed. Philadelphia: Lea & Febiger; 1986.

20. Hatoum, H.T., Catizone C, Hutchinson R.A., Purohit A. An eleven-year review of the pharmacy literature: Documentation of the value and acceptance of clinical pharmacy. *Drug Intell Clin Pharm* 1986; 20:33–48.

21. Stolar, M.H. National survey of selected hospital pharmacy practices. *Am J Hosp Pharm* 1976; 33:225–230.

22. Stolar, M.H. National survey of hospital pharmaceutical services—1978. *Am J Hosp Pharm* 1979; 36:316–325.

23. Stolar, M.H. National survey of hospital pharmaceutical services—1982. *Am J Hosp Pharm* 1983; 40:963–969.

24. Stolar, M.H. national survey of hospital pharmaceutical services—1985. *Am J Hosp Pharm* 1985; 42:2667–2678.

25. Crawford, S.Y. National survey of hospital pharmaceutical services—1990. *Am J Hosp Pharm* 1990; 47:2665–2695.

26. McKenney, J.M, Rabin, D.l., Heltzer, N.E. The pharmacist's role in community preventive health care. *Am Pharm* 1983; NS23:16–22.

27. Morton, M.R, Spruill, W.J., Cooper, J.W. Pharmacist impact on pneumococcal vaccination rates in long-term care facilities. *Am J Hosp Pharm* 1988; 45:73.

28. Casto, D.T. Recent developments in vaccines and immunization practices. *Pharmacotherapy* 1992; 12:945–1035.

29. Williams, D.M., Daugherty, L.M., Azcock, D.G., et al. Effectiveness of improved targeting efforts for influenza immunization in an ambulatory care setting. *Hosp Pharm* 1987; 22:462–464.

30. Spruill, W.J., Cooper, J.W., Taylor, W.J. Pharmacist-coordinated pneumonia and influenza vaccination program. *Am J Hosp Pharm* 1982; 39:1904–1906.

31. Huff, P.S., Had, S.H., Calola, S.M. Immunizations for international travel as a pharmaceutical service. *Am J Hosp Pharm* 1982; 39:90–93.

32. Grabenstein, J.D., Smith, L.J., Carter, D.W., et al. Comprehensive immunization delivery in conjunction with influenza vaccination. *Arch Intern Med* 1986; 146:1189–1192.

33. Grabenstein, J.D. Pharmacists and immunizations: Advocating preventive medicine. *Am Pharm* 1988; NS28:25–33.

34. Madejski, R.M., Madejski, T.J. Cholesterol Screen-

ing in a Community Pharmacy. *JAPHA* 1996; NS36: 243–248.

35. Pearson, J.R., Dusenbury, L.J., Bakes-Martin, R., et al. Evaluation of a simple method for measuring blood cholesterol levels using non-laboratory observers. *Am J Med* 1988; 85:369–374.

36. Pharmacists' "Helping Smokers Quit" program. *Am Pharm* 1986; NS26:25–27, 28–33.

37. Houghton, J., McKenna, J., Ferguson, S.A. Pharmacist's role in smoking cessation. *Am Pharm* 1986; NS26:21–24.

38. Fincham, J.E., Smith, M.C. Pharmacist's views about health promotion practices. *J Comm Health* 1988; 13:115–123.

39. Hill, M. Hendeles, L. Evaluation of an office method of measuring theophylline serum concentrations. *J Allergy Clin Immunol* 1988; 82:30–34.

40. Shaw, K.N., Fleisher, G.R., Schwartz, J.S. Comparison of two methods of rapid theophylline testing in clinical practice. *J Pediatr* 1988; 112:131–134.

41. Clouse, E., Celestin, C. Development of a laboratory center in community pharmacies. *Florida Pharm Today* 1988; 55:7–8.

42. Connell, C.M., Crawford, C.O. How people obtain their health information: A survey in two Pennsylvania counties. *Public Health Rep* 1988; 103:189–195.

43. Martin, S. Medicaid drug rebate law is working to change reimbursement. *Am Pharm* 1991; NS31: 24–26.

44. Chrischilles, E., Sorofman, B., Zieglowsky, M.B., Davis, C. Iowa on-line prospective drug utilization review (OPDUR) demonstration project: study, design, system design, and conceptual models. *Journal of Research in Pharmaceutical Economics* 1997; 8(1): 171–191.

45. Gibson, P.A., Cloutier, G. Epilepsy: Patient education and services. *Am Pharm* 1984; NS24:39–43.

46. Chrisman, C.R., Self, T.H., Rumbak, M.J. Use of peak flow meters in asthmatics. *Am Pharm* 1991; NS31:24–28.

47. Martin, S. Traditional values, inovative practices: Pharmacists who provide cognitive services: Margaret C. Yarborough Diabetes Care Specialist. *Am Pharm* 1990; NS30:25–27.

48. Larrat, E.P., Taubman, A.H., Willey, C. Compliance-related problems in the ambulatory population. *Am Pharm* 1990; NS30:18–23.

49. McCormick, M.A., Easom, J.M. the pharmacist's role in counseling patients on the care and prevention of painful stings. *NARD J* 1981; 103:51–55.

50. Meade, V. A pharmacist helps dying patients. *Am Pharm* 1991; NS31:49–52.

51. Small, R.E., Moherman, L.J. Geriatric education: A fundamental requirement for pharmacy practice. *Am Pharm* 1990; NS30:42–44.

52. Lundin, D.V., Eros, P.A., Melloh, J., et al. Education of independent elderly in the responsible use of prescription medication. *Drug Intell Clin Pharm* 1980; 14:335–342.

53. Witte, K.W., Bober, K.F. Developing a patient education program in the community pharmacy. *Am Pharm* 1982; NS22:28–32.

54. Fudge, R.P., Vlasses, P.H. Third-party reimbursement for pharmacist instruction about antihemophiliac factor. *Am J Hosp Pharm* 1977; 34:831–831.

55. McKenney, J., Slining, J., Henderson, H. The effect of clinical pharmacy services on patients with essential hypertension. *Circulation* 1973; 48:1104–1111.

56. Reeder, C.E. Patient medication counseling: A practical perspective. *Pharm Times* 1989; 55:57–67.

57. Setting up a diabetic patient education program. *Am Pharm* 1984; NS24:61.

58. Smith, D.L. Patient counseling: Your competitive edge. *Am Pharm* 1991; NS31:53–56.

59. Rupp, M.T. Evaluation of prescribing errors and pharmacist interventions in community practice: An estimate of "value added" *Am Pharm* 1988; NS28:22–26.

60. Rupp, M.T., DeYoung, M., Schondelmeyer, S.W. Prescribing problems and pharmacist interventions in community practice: *Med Care* 1992; 30:926–940.

61. Stanaszek, W.F., Baker, D. Drug monitoring in the geriatric patient. *Am Pharm* 1983; NS23:32–37.

62. Einarson, T.R., Bootman, J.L., Larson, L.N., McGhan, W.F. Blood level testing in a community pharmacy: consumer demand and financial feasibility. *Am Pharm* 1988; NS28:76–79.

63. Einarson, T.R., Bootman, J.L., McGhan, W.F., et al. Establishment and evaluation of a serum cho-

lesterol monitoring service in a community pharmacy. *Drug Intell Clin Pharm* 1988; 22:45–48.

64. The Dichter Institute for Motivational Research. Communicating the value of comprehensive pharmaceutical services to the consumer. Washington, D.C.: American Pharmaceutical Association, 1973.

65. Monsanto, H.A., Mason, H.L. Consumer use of nondispensing professional pharmacy services. DICP, *Ann Pharmacother* 1989; 23:218–223.

66. Gagnon, J.P. Pharmaceutical Services: Consumer perceptions. *Am Pharm* 1976; NS16:137–142.

67. Mason, H.L. Clinical services in an independent community pharmacy. NARD Foundation Grant Report, Washington, D.C. 1984.

68. Hirsch, J.D., Gagnon, J.P., Camp, R. Value of pharmacy services: perceptions of consumers, physicians, and third party prescription plan administrators. *Am Pharm* 1990; 30:20–25.

69. Theophylline pharmacokinetic consultation in a community pharmacy. *Consult Pharm* 1988; (January/February):54–57.

70. Robinson, B. Cardiac risk screening gets Florida pharmacy test. *Drug Topics* 1988; (Feb 15); 12.

71. Schondelmeyer, S.W., Trinca, C.E. Consumer demand for a pharmacist-conducted prescription counseling service. *Am Pharm* 1983; NS23:65–68.

72. APhA National Survey: Willingness of consumers to pay for pharmacists' clinical services. *Am Pharm* 1983; NS23:58–64.

73. Strandberg, L.R., Stennett, D.J., Simonson, W. Payment for nondistributive hospital pharmacy services: A regional survey. *Drug Intell Clin Pharm* 1978; 12:410–412.

74. Brown, G.H., Kirking, D.M., Ascione, F.J. Patient willingness to pay for a community pharmacy based medication reminder system. *Am Pharm* 1983; NS23:69–71.

75. Marion Merrell Dow, Inc. Consumer pharmacists rate Marion Merrell Dow's "Value added pharmacy services" program a success. News Release, Kansas City, Missouri, June 12, 1991.

76. Berardo, D.H., Kimberlin C.L., Barnett, C.W. Observational research on patient education activities of community pharmacists. *J Soc Admin Pharm* 1989; 6:21–30.

77. Mason, H.L., Svarstad, B.L. Medication counseling behaviors and attitudes of rural community pharmacists. *Drug Intell Clin Pharm* 1984;18:409–414.

78. Martin, S. Teaching pharmacists to provide and bill for clinical services. *Am Pharm* 1990; NS30:24–26.

79. Klotz, R. Written documentation in the provision of cognitive pharmacy services. *APPM Update* 1990; 25:2.

80. ASHP Guidelines for implementing and obtaining compensation for clinical services by pharmacists. *Am J Hosp Pharm* 1985; 42:1581–1582.

81. Fee paid cholesterol screening program introduced. *Am Pharm* 1987; NS27:18.

82. Apple, W.S. Prescription pricing. *Wisconsin Commerce Rep* 1952; 3:3.

83. Martin, S. Traditional values, innovative practices: Pharmacists who provide cognitive services: Richard Brychell: Patient oriented pharmacist. *Am Pharm* 1990; NS30:22–27.

84. Martin, S. Making cholesterol screening work in small town America. *Am Pharm* 1990; NS30:42–43.

85. Two for-fee pharmacist consulting services begin operations. *Consult Pharm* 1987; 2:369–370.

86. Zemke, R., Schaaf, D. *The Service Edge: 101 Companies that Profit from Customer Care.* New York: New American Library, 1989.

87. Goldzimer, L.S. *I'm First: Your Customers Message to You.* New York: Rawson Associates; 1989.

88. Shepherd, M.D. Product differentiation: Its role in pharmacy marketing. *Am Pharm* 1986; NS26:34–39.

89. Kalman, S.H., Schlegal, J.F. Standards of practice for the profession of pharmacy. *Am Pharm* 1979; NS19:21–23.

90. American Medical Association. *Medicare Physician Payment Reform: The Physicians' Guide.* Chicago: American Medical Association, 1992.

91. Hsiao, W.C., Braun, B., Becker, E.R., Thomas, S.R. The resource based relative value scale. Toward the development of an alternative physician payment system *JAMA* 1987; 258:799–802.

92. Lee, P.R., Ginsberg P.B. Physician payment reform: An idea whose time has come. *JAMA* 1988; 260:2441–2443.

93. Tomechko, M.A., Strand, L.M., Morley, P.C., Cipolle, R.J. Q and A from the Pharmaceutical Care Project in Minnesota. *Am Pharm* 1995; NS35:30–39.

94. *Physicians' Current Procedurial Terminology, CPT '94.* Chicago: American Medical Association; 1994.

RECOMMENDED READINGS

Bergthold, L. *Purchasing Power in Health.* NJ: Rutgers University Press; 1990.

Bodenheimer, T.S., Grumbach, K. *Understanding Health Policy, a Clinical Approach.* Stamford, CT: Appleton and Lange; 1995.

Casalino, L.P. Balancing Health Incentives: How Should Physicians be Reimbursed? *JAMA* 1992; 267:403.

Reinhardt, V.E. Reorganizing the financial flows in US Health Care. *Health Aff,* 1993; 12 (Suppl):172.

CHAPTER NINE

PREPARING THE PHARMACEUTICAL CARE PRACTITIONER

This chapter is written for practitioners, teachers, and students alike. We firmly believe that all those engaged in pharmaceutical care must face the learning process—its substantive content, its values, its ideological/political substrates, and its many conflicts—openly and as partners in this transformative mission. Students, in particular, should be exposed to all the nuances of the educational context and the processes affecting their education and their future.

TEACHING THE PRACTICING PHARMACIST

An important means of extending pharmaceutical care to patients is to educate those pharmacists who have already graduated from an accredited college of pharmacy and are licensed to practice. These individuals have access to the patient and a solid knowledge base on which to build a new patient care practice. With an expenditure of energy, time, and a few strategically placed financial resources, practicing pharmacists can change the "business" they are in. However, this sounds much easier than it has proved to be. Changing one's paradigm is not easy, and this change requires a major shift in focus from the drug product to the patient. We have discussed some of the principles of building a pharmaceutical care practice in Chap. 7, and now we will discuss what is required to prepare a practitioner, beginning with the practicing pharmacist and then describing the preparation of the pharmacy student.

Pharmaceutical care requires a major shift in focus—from drug product to patient.

THE PHARMACEUTICAL CARE CERTIFICATE PROGRAM

In societies in which special privileges are granted to health care practitioners, certificate programs have emerged as mechanisms to provide the practitioner with certain new competencies in a given field. Third-party payers, insurers and provider groups who employ practitioners and/or pay for services, as well as the public at large, use certificate programs as a way of making certain that the personnel providing care have the necessary preparation. We have developed a certificate program for pharmacists who want to provide pharmaceutical care. Similar to many certificate programs within health care, the Pharmaceutical Care Certificate Program, developed by personnel at the Peters Institute of Pharmaceutical Care in the College of Pharmacy at the University of Minnesota, consists of an approved educational program, a required practice period, and a competency assessment examination.

The Pharmaceutical Care Certificate Program aims to provide practicing pharmacists with the knowledge, understanding, skills, and initial practice experience required to provide pharmaceutical care in their communities. Many programs today purport to accomplish the same objectives, so it is important to understand the principles underlying this particular program. First, this program is based on a very specific and comprehensively defined practice of pharmaceutical care. Second, this program integrates didactic learning with patient care practice, writing activities, reading exercises, interactions with experienced practitioners, and the skills and knowledge required to develop a lifelong learning approach. Third, this program is designed to accommodate the full-time practicing pharmacist and is of a length that is manageable yet allows a significant practice period for achieving the goals of the program. Fourth, it was designed by those who developed the practice and have taught many professional students and pharmacists the practice of pharmaceutical care.

The Pharmaceutical Care Certificate Program is summarized in Table 9-1. This program is described here to serve as a prototype for how to teach practitioners to provide pharmaceutical care.

> The certificate program is designed to prepare the individual practitioner to provide pharmaceutical care.

This certificate program does not require that the participant be practicing in a pharmacy that presently provides pharmaceutical care, nor is it necessary that all pharmacists at a site be enrolled. This is not a program for conversion of traditional dispensing pharmacies into practices supporting pharmaceutical care. Rather, it is an eight-week educational program designed for the individual practitioner. Upon completion, pharmacists will have the knowledge and skills necessary to practice pharmaceutical care and, therefore, will be able to decide whether or not they wish to practice pharmaceutical care on a full-time basis.

This program prepares the practitioner for successful completion of competency-based examinations such as those developed by the Minnesota Pharmacists Association. It introduces participants to the basic requirements for site accreditation, which are also included in the Pharmaceutical Care Competency Assessment Tool.[1]

This is an *intensive* eight-week program. It includes 30 hours of didactic workshops, 30 hours of self-directed home study, and 60 hours of direct patient care, for a total of 120 hours of continuing education for pharmacists.

The program consists of six learning units, all of which must be completed to receive credit. The learning units are organized to accomplish the following general goals:

1. motivate the practitioner to devote time and energy to meeting patients' drug-related needs
2. learn the practice of pharmaceutical care
3. engage in the initial patient care experience
4. learn the common diseases, drug therapies, and patient characteristics frequently associated with drug therapy problems
5. acquire patient care practice skills, and
6. complete the evaluation process

Each of the learning units is described below. The description presents the goals and objectives for each unit and a general description of the activities required of participants. Successful completion of the program requires that all six learning units be undertaken and all activities for each unit be completed. Each unit has a number of different learning activities so that individual learning styles can be accommodated. There are writing, reading, and practice activities in each unit.

Learning Unit I: Getting Started

This learning unit is designed so that participants can experience pharmaceutical care from the beginning. This requires the participants to critically examine pharmaceutical care, and determine its significance. Specifically participants are expected to explore what it means to take responsibility for a patient's drug therapy.

Pharmaceutical care begins with the patient.

This learning unit occurs during the week before the first group meeting. It is completed as a self-study unit. It involves three different assignments: one written, one patient care, and one reading assignment. All must be completed before the first group meeting.

The following goals and specific objectives will be met by participants completing this learning unit. They will

1. Critically examine what is currently understood about pharmaceutical care. Participants will
   • Comparatively define pharmaceutical care, patient education, OBRA counseling regulations, generic substitution, formulary management, drug use review, and disease-state management.
   • Compose a personal working definition for pharmaceutical care.
2. Critically examine what is presently motivating the participant's professional behavior. Participants will

(*Text continues on page 302.*)

TABLE 9-1 PHARMACEUTICAL CARE CERTIFICATE PROGRAM SUMMARY[a]

LEARNING UNIT	LEARNING OBJECTIVES	ACTIVITIES	SCHEDULE
I: Getting Started	• Determine what is currently understood about pharmaceutical care. • Critically examine what is presently motivating professional behavior. • Discover what it means to provide pharmaceutical care.	1. Answer questions that stimulate ideas about pharmaceutical care. 2. Take responsibility for the drug-related needs of three patients and record the experience in narrative form. 3. Complete a reading assignment.	• Receive mailed materials no later than one week before Workshop #1. • *Complete activities during the week as independent study.*
II: Workshop #1	• Learn to present patient cases for the purpose of pharmaceutical care. • Identify drug therapy problems. • Complete the patient care process for simulated patients. • Understand the discipline implicit in the practice and its documentation	1. Attend a three-day workshop. 2. Discuss with the group one of three patient experiences. 3. Complete a reading assignment.	**Workshop #1** **Sunday, 12N–6 p.m.** **Monday, 6–9 p.m.** **Tuesday, 6–9 p.m.**
III: Patient Care Experience #1	• Gain experience at providing pharmaceutical care. • Learn to utilize colleagues to help with patient issues, gain support, and provide feedback. • Understand issues of implementing professional activities to provide pharmaceutical care.	1. Provide pharmaceutical care to one new patient each work day and document the care. 2. Attend weekly practitioner meetings to present patient cases and receive and provide feedback. 3. Implement three new "professional" activities into practice. 4. Gain experience in a pharmaceutical care practitioner's practice. 5. Complete a reading assignment.	• Attend weekly practitioner meetings on Tuesday evenings of the next two weeks. • *Complete activities during the next two weeks as independent study.*

IV: Workshop #2	• Learn the ten most common diseases, drug therapies, and patient characteristics in community practice. • Understand the patient, disease, and drug information needed to provide pharmaceutical care. • Establish a personal learning plan to acquire the necessary knowledge and skills. • Understand basic concepts of building a practice, obtaining reimbursement, and documenting patient care.	1. Attend a three-day workshop. 2. Present a patient case. 3. Provide patient care documentation (without patient identifiers) to program faculty. 4. Complete the reading assignment.	**Workshop #2** **Sunday, 12N–6 p.m.** **Monday, 6–9 p.m.** **Tuesday, 6–9 p.m.**
V: Patient Care Experience #2	• Gain experience at providing pharmaceutical care. • Learn to utilize colleagues to help improve practice. • Understand issues associated with building a practice.	1. Provide pharmaceutical care to two new patients each work day and document the care. 2. Attend weekly practitioner meetings. 3. Implement three new "professional" activities into practice. 4. Gain experience from a pharmaceutical care practitioner, meeting in participant's practice. 5. Complete the reading assignment.	• Attend weekly practitioner meetings on Tuesdays during these three weeks. • *Complete activities during the next three weeks as independent study.*
VI: Workshop #3	• Write the examination to complete the requirements. • Discuss new patients with colleagues. • Design a mechanism for continued practice. • Provide program faculty with evaluation feedback.	1. Attend a one-day workshop. 2. Present one new patient case. 3. Provide patient care documentation (without patient identifiers) to program faculty. 4. Complete the written examination. 5. Complete the program evaluation. 6. Attend completion ceremony.	**Workshop #3** **Sunday, 12N–6 p.m.**

[a]This represents a template for the content, assignments, and schedule for the eight-week program.

- Determine what influences current decision making and actions.
- Assess priorities and how they are set.

3. Discover what it means to provide pharmaceutical care. Participants will
   - Identify the responsibilities involved.
   - Describe the work included.
   - Determine the knowledge, skills, and values that are needed to provide pharmaceutical care.

Participants will have successfully completed this unit when they have

1. Prepared written responses to questions that stimulate participants to think about the meaning of pharmaceutical care and the responsibilities of practitioners.
2. Taken responsibility for the drug-related needs of three patients familiar to the participant and recorded each experience as a narrative writing assignment.
3. Completed the reading assignment (Chap. 1 of this text).

Learning Unit II: Workshop #1, Understanding Pharmaceutical Care

This learning unit is designed so participants can learn the practice of pharmaceutical care, what skills are required, and how it is provided to individual patients. This is accomplished by discussing experiences with patients, working up and documenting simulated patients, and completing vocabulary exercises.

The following goals and specific objectives are to be met by the participants completing this learning unit. They will

1. Learn to present patient cases to colleagues for the purpose of providing pharmaceutical care. Participants will
   - Understand the components of a patient case presentation.
   - Formulate and present an actual patient case to other practitioners, using the patient case presentation format.

Participants learn to identify drug therapy problems.

2. Learn to identify drug therapy problems. Participants will
   - Describe the relationship between drug-related needs and drug therapy problems.
   - Learn the seven different categories of drug therapy problems.
   - Understand the various causes of drug therapy problems and their relationship to interventions and resolutions.
3. Complete the patient care process for simulated patients. Participants will
   - Learn the three major components of the patient care process.
   - Explain how to conduct each component of the patient care process.
   - Demonstrate the process on simulated patients.

4. Understand the discipline implicit in standards of practice that are represented by patient care documentation. Participants will

- Learn the level of discipline expected in a standard of practice.
- Learn to use standards of practice.
- Demonstrate documenting the patient care process.

Participants will have successfully completed Learning Unit II when they have

1. Attended the three half-day workshops containing didactic teaching, small group discussions, and written and reading assignments.
2. Discussed with the group one of the initial three patient experiences completed during Learning Unit 1.
3. Completed the reading assignment (Chaps. 3 and 4 of this text).

Learning Unit III: Patient Care Experience #1

The major focus of this learning unit is to acquire experience with patient care and to establish relationships with other practitioners for the purpose of taking care of patients. This is necessary to gain the confidence, skills, and experience required to provide pharmaceutical care.

This experience will be acquired by working up and providing pharmaceutical care to one new patient each day, attending weekly practitioner meetings, engaging in nonclinical professional activities, and interacting with an experienced practitioner in a pharmaceutical care practice.

The following goals and specific objectives are to be met by participants completing Learning Unit III. They are

1. To acquire experience in providing pharmaceutical care to different types of patients with varying medical conditions and requiring different drug therapies. Participants will learn to

    Acquire experience providing pharmaceutical care everyday.

    - Employ communication techniques for interaction with patients and other health care providers.
    - Practice the decision-making process required to provide pharmaceutical care.
    - Understand the differences between the practice and documentation of the practice.
2. To learn to effectively utilize other pharmacist colleagues to help with patient issues, to gain support, and to provide feedback so that practice can be improved. Participants will
    - Present patient cases to other practitioners to seek advice on complex patient problems and issues.
    - Practice giving and receiving critical comment regarding the practice of pharmaceutical care.
3. To understand the issues associated with implementing the nonclinical professional activities required to provide pharmaceutical care in a community practice setting. This requires that participants

- Understand the support needed to provide pharmaceutical care.
- Evaluate the challenges associated with the implementation of the necessary nonclinical professional activities.

Participants will have successfully completed this unit when they have

Meet with colleagues and discuss patient care.

1. Attended weekly practitioner meetings, presented patient cases, received comment and advice from colleagues, and provided feedback to other practitioners.
2. Implemented the following nonclinical professional activities required to provide pharmaceutical care:
   - Identify three physician prescribers in their practice and make appointments to introduce themselves, discuss what they can do for patients, and identify patients with drug therapy problems the prescribers would like resolved.
   - Identify three nonphysician prescribers (physician assistants, dentists, nurses, veterinarians) in their practice and make appointments to introduce themselves, discuss what they are able to do for them, and identify patients with drug therapy problems that these prescribers would like resolved.
   - Create filing system to keep records of the drug, disease, and patient information to be used in practice.
   - Create a resource library to help patients receive additional information about their illness, drug therapy, and/or other health care needs.
   - Use the dispensing computer system and/or purchasing records to identify the ten most frequently prescribed drugs (not products) in the practice, identify how many "active" patients are presently in the practice, and identify the ten most frequently purchased nonprescription medications.
   - Learn how to gain access to the Internet and how to search for and use drug and disease Web sites.
   - Identify the three references that are the most useful (see Table 7-3) and obtain access to current editions.
   - Identify and make a list (name, telephone number, fax number, E-mail address, area of interest/experience) of a minimum of five pharmacist colleagues to be contacted for consultation on complex patient problems.
   - Create a registry (list) of common drug therapy problems identified in practice. For each entry, describe the drug therapy problem, how it was resolved or prevented, references used to learn about it, and colleagues contacted for assistance.

Learn from experienced practitioners.

3. Interacted with an experienced pharmaceutical care provider by observing direct patient care, and completing a number of exercises with the practitioner, in the experienced practitioner's practice setting.
4. Completed the reading assignment (Chaps. 2 and 5 of this text).
5. Provided pharmaceutical care for one new patient each working day, and documented this care (patient case load of 14 active patients). This documentation will be evaluated using the two evaluation tools described in Tables 9-2 and 9-3.

TABLE 9-2 INFORMATION INCLUDED IN THE ASSESSMENT, CARE PLAN, AND EVALUATION	
Completeness of patient demographics in assessment	• Weight, height, and age (birth date) of patient must be documented to determine appropriateness of drug and dosage selections. • Current phone number preferred by patient should be recorded to support follow-up patient contact. • Current mailing address for each patient should be recorded to facilitate follow-up patient contact and to support billing systems. • Insurance carrier should be recorded to support billing processes; if none, write "self," indicating self-pay. • Allergies to medications or other substances and any adverse reactions to past medications must be documented to ensure patient safety. • Alerts describing patient-specific information required to ensure safe and effective drug therapy should be recorded, including alcohol, tobacco, or heavy caffeine use. • Medical devices needed by the patient, such as canes, wheelchairs, or contact lenses, should be recorded to support patient comfort and safety.
Appropriateness of care plan	• All medications the patient is taking must be documented, including prescription drugs, nonprescription drugs, samples, and others. • An appropriate indication must be documented for each medication the patient is taking. • For each medication, the dosage schedule must be documented. • For each prescription medication, the prescriber should be recorded. • For each care plan, all drug therapy problems must be documented. "None known at this time" is used to document that the patient does not have any drug therapy problems. • For all drug therapy problems identified, when and how each problem was resolved should be documented. • The specific services provided including patient consultation and education should be documented. • For each patient, directives including follow-up plans must be documented. • Follow-up dates should be recorded to facilitate follow-up contact to monitor patient progress and outcomes. • Follow-up dates for a patient's various care plans should be synchronized to ensure that the pharmacist can assess the patient's drug therapy in a comprehensive manner.
Clarity of follow-up evaluation	• For every episode in which pharmaceutical care services are provided, the pharmacist's evaluation of the status of each patient problem and/or the overall status of the patient must be documented. • Each evaluation of patient status must be dated, and the pharmacist (initials) making the evaluation must be documented. • If no professional evaluation was made, but the patient's status demands a note in the pharmacy chart, a status "note" should be recorded. • Written descriptions, explanations, and any other comments germane to the patient's condition or progress should be recorded in the "evaluation" field.

TABLE 9-3 Pharmaceutical care patient chart scoring

ABSOLUTELY NECESSARY INFORMATION	REQUIRED PATIENT-SPECIFIC INFORMATION	NEEDED INFORMATION
In order to provide pharmaceutical care.	Due to patient-specific nature of the medical or drug therapy problem(s).	In order to effectively and efficiently provide services to patients.
Demographics (5 points each)	**Demographics** (3 points each)	**Demographics** (2 points each)
Patient demographic information must include patient's age, gender, weight, drug allergies, and any history of adverse drug reactions in order to provide pharmaceutical care.	Patient demographic information such as height, medical devices, food allergies or alerts must be included, depending on the specific medical or drug therapy problem(s) present.	Patient demographic information such as address, phone number, and financial data are required to facilitate follow-up and to fully assess patient need for continued services and reimbursement.
Demographics Age, weight, and gender of the patient are documented.	Height, weight, age, and pregnancy status are often necessary to ensure safe and effective drug therapy.	Current mailing address is recorded.
Allergies Drug allergies are documented to avoid rechallenge.	Food allergies are documented to avoid rechallenge.	Preferred phone number for follow-up contact is recorded.
Adverse Reactions Reactions to past medications are documented to avoid reoccurrence.	Devices required by patients to support their care are recorded.	*Financial* Insurance carrier and financial information is recorded to support billing systems.
Alerts Alerts concerning alcohol, caffeine, and tobacco use are documented.	Alerts or devices describing medical, social, or other special patient needs are recorded.	

Care Plans (5 points each)	**Care Plans** (3 points each)	**Care Plans** (2 points each)
Care plans must contain complete drug indications, drug therapy problems, patient consultation provided, and follow-up plans in order to provide pharmaceutical care.	Care plans must contain resolutions for any problems that are identified.	Care plans that include complete prescriber information and coordinated follow-up dates will facilitate providing services for numerous patients efficiently.
Medication Record All prescription, nonprescription, sample, and herbal medications are documented.		For each prescription medication, the prescriber is recorded.
For each medication, the dosage schedule is documented.		For each sample medication, the source is recorded.
Indications Appropriate indication is documented for every medication.		
Drug Therapy Problems For each care plan, all drug therapy problems are documented.	*Resolution Code* When and how each drug therapy problem was resolved is recorded.	
Interventions All interventions made are recorded	Nonapplicable interventions are removed from standard care plans.	
Follow-up Plans and appropriate dates for follow-up are recorded.		Follow-up dates are synchronized.

(continued)

TABLE 9-3 (CONTINUED) PHARMACEUTICAL CARE PATIENT CHART SCORING

Evaluation (5 points each)	Evaluation (3 points each)	Evaluation (2 points each)
Evaluations must include the status of the patient's problems at follow-up.	Evaluations may require written explanations depending on the specific patient problems.	Evaluations that contain informational notes may facilitate future care for that patient.
Evaluation Patient follow-up is completed, and the status of each patient problem is documented.	Written description of the details of drug therapy problem is recorded.	Notes describing the patient's initial status are recorded.
The pharmacist making the evaluation and the date of the evaluation are documented.	Written explanation describing the status of the patient's problem is recorded.	Notes are recorded as an update of the patient's status at the follow-up evaluation.
Subtotal points (60 max)	Subtotal points (24 max)	Subtotal points (16 max)
	TOTAL out of 100 points =	
	18 to 74 points 75 to 92 points 93 to 100 points	Inadequate performance Required performance Excellent performance

Learning Unit IV: Workshop #2, Providing Pharmaceutical Care

The purpose of this learning unit is to understand the common patient, disease, and drug characteristics that can influence decisions when providing pharmaceutical care. The participant will understand the knowledge and skills to provide pharmaceutical care, and will learn how to use a personal learning plan. In addition, discussion of how to build a practice, what is required to obtain reimbursement, and how to document pharmaceutical care is presented. This unit utilizes the workshop, patient case presentations, the personal learning plan, and practice guidelines to prepare the participant.

The following goals and specific objectives will be met by the participants completing this learning unit. They will

1. Learn the ten most common medical conditions associated with drug therapy problems, as well as the drug therapy and patient characteristics associated with them. Participants will

   Learn common medical conditions, drug therapies, and patient characteristics first.

   - Identify patients with specific drug therapy problems.
   - Present patient cases with specific drug therapy problems to colleagues.

2. Understand the scope of patient, disease, and drug information required to provide pharmaceutical care. Participants will

   - Learn a common organizational framework for the information needed to provide pharmaceutical care.
   - Develop a disciplined method for organizing and synthesizing the information required.

3. Establish a personal learning plan to accumulate the necessary knowledge and skills. Participants will

   - Utilize the personal learning plan to acquire the necessary information about a new disease or illness.
   - Utilize the personal learning plan to acquire the necessary information about a new drug therapy.
   - Utilize the personal learning plan to acquire the necessary information about patient characteristics that influence drug therapy decisions.

4. Understand the basic concepts involved in building a practice, obtaining reimbursement, and documenting patient care. Participants will

   - Apply the steps of building a practice to the participant's current practice setting.

     Learn to build a practice.

   - Outline the steps in achieving reimbursement for a patient care service.
   - Define the requirements of a functional patient care documentation system.

Participants will have successfully completed this unit when they have

1. Attended the three one-half day workshops containing didactic teaching, small group discussions, and written and reading assignments.

2. Presented one patient from practice to the group as a patient case presentation.

3. Provided copies of the patient care documentation to program faculty (without patient identifiers) for evaluation and feedback.

4. Completed the reading assignment (Chaps. 6, 7, and 8 of this text).

Learning Unit V: Patient Care Experience #2

The major focus of this learning unit is on acquiring additional experience with patient care and further establishing relationships with other practitioners for the purpose of taking care of a variety of patients. This is necessary in order to gain the confidence, the skills, and the experience required to provide quality pharmaceutical care.

This experience will be acquired by working up *two* new patients each day, attending weekly practitioner meetings, engaging in nonclinical professional activities, and interacting with an experienced pharmaceutical care practitioner.

The following goals and specific objectives are to be met by participants completing this learning unit. They will

1. Provide pharmaceutical care for different types of patients with different medical conditions and requiring different drug therapies. Participants will
   • Identify additional drug therapy problems, including examples of patient conditions of common types, and including both chronic and acute diseases, pediatric and geriatric patients, females and males, organic and behavioral/psychological disorders, and curable and palliative indications for drug therapy.

Establish a personal learning plan.
   • Apply the personal learning plan in practice to learn the different diseases, drug therapies, and patient types.

2. Learn to consult with pharmacist colleagues to assist with patient care problems, to gain support, and to provide feedback so that practice can be improved. Participants will
   • Learn to present patient cases to other practitioners to seek advice on complex patient problems and issues.
   • Practice giving and receiving critical comment regarding the practice of pharmaceutical care.

3. Understand the issues associated with implementing the professional activities required to provide pharmaceutical care in a community practice setting. Participants will
   • Determine what technical and personnel support is needed in order to provide pharmaceutical care.
   • Discuss the problems associated with the implementation of the necessary professional activities.

Participants will have successfully completed this learning unit when they have

1. Provided pharmaceutical care to two new patients each working day and documented the care provided (total patient case load of 44 active patients).

2. Attended weekly practitioner meetings, presented patients, received comment, and provided feedback to other practitioners.

3. Implemented the nonclinical professional activities required to provide pharmaceutical care (see Learning Unit III for list of activities).

4. Benefited from an experienced pharmaceutical care provider by having the practitioner observe the participant provide direct patient care and completing a number of exercises with the practitioner in the participant's practice setting.

5. Completed the reading assignment (Chap. 2 of this text).

Document the care provided for two new patients a day.

Learning Unit VI: Workshop #3, Completing the Program

This learning unit completes the certificate program. Completion of the program includes writing an examination, discussing new patients cared for since the last workshop, evaluating the program, and accepting the Pharmaceutical Care Certificate.

The following goals and specific objectives will be met by participants completing this learning unit. They will

1. Discuss new patients with colleagues to obtain and provide feedback.
2. Provide program faculty with evaluation feedback.
3. Pass the examination to complete the program requirements.

Participants will have successfully completed this final unit when they have

1. Attended the entire one-day workshop.
2. Presented one new patient case at the workshop.
3. Provided copies of the patient care documentation to program faculty (without patient identifiers) for evaluation and feedback.
4. Completed a program evaluation.
5. Completed the written examination with an average score of 80 percent or greater. The examination process for the patient care portion of the examination is described in Table 9-4.

Demonstrate competency at providing pharmaceutical care.

The successful execution of this program results in a certificate of completion and 120 credits of continuing pharmacy education. At the conclusion of the program, participants will not only understand the practice of pharmaceutical care and how to provide it to patients, but also understand the basic concepts involved in building a pharmaceutical care practice. All three of these objectives must be accomplished before a lasting, professionally rewarding practice can become a reality. It takes a significant amount of effort, commitment, and risk-taking to accept the challenge of changing from a dispensing pharmacist to a pharmaceutical care practitioner.

TABLE 9-4 THE PATIENT CASE PORTION OF THE PHARMACEUTICAL CARE EXAMINATION	

Format of the exam	*This examination will*
	• Use a patient case format and require written responses for each of the four patient cases.
	• Be a maximum of 2 h in length.
	• Allow the pharmacist to demonstrate the ability to
	  1. Identify and describe drug therapy problems.
	  2. Construct a patient-specific care plan to ensure appropriate, effective, safe, and convenient drug therapy.
	    a. Design interventions to meet patient-specific needs for drug information and care plan instruction.
	    b. Design follow-up plans to evaluate actual patient outcomes and status, and monitor progress in meeting therapeutic goals.

Directions for the exam	*Directions* 1. Each case has *at least one* drug therapy problem. *Prioritize* the drug therapy problems by urgency and list the most urgent ones first. 2. Describe all active and potential drug therapy problems *for which you will assume professional responsibility.* 3. Document and prioritize the interventions required. List the most urgent and important interventions first. 4. Write an evaluation of the patient (include the questions or issues to address at the follow-up and recommend a schedule for follow-up evaluation). 5. For each written case used in the examination **"the reason for the patient's visit to your pharmacy"** is clearly stated in the *"Background"* section of the Pharmaceutical Care Patient Chart.
Grading of the exam	*Grading* Points for each case will be distributed in the following manner: Drug therapy problems 60% Interventions 24% Evaluation 16% To receive a passing grade on the examination, a score of 80% is required.

ACCREDITATION OF THE PRACTICE SITE

An accredited practice site is essential.

The preparation of the pharmacist is the first step to becoming recognized as a qualified pharmaceutical care provider. However, most third-party payers, government personnel, and managed care representatives also require accreditation of the practice site at which pharmaceutical care is provided. This is necessary because a practitioner can become incapacitated if the environment is not supportive of pharmaceutical care. The accreditation process is necessary to demonstrate that the practice site has all the elements necessary to facilitate pharmaceutical care practice. These include the following:

- A qualified pharmaceutical care practitioner
- A semi-private space designated for patient care
- A documentation system that can be audited for quality and reimbursement purposes
- The necessary educational and practice resources (up-to-date references, access to experts, and sufficient support personnel)
- Patient access to practitioner when care is required.

All of the criteria listed must be met to be accredited. Each of these criteria is described in detail in other sections of this book.[1]

TEACHING THE PHARMACY STUDENT

We may find that a significant portion of pharmacists currently in practice choose not to provide pharmaceutical care. This may occur for very understandable reasons. For example, the change may be too dramatic for many to accept; their investment in the commercial pharmacy business may be too great; they may have so little time remaining before retirement that they consider it senseless to contemplate such a transition; or they may simply not be interested in taking care of patients. All of these reasons are realistic and may explain why as few as 20 to 25 percent of current pharmacists may choose to provide pharmaceutical care in the near future. Therefore, it is necessary to devote significant time and energy to discovering what is required to prepare the next generation of pharmacy students to practice pharmaceutical care.

The next generation of pharmacy students will provide pharmaceutical care.

It would be presumptuous to claim that anyone knows how to teach a pharmacy student to become a qualified practitioner of pharmaceutical care, since this work is yet to be completed. However, we have gained considerable insight into some of the fundamentals of this process. We intend to discuss these beginnings, not in the context of existing pharmacy curricula, but by proposing a way to begin conceptualizing a new program. The program we are proposing refers not only to the curriculum involving its didactic and experiential courses, but also to the environment, culture, socialization processes, and relationships that must be developed between faculty, students, practitioners, and patients.

The building of a new conceptual framework, or program, means to begin with a different set of assumptions from those presently in place. These new assumptions are as follows:

1. The primary objective of this program is the preparation of a health care practitioner who can contribute to society in a meaningful, measurable manner, and those responsible for the program are to be held accountable for meeting this objective.

The product of a pharmacy curriculum must be a generalist practitioner who has the skills and knowledge to provide pharmaceutical care.

2. The program has as its focus a single, specific, professional practice which can be explicitly and clearly articulated. Faculty must understand and teach to the same practice.

The curriculum must teach to a single practice.

3. The specific practice is pharmaceutical care, as it is described here. It must be understood completely and at an intellectually sophisticated level by both faculty and administration. This practice must be agreed to and accepted by faculty and practitioners as the *basic* generalist practice, a primary care practice. Only then can it become the standard of practice.

4. The content of the program must reflect practice as described by experience and data generated by practitioners providing pharmaceutical care.

The care of patients must serve as the organizing force for the curriculum.

5. The program should be constructed in an orderly, logical, systematic, and comprehensive manner. This is necessary for the program to be internally consistent and for those responsible to be held accountable.

6. To be complete, and to succeed at producing a practitioner who can care for patients, the program must have the following:

- A clearly defined and consciously constructed culture
- Relevant and complete content
- Appropriate teaching/learning methods designed for the specific content of the program
- An appraisal process that holds all participants accountable

These six concepts are neither original nor new, nor are they unique to pharmacy, and few would disagree with them outright. However, forming a consensus on these concepts and acting to implement them in academe are two completely different challenges. We believe Aristotle summed up the task well when he stated: "A whole is that which has a beginning, middle and end." In this case it is especially important that we start at the beginning of how to create a program to prepare pharmaceutical care practitioners.

TRIANGLES TO REPRESENT PHARMACEUTICAL CARE PRACTICE AND EDUCATION

Throughout this book you may have noted our use of the triangle to represent the different components of practice. We will use another series of triangles to represent many of the concepts related to education. We have chosen the triangle for a number of reasons. First, as Michael S. Schneider observes: "A triangle is a most astringent shape. In contrast with the circle, which encloses the greatest area within the smallest perimeter, the triangle has the opposite property; it encloses the smallest area for the greatest perimeter."[2]

Applied to pharmaceutical care, this suggests that it is necessary to understand what is within the domain of practice and what is not. Toward this end, we have tried to describe the practitioner's responsibilities as distinct, known, and having identifiable boundaries.

The triangle also represents the first area enclosed by straight lines, thereby combining content with structure. Like the triad, every whole event inherently comprises a trinity of two opposites and an outside third element that brings about a new whole. Physicists call this trinity "action, reaction, and resultant." In pharmaceutical care, the practitioner must attend to patient needs while balancing social demands. Similarly, the philosophical underpinnings of the practice serve to balance and even counteract the polarization that practitioners caring for patients often encounter when faced with certain management decisions.

We will discuss the educational experiences preparing the pharmaceutical care practitioner. This discussion is necessary to develop of the concept of practice in an educational context. Finally, we discuss developing the program components themselves (culture, content, methods, and appraisal processes). These ideas are the developmental work that will form the foundation for the final task at hand: the development of the educational program preparing pharmacists to provide pharmaceutical care.

THE EDUCATIONAL EXPERIENCE: STARTING WITH THE "BIG PICTURE"

The triumvirate of academe is always given as teaching, research, and service, as illustrated in Fig. 9-1. Moreover, *service* usually refers to the service provided at the institutional level. The priority actually given to each of these three activities often reflects the individual speaker's personal priorities. It is no secret that in many large universities the order of priorities is research, service, and teaching. These three categories of activities are usually discussed as ends in themselves, and certainly it may be argued that the university rewards them in this manner. However, as a professional program, pharmacy is ethically bound to address this triumvirate differently.

Pharmacy, like all other professional programs, is responsible for preparing practitioners to perform licensed (regulated) activities in the public domain. For this reason, pharmacy educators are responsible for producing graduates who will contribute to society in a unique, meaningful, and measurable manner. In fact, this is the raison d'etre of all professional programs, especially health care professional programs. It is

> In a professional program, practice creates the relationship and defines the balance between teaching and research.

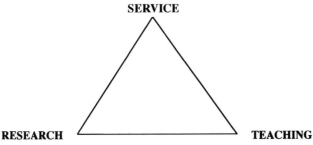

•**Figure 9-1** The components of the educational experience.

interesting that those outside of the university see this more clearly than do many located inside the academy.

This makes the triumvirate take on a different function. First, research, teaching, and service cannot serve as ends in themselves, but must function together to produce a product that clearly has a purpose and can contribute meaningfully to society. Second, service takes on a different meaning when graduates are expected to serve patients and society through the practice of pharmaceutical care. Service to the institution remains important, but service in the form of patient care becomes of paramount importance. This conceptualization of service must become the major focus of the educational endeavor—to care for the needs of patients in society.

Graduates from colleges of pharmacy will ultimately make decisions and exercise judgments that affect people's lives. Students presently commit themselves to a lengthy curriculum with demanding, complex content. Such an undertaking requires hard work, high energy levels, and a determination to "make sense of it all." Increasingly, students earnestly engage in discourse on relevance. Few faculty members join this conversation. The length of the programs, the cost, and the question of public interest raise important issues. One of these is the legitimacy of programs that continue to produce graduates who lack a clear conceptualization of practice.

Paradoxically, when discussing curricular changes or improvements, the professoriate tends to quite readily agree that it must reconceptualize purpose and "mission," and it avers that patient care is important. All members of this body declare their knowledge and expertise to be relevant. However, too often, when pharmacy faculty actually design and negotiate their own course content and course sequencing, the goal of producing qualified practitioners of pharmaceutical care becomes secondary to personal and research interests.

Before we begin to understand how the practice of pharmaceutical care can become and remain the primary focus of the new pharmacy program, it is necessary to understand how the triumvirate, and the participants in the triumvirate, can ultimately influence the design of the program. First, we need to consider what each of the participants in this triumvirate contributes. Figure 9-2 illustrates the major contributions of each component of the triumvirate.

Figure 9-2 is meant to communicate a number of concepts. First, practice is the most important component of the triumvirate in a professional (health care) program because it serves as the social nexus between the faculty's research and their teaching. Second, research and teaching provide the foundation for practice and supply the tools with which to provide care. All three components, focused on the same priority, are necessary to prepare a practitioner to care for others.

Each of the participants in the academic experience brings to it significant history and disciplinary bias. This cannot be ignored when

Practice is the most important component in a health care professional program.

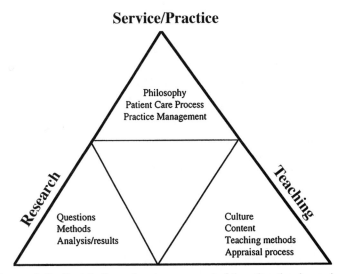

•**Figure 9-2** Contributions of each component of the educational experience.

designing a new program. Figure 9-3 raises our consciousness about the existence of these factors.

We often fail to understand that in the pharmacy education process, the three must be working on the same agenda, with the same primary vision in place. Each of the three can have other priorities, but for the purpose of educating the pharmacy student, the components in

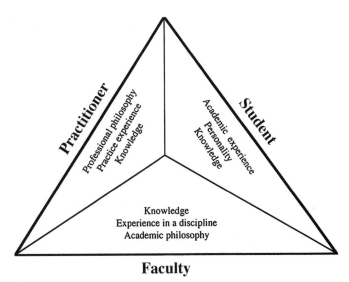

•**Figure 9-3** Participants and their influence on the educational experience.

Fig. 9-3 have to be elaborated, accepted, and promoted by all groups as they collaborate to prepare practitioners capable of providing pharmaceutical care *in any practice setting*.

If any one of the three areas (practice/service, research, or teaching) is not clearly articulated and its role prioritized, or if the individual participant (student, faculty, or practitioner) is allowed to exercise his or her discretion about participation, then the relationships among the three components and participants disintegrate into weak liaisons that do not create a well-defined system in which all can function optimally. If the integrity of the collective enterprise is lost, then growth and program development, along with purpose, are seriously compromised.

Figure 9-4 presents common situations that provide suboptimal educational experiences. We present them as cautions to consider during the developmental phase of the new program. Figure 9-4*A* presents the situation in which teaching is directed more at research interests than at practice goals. This can cause significant confusion on the part of the student in terms of what to practice and how to practice it. It leads to the preparation of an incompetent practitioner.

Figure 9-4*B* illustrates a situation in which research is the major interest and its application in the classroom is of minor importance. In this common situation, a faculty member neither understands nor accepts the responsibility to make the material taught relevant and useful to the student's ultimate application of the knowledge—that of practice. This is especially important in the practice of pharmaceutical care, in which the student is responsible to apply his or her knowledge for the benefit or to the detriment of another human being. This scenario may be putting the student (and potential patients) at significant risk.

> Teaching, research, and practice must all contribute to the pharmaceutical care program.

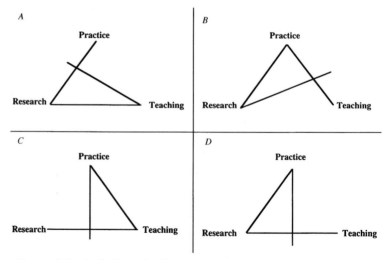

•**Figure 9-4** Ineffective educational experiences.

Figure 9-4*C* represents a situation in which practice suffers from the absence of the constant input of new knowledge generated through the research endeavor and applied to maintain the highest practice standards achievable. This situation can create a practice that does not serve the interests of patients experiencing drug-related illness. If this persists, the academic institutions preparing these practitioners will be replaced by vocational training centers or will disappear completely.

The last example of an ineffective educational experience for the student, represented in Fig. 9-4*D*, is the situation in which the practice becomes a research unit. The primary purpose for practicing becomes the completion of one research project after another. In this situation, the service to the patient is not driving the practice. Again, this is not to suggest that research is unimportant; however, when it becomes primary, teaching is compromised.

Obviously there are many more combinations that result in less than optimal educational and practice outcomes. The strongest and best situation is when all components of the academic experience are clearly defined and articulate with one another for the overall purpose of educating pharmaceutical care practitioners. This does not mean that academic freedom is sacrificed. In fact, it is quite the opposite. This triadic configuration is meant to provide just enough structure so that all are free to contribute to the "defined whole" in the manner they choose.

TEACHING TO A SPECIFIC PRACTICE

We have been saying in a number of different ways that the practice must serve as the focus of the new program. Schneider helps to make our point: "An idea . . . is considered 'pointless' not because it leads nowhere but because it has no center holding it together."[2]

This is frequently difficult for those in contemporary pharmacy schools to understand, for two reasons. First, programs in pharmacy have never taught to a *particular*, or specific, practice that is clearly articulated and accepted as a uniform, normative standard by faculty, administration, practitioners, and students. Pharmacy is the only health care profession in which this is the case. One can only imagine the disarray medicine, nursing, or dentistry would be in without a commonly understood practice in each profession.

Moreover, pharmacy educators appear to misunderstand what is meant by a *practice* as defined by other health care practitioners. There are very specific standards and rules that must be met to qualify as having a practice. Pharmacy educators frequently do not ask what those rules are, and yet other health care educators use them as the basis for their teaching programs. Pharmacy educators have been teaching to many different "practices," usually defined by a list of activities, usually differentiated by practice setting and settled on by the individual practi-

A practice has specific standards, rules, and responsibilities.

tioner, and usually defined based on a particular drug category, disease state, or patient characteristic. This is very confusing to the pharmacy student and to the rest of the participants in the health care system, and provides little direction for those who teach. When practice is not specifically defined, or is ill defined or assumed or allowed to be whatever the individual does on a day-to-day basis, it is impossible to teach to a unifying practice, to expect quality from students, or to achieve excellence in practice. An example may be helpful.

Clinical pharmacy was not clearly defined at the outset, nor has it been during the past 30 years, at least according to traditional definitions of a patient care practice. This was intentional in many cases, since the argument was that to define it would limit it. However, not clearly defining clinical pharmacy has made it difficult to teach, cumbersome to articulate to other health care professionals, and virtually impossible for managers to support and payers to reimburse. Perhaps most devastating of all, far too many patients have not been able to experience it. All of this and more prevented clinical pharmacy from developing and receiving widespread acceptance. Neither the time nor the resources will be made available to make the same mistakes with pharmaceutical care. It is necessary to define pharmaceutical care so clearly that it can be subjected to rigorous critique and improvement.

Practice must be the focus of the new program.

With this in mind, pharmacy educators must first come to accept that *practice*, a particular practice, is the focus of the new program. Second, all teaching faculty must understand and accept that pharmaceutical care will be the specific practice that drives the teaching efforts. Understanding something as complex as a professional practice is time-consuming and challenging. It is particularly difficult in the case of pharmaceutical care, since many pharmacists and those in education believe that they share a common understanding of this term. However, our experience is that those in the profession have been using the term to mean many different things. It is also common to find administrators and faculty who feel that they understand pharmaceutical care as well as they understand many other "topics" in the curriculum—rather superficially, but adequately for their own purposes. If pharmaceutical care is the focus of the program and not simply another topic to be taught in the classroom, then it must be understood completely, at an intellectually sophisticated level, by all faculty and administrators involved in delivering the program. This is a new standard for pharmacy educators.

Pharmaceutical care must be more than a class in the curriculum.

Placing Practice in an Educational Context

In this section we introduce the conceptualization of pharmaceutical care practice within the framework of the educational experience. This process may seem a bit tedious, but so much of this is missing from existing pharmacy programs that it is important to highlight these foundational concepts before we discuss building the new program.

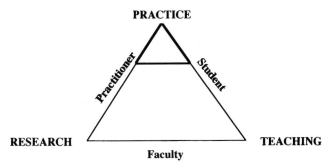

•**Figure 9-5**   Practice as the focus of the educational experience.

Directing educational efforts toward a uniform practice requires a level of understanding of that practice that is unfamiliar to pharmacy. The practice itself must be commonly understood, but perhaps more importantly, the practice must be understood in the broad context of the educational experience and in the broad context of the health care system and society. Because all those who find themselves teaching to this practice should share this common vision, it is necessary to place the practice of pharmaceutical care in all of these contexts, one at a time. With this information and the vocabulary that accompanies it, pharmacy will have a vision that will help to develop the methods needed to navigate changes within the health care system in the new millennium.

To begin, we place the practice of pharmaceutical care within the educational experience discussed earlier. This is depicted in Figure 9-5. Although quite simple, this figure illustrates the coordination, the "fit," that must exist to produce a positive experience for all involved. Making progress toward the development of a new program, however, requires that this practice be developed in more detail.

Figure 9-6 adds detail to the practice triangle introduced in Fig. 9-5. The principal participants in the practice of pharmaceutical care are the

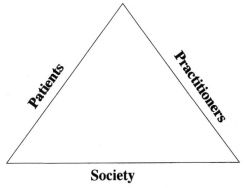

•**Figure 9-6**   Participants in the practice experience.

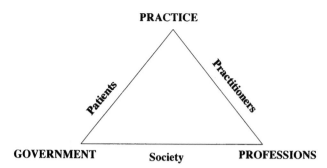

•Figure 9-7 Interactions of the participants in practice.

A health care professional practice exists in a social context. Therefore, the practice must be understood broadly to include the influences of the profession, the health care industry, and the government.

patient, the practitioner, and society. The practitioner must have access to, and interact with, the patient in order to provide direct patient care. Practitioners interact in society to form professions. Society can recognize only groups of health care practitioners who contribute in a meaningful, valuable way to the overall health and well-being of the general public. Remember, this group of practitioners is afforded special recognition (licensure, titles, exclusivity), rewards (salary, promotion), and support (subsidized education, government payment) as long as it continues to meet a recognized and valued social need. Patients, their families, and other members of the public form governments. In so doing, they regulate, protect, and reimburse professional practitioners in order to make certain that the public has access to competent, quality services. These dynamic interactions are depicted in Figure 9-7.

Each element of pharmaceutical care practice and the context in which it exists can be developed with another level of detail. The next series of figures accomplishes this. We have tried to look at each category of variable (practice, patient, practitioner, and so on), and to organize the knowledge about that variable that a pharmacy student needs to possess in order to provide pharmaceutical care. This organization of knowledge will ultimately become the defining force, along with data from practice itself, for the new program's content and structure. It is not our intention to prescribe the "right" answers in this development process. This vision is presented as a starting place for those interested in preparing the next generation of pharmaceutical care practitioners.

The impact of a practice is measurable at the individual patient level and collectively, across populations.

Figure 9-8 adds the detail of the practice components and their elements. The practice is shown as the center pillar connecting patients to practitioners. The scale on the left of this figure indicates that decisions are made and data are managed at two different levels: the patient-specific or individual level and the group or population level. This can be confusing, since we often present these two categories as mutually exclusive when, in fact, the student must learn to process and apply information at both levels simultaneously.

The next diagram, Figure 9-9, provides additional definition of practice variables. This organization allows students to understand the

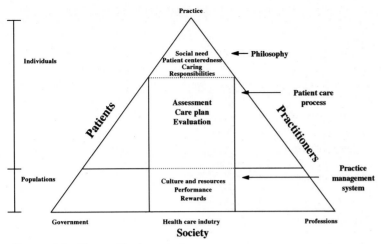

•**Figure 9-8** The practice in context.

scope of the knowledge needed to provide pharmaceutical care. It also introduces students to the disciplined way they must think about practice. All of these content areas describe the knowledge students require to learn in order to provide pharmaceutical care.

BUILDING A NEW PROGRAM

With this as background, it is now possible to discuss the nature of a program that will successfully prepare a practitioner to provide pharmaceutical care. We should reiterate that we are not discussing this mater-

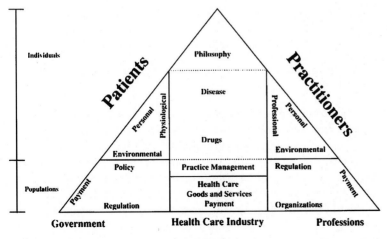

•**Figure 9-9** Components of the educational experience.

TABLE 9-5 COMPONENTS OF THE PHARMACEUTICAL CARE PROGRAM		
DIMENSION OF CURRICULUM	CHARACTERISTICS OF DIMENSION	HOW IT IS DETERMINED
Culture/context	• Core values, expectations, goals, rites, rituals • Needs to be transmitted to next generation • Development of a team philosophy • Defined by a generalist practice • Patient-centered • Caring philosophy of practice • Focused on pharmacist responsibilities • Determines teaching methods • Applies to faculty and students	Decided and agreed upon by dean/faculty, etc.
Content	• Core knowledge is defined by patient drug-related needs • Common problems define content, timing, and amount delivered	Negotiated
Teaching methods	• Determined by the culture • Team approach • General approach is problem-based (knowledge is problem-bound) • Student responsibility for education • Very active process • Personal (one-on-one) • Specific approach determined by content and teaching method • Information availability through technology • Applies knowledge and skills unique to site • Requires strong "core" knowledge and skills	Fixed list of effective alternatives Data-driven and futuristic Data-driven in practice
Evaluation	• Student performance • Faculty performance • Assess application to practice (from need to outcome)	Consistent with the program objectives

ial in the context of existing programs, but as though we are designing the program with a new beginning. The ideas presented here are provided for discussion purposes to begin the development process.

Table 9-5 presents the major components of the program, their characteristics, and how we believe each should be derived. This is quite basic information, and the initial reaction might be that it is obvious. However, each component is as important as the others, and too frequently, content is the preoccupation of those building such a program. Each component, although perhaps not necessarily implemented or achieved in the order presented, must be thought about in this logical order as the program's conceptual framework is developed.

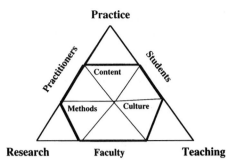

•**Figure 9-10** Components of the program.

Figure 9-10 places the components of the program in the midst of all the educational experience influences discussed earlier.

Creating the Desired Culture

The culture of the program includes all core values, behavior patterns, goals, expectations, rites, and rituals involved in the preparation of the student to practice pharmaceutical care. This set of understandings, or meanings shared by practitioners, must be passed on to the next generation. This is an active, explicitly stated process engaged in by faculty, students, mentors, preceptors, and administrators. In the pharmaceutical care program, the core values must be communicated early and repeated so that a commitment to patient care and accountability can be achieved. In essence, the culture of pharmaceutical care will promote norms and values that define professional identity and legitimize performance.

> The practitioner created is a direct reflection of the culture created in the program.

Too frequently, the culture is allowed to become whatever evolves when a program exists for an extended time. Such a passive method of determining the student values and goals results in less than optimal outcomes. The discussion that defines the desired and consistent culture for a program should be thorough and involve explicit plans for achieving it.

Identifying Appropriate Content

The pharmaceutical care practitioner has very explicit responsibilities that must be met during every patient care encounter. This set of patient care responsibilities must be taught and clearly understood by all students. Meeting these responsibilities and being held accountable for all clinical decisions made will serve as a fundamental driving force, leading students to be *active* learners and to further develop their knowledge and skills.

The practice of pharmaceutical care occurs in a community, a place where people live and interact. This community may be a neighborhood, a group of acutely ill patients requiring hospitalization, a group

> Experience and data from practice will provide the criteria with which to determine relevancy of content.

requiring hospice care, a group of families living on a reservation, a group of prisoners, or elderly or disabled individuals living in a long-term-care facility. Therefore, the content of the curriculum should be determined by the common drug therapy problems and needs of individuals in the community. These epidemiological data (common patients, their diseases, and their medication needs) will determine the nature, the amount, and timing of core knowledge and required material delivered throughout the curriculum. This core must also serve as an adequate foundation for those who choose to specialize later in their education.

To make progress in the area of content development, and to avoid making decisions based on tradition, emotion, or politics, an organizational framework is required. Within this framework, the patient is central. We begin teaching with a fundamental question: "What does the student need to know about the patient?" Program content, then, should be organized around the patient. The second question is: "What knowledge does the student need to meet patient needs?"

If you refer back to Fig. 9-9, you will be reminded of all the factors that can influence practice. We have evaluated what the student has to know about each of these factors to begin to define the scope of the program content. A structure for organizing the knowledge associated with each of these major factors follows, first for the patient (Table 9-6),

TABLE 9-6 LEARNING TO USE PATIENT INFORMATION TO PROVIDE PHARMACEUTICAL CARE

DIMENSION	TIME FRAME		
		HISTORY OF PRESENT	
	PRESENT	CONDITION	BACKGROUND
Personal	Health concerns	Change in mood or behavior	Personality traits
	Expectations of treatment outcomes	Change in habits	Coping mechanisms
		Change in mental outlook	
	Understanding of diseases and therapies		
Environmental	Who lives with patient	Change in a living situation	Socioeconomic status
	Who cares for patient	Change in physical environment	Cultural influences
	Living situation		Job/employment
			Insurance benefits
			Personal relationships
Physiological	Indications for drug therapy	Change in signs and symptoms	Risk factors
	Diagnosis, conditions	Change in physical condition	Allergies/alerts
	Signs, symptoms	Change in medications	Family history
	Medications		Hereditary factors
	Laboratory values		Cultural traits

Source: Adapted from Norman, 1995.[3]

DIMENSION			
Characteristics of the disease	**Definition of the disease** Mechanism of the disease: • Structural abnormalities— disturbances of the normal anatomic and/or biochemical conformation of the body • Functional abnormalities— disturbances in the normal performances and actions of cells, tissue, and/or organs • Results in signs, symptoms, and laboratory abnormalities (clinical presentation)	**Cause/etiology:** • What brings about the condition or produces the effect • Sum of knowledge regarding cause **Epidemiology:** • Frequency and distribution of causes • Incidence—rate at which a disease occurs (#/time) • Prevalence—total number of cases in existence at a given time	**Natural course:** • Onset •Severity/intensity •Prognosis
Intent of treatment	**Specify:** • Drug treatment • Nondrug treatment	**For the following purposes:** • Curative • Preventive • Palliative • Diagnostic	
Therapeutic goals	Physiological (physical) Behavioral (psychological) Economic	Presenting signs and symptoms laboratory findings	Functional Symptoms/sequelae Global

TABLE 9-7 LEARNING TO USE DISEASE INFORMATION TO PROVIDE PHARMACEUTICAL CARE

then for the disease process (Table 9-7), and then for drug therapy (Table 9-8). These three tables organize the information the student needs to learn in order to provide pharmaceutical care. The next series of tables presents the broad scope of knowledge needed to place practice in context. Table 9-9 describes the relevant information about the practitioner, and Table 9-10 describes the important components of society. The next series of tables adds detail to each of the components of society. Table 9-11 describes the information about the profession that is relevant to practice, Table 9-12 presents health care industry information, and Table 9-13 presents the government portion of society. This information is presented to demonstrate that those teaching and learning the information need to have a clear picture of how the information is organized, an understanding of its relevance to practice, and experience with applying it in practice. The development of critical thinking skills, problem-solving expertise, and good clinical judgment depends on this.

Applying Optimal Teaching Methods

The culture of the pharmaceutical care program and the content to be taught will determine the teaching methods that are appropriate to de-

TABLE 9-8 LEARNING TO USE DRUG INFORMATION TO PROVIDE PHARMACEUTICAL CARE

DIMENSION

Characteristics of the drug	Description of the drug Action of the drug: • Mechanism of action • Site of action	Efficacy for an indication: • Differential approach Toxicology: • Precautions • Contraindications • Adverse effects	Dosage of the drug
The drug in the patient	Pharmaceutical process (getting the drug into the patient): • Bioavailibility • Patient compliance • Physicochemical properties • Formulations and dosage forms • Methods of drug administration	Pharmacokinetic process (what the body does to the drug): • Absorption • Distribution • Metabolism • Elimination	Pharmacodynamic process (what the drug does to the body): • Molecular and cellular pharmacological action of a drug on cell tissue or organ
The outcome of the drug in the patient	Therapeutic process: • Effectiveness (the therapeutic effect): beneficial pharmacological effect of drug on pathophysiology of disease • Safety: detrimental pharmacological effect of drug on pathophysiology of disease		

TABLE 9-9 LEARNING TO USE INFORMATION ABOUT PRACTITIONERS TO PROVIDE PHARMACEUTICAL CARE

DIMENSION	CHARACTERISTICS OF THE DIMENSION
Personal	Professional philosophy Ethical framework Personality traits Expectations Career satisfaction
Environmental	Culture of the practice setting Practice support (personnel, technology, rewards, time) Authority/autonomy
Knowledge and skills (didactic and experiential)	Internalization of the practice (process) Knowledge of drugs, diseases, patients Understanding of society, the health care industry, and professions Practice skills (assessment, care planning, evaluation, communication, analysis, interpretation, research) Practice experience Limitations of knowledge/skills/experience

TABLE 9-10 LEARNING TO USE INFORMATION ABOUT SOCIETY TO PROVIDE PHARMACEUTICAL CARE			
Dimension	**Components**		
Government	Policy	Regulation	Payment for goods and services
Health care industry	Suppliers of health care goods	Providers of health care services	Payment for goods and services
Professional	Organizations	Regulation	Educational systems

liver the relevant content. The culture consistent with the practice of pharmaceutical care requires (1) teaching methods that are organized in a more problem-based format, (2) enrollment of students who are willing to actively assume responsibility for their own education, and (3) employ faculty who are student advocates, friends, and colleagues. Methods that truly engage the students as well as challenge them intellectually must be developed for this program.

This type of instruction will require substantial personalized, active, and problem-based student educational approaches. With these general approaches, specific teaching and learning opportunities can be designed.

Many methods will be used to teach students to provide pharmaceutical care—for example, didactic courses, laboratories, and computer

TABLE 9-11 LEARNING TO USE INFORMATION ABOUT THE PHARMACY PROFESSION TO PROVIDE PHARMACEUTICAL CARE	
Component	**Characteristics**
Organizations	Practice standards
	Peer review
	Educational programs
Regulations	Enabling
	Restrictive
	Standards for practice
Educational systems	Didactic curricula
	Experiential education
	Self-learning/teaching
	Diploma programs
	Certificate programs

TABLE 9-12 LEARNING TO USE INFORMATION ABOUT THE HEALTH CARE INDUSTRY TO PROVIDE PHARMACEUTICAL CARE	
COMPONENT	CHARACTERISTICS
Suppliers of health care goods	Pharmaceutical industry
	Technology and medical device supplies
	Alternative medical providers
	Wholesalers
	Retail pharmacies
Providers of health care services	Other health care providers
	Health care institutions
	Managed care organizations
Payment for goods and services	Payment for product
	Payment for services
	Pharmacy benefit managers
	Third-party payers (insurers, managed care)

Culture and content determine optimal teaching methods.

technology. The most appropriate structure will be determined by the specific content and the ultimate application of the content. New technologies that represent futuristic informational retrieval support systems should be incorporated into classroom teaching as well as into laboratory courses in order to prepare students to be efficient lifelong learners. The general purpose of the didactic courses and laboratory exercises is to prepare the students with the core knowledge and skills they need for the experiential portion of their curriculum.

Courses should be taught with methods that enable students to develop critical thinking, decision making, and communication skills.

TABLE 9-13 LEARNING TO USE INFORMATION ABOUT GOVERNMENT TO PROVIDE PHARMACEUTICAL CARE	
COMPONENT	CHARACTERISTICS
Policy	Access to services
	Enabling policy
	Economic policy
Regulation	Restrictive policies
	Practice guidelines
Payment	Payment for products and services
	Methods of payment
	Level of payment

Respect for patients, trust, cooperation, empathy, sensitivity, caring, and commitment are attributes that students must acquire and incorporate into their approach to patient care. These values need to be modeled and reinforced continually by faculty and preceptors.

Experiential education, in terms of pharmaceutical care practice sites, must be developed and utilized by pharmacy programs. The practice at these teaching sites will serve as the basis for the educational experience of the students. It is imperative that experiential education be consistent with the culture and content of the pharmaceutical care program. The goal of the experiential portion is to facilitate the students' ability to apply what they have learned in the didactic program. The experiential portions represent the application of knowledge and skills to patients in specific settings. Additionally, students will use this portion of their program to learn from patients—their health care beliefs, understanding, expectations, and concerns about their drug therapy.

The program's success can be measured in terms of the patient's well-being.

Over the past two decades, virtually all pharmacy programs have added clinical practitioners to their faculty payrolls as well as to their "volunteer" preceptor rosters. Despite significant efforts to assist these extremely diverse preceptors in their pedagogical pursuits, much of the experiential education in pharmacy is still based on the time-honored "see one, do one, teach one." Thus far in this text, we have addressed the "see one" and the "do one" portions of preceptorship. Teaching pharmaceutical care to students is extremely important to the future of this practice. In fact, history tells us that the transmission of specific practices is almost solely dependent on the one-to-one, generation-to-generation handing down of acquired and acceptable attitudes, approaches, skills, language, and behaviors. Therefore, it is essential that preceptors charged with the generational burden of perpetuating, improving, and expanding pharmaceutical care practice be mindful that their actions, inactions, decisions, words, and performance while providing pharmaceutical care to patients are all observed and learned by their students. Temptations to make things easier, more efficient, more practical, or more like "real life" can make it impossible for students to learn for themselves. Every practitioner learns through experience the risks and benefits, to both patients and pharmacist, of taking short-cuts, jumping to conclusions, or being less than comprehensive in certain situations. However, to use this type of less than optimal experience to teach students can be a great disservice. Students require and deserve a learning experience in which they can personally develop their own problem-identification and problem-solving skills. To develop these skills requires special knowledge and personal experience in the application of that knowledge. A certain amount of trial and error is required to acquire a clinically useful database which has relevant information and which has discarded information, that, while interesting, is not clinically useful.

"Practice makes perfect." This commonly used quote is often inaccurately attributed to the great American football coach Vince Lombardi. Many faculty and preceptors have used this quote to support adding more and more clinical experience to professional pharmacy teaching programs until they now require 6 to 7 years of full-time college study at a cost of $30,000 to $175,000. The actual quote was, "Perfect practice makes perfect." This message is very different and is directly applicable to clinical preceptors in pharmacy who accept the responsibility of helping to teach the practice of pharmaceutical care. In pharmaceutical care terms, early in a student's experiential studies, "perfect practice makes perfect" means that students must experience (see, observe) examples of perfect (complete, comprehensive) pharmaceutical care practice. Effectiveness must be the primary goal when the student is taking care of his or her first few patients. Efficiency can and will come later, but efficiency without effectiveness is harmful to patient care and obstructive to learning.

Experienced practitioners know that even if one is taught at a "100 percent" level, practice is often at an "80 percent" level as a result of day-to-day time and resource constraints. If that 80 percent level of practice is used to prepare the next generation of pharmaceutical care practitioners, they are likely to perform at 80 percent of 80 percent, or 64 percent, which is unacceptable by most health care standards. Therefore, it is essential that preceptors have the capacity, resources, and willingness to demonstrate and teach pharmaceutical care practice at an exemplary 100 percent level.

Although we are teaching pharmacy "practice," not pharmacy "perfect," there are several ways in which preceptors can maximize their students' ability to understand and learn the practice of pharmaceutical care. As described earlier in this text, the language used is essential to understand and communicate the practice of pharmaceutical care. Preceptors must use, describe, and demonstrate terms such as *assessment, care plan, evaluation, drug therapy problems, intervention,* and *therapeutic relationship* in a way that is consistent with the practice of pharmaceutical care and understood by their students.

Preceptors have an additional obligation in the preparation of the next generation of pharmaceutical care practitioners: the demonstration of a caring philosophy and attitude toward patients with drug-related needs. Preceptors in their roles as teachers must bring the caring portion of pharmaceutical care to life for the student. The student must be able to observe the preceptor taking sufficient time with patients to determine all of the patients' drug-related needs. The student must be able to observe the preceptor gathering the resources (information, products, devices) necessary to help patients meet their goals. The student must also be able to observe the preceptor keeping in personal contact with patients to evaluate the impact of the care provided, and to gather pa-

Preceptors must use vocabulary consistent with the practice.

tient feedback as to the quality of that care. Finally, the preceptor must teach the student the value of accurate and complete documentation, not only to support patient care but to use to critically evaluate one's own practice performance.

The didactic portion of the program will teach common material to the student—the practice itself, essential patient information, drug-related knowledge, and disease and illness information—whereas the experiential portion of the curriculum should teach the particular knowledge and skills specific to the provision of care in a particular patient setting. This includes the management of the practice, communication, and documentation required to care for many patients over time. The student's experiential learning should include a variety of patients, including both those with common drug-related needs and those with more complex problems. Standards for the number of patients cared for by the students should be established to ensure that students have sufficient breadth and depth of practice experience upon graduation. Experiential education will also instruct the student how to deal with legal concerns, ethical issues, financial issues, and personnel management. This can happen only when students come to a practice site prepared with the basic knowledge and skills of pharmaceutical care practice. It will be very important to develop "core" sites to teach the basic knowledge and skills of pharmaceutical care. Students can then use the basic tools to develop new sites and expand their experiences. Although many in pharmacy education profess these standards are already being met, it is only necessary to compare practice care skills of pharmacy students with those in medicine, nursing, or dentistry to realize what a great distance remains to be traveled.

Core sites are needed to teach basic practice skills.

A Meaningful Appraisal Process

Evaluation will be designed to reflect student performance in practice. A pharmaceutical care portfolio of student activities and performance should be developed to facilitate evaluation of students by their patients, faculty, and colleagues. Documentation of the care provided for certain patients must be reviewed and evaluated by mentors. Systematic, consistent, and constructive evaluation instruments should be developed to ensure that student performance can be fairly evaluated and areas requiring strengthening can be identified. The student pharmaceutical care portfolio would also include self-assessment, in which each student describes his or her knowledge, skills, accomplishments, growth, areas of weakness, areas of concern, and goals. Peer evaluation is important in a culture in which collegiality and mutual support thrive. To support peer evaluation, an evaluation rubric for completeness should be developed (refer to Table 9-2 of this chapter for an example). This should include expectations about appropriate content to be reviewed and critiqued by student colleagues. This notion was introduced in the "certificate" section of this chapter. The student's pharmaceutical care portfolio should be available to all students and mentors at all times. Electronic documentation systems can be employed for this purpose.

Program evaluation is necessary in order to ensure that commonly required knowledge and skills are being taught effectively and efficiently. Faculty evaluation should be based on the faculty's responsibility to prepare students with the knowledge and skills they need in order to practice and provide pharmaceutical care. Therefore, in addition to standard teaching evaluation methods, an important element in faculty evaluation in a pharmaceutical care program will be *student performance in practice*. Most standard evaluation techniques measure faculty output, whereas in a practice-based program, outcomes must be measured in the form of student performance. It is through performance that, in the final analysis, the profession itself will be judged.

> Program evaluation is based on student performance in practice.

We have presented what we consider to be the fundamental ideas needed to develop the educational program for pharmaceutical care providers. To succeed, it will be necessary to start at the beginning in a logical manner, learn the practice, describe the desired culture, decide on the content, develop the appropriate teaching and learning methods, and ensure that a consistent and comprehensive appraisal process is in order. This will position educators to attract those who are interested in taking responsibility for patients' drug-related needs. Society will benefit greatly from such an accomplishment.

As Marcel Proust (1871–1922) said, "the real voyage of discovery consists not in seeking new lands but seeing with new eyes."

REFERENCES

1. Bond, W.E. *Pharmaceutical Care Competency Assessment Tool.* St. Paul, MN: MPhA; 1997.
2. Schneider, M.S. *A Beginner's Guide to Constructing the Universe, The Mathematical Archetypes of Nature, Art, and Science. A Voyage from 1 to 10.* New York: HarperCollins; 1995.
3. Norman, D.D. Perceptions of the elderly regarding the medicating experience: A discourse analysis of the interpretation of medication usage. Ph.D. thesis, University of Minnesota, 1995.

RECOMMENDED READINGS

Barrows, H.S., Tamblyn, R. *Problem-Based Learning: An Approach to Medical Education.* New York: Springer-Verlag; 1980.

Beare, H. and Slaughter R. *Education for the Twenty-First Century.* London: Routledge, 1993.

Brandes, D., Ginnis, P. *A Guide to Student-Centred Learning.* Oxford, England: Blackwell; 1986.

Isbister, J.P., Harmening, P.D. *Clinical Hematology: A Problem-Oriented Approach.* Baltimore: Williams & Wilkins, 1988.

Kaufman, A., (ed.) *Implementing Problem-Based Medical Education: Lessons from Successful Innovations.* New York: Springer-Verlag; 1985.

Kettner, P.M., Moroney, R.M., Martin, L.L. *Designing and Managing Programs: An Effectiveness-Based Approach.* Newbury Park, CA: Sage; 1990.

Ross, R.H., Fineberg, H.V. *Innovations in Physician Education.* New York: Springer-Verlag; 1996.

Tindall, W.N., Beardsley, R.S., Kimberlin, C.L., *Communication Skills in Pharmacy Practice.* Philadelphia: Lea and Febiger, 1994.

GLOSSARY

adherence

to follow medication and care plan instructions as intended

a term used synonymously with *compliance*, but has less authoritarian connotations

preferred to compliance

assessment

a systematic review of the patient's drug-related needs performed by the practitioner with the patient

completed for the purpose of insuring that all the patient's drug therapy is *indicated, effective, safe,* and *convenient*; and to identify any drug therapy problems

involves the collection of information (e.g., interviewing the patient, contacting the prescriber, reviewing patient medication charts, etc.), decision making, and problem solving

one of three components of the patient-specific care process in the practice of pharmaceutical care (the *care plan* and the *follow-up evaluation* complete the process)

bioavailability

the degree to which a drug or other substance becomes available to the systemic circulation after administration

care plan

a detailed schedule outlining the practitioner's and the patient's activities and responsibilities

completed by the practitioner, with the input and participation of the patient

designed for three different purposes: (1) to resolve any drug therapy problems, (2) to successfully achieve the therapeutic goals of the patient, and prescriber, and (3) to prevent any potential drug therapy problems

includes (1) a statement of the goals to resolve any drug therapy problems present, meet the therapeutic goals of the patient and prescriber, and to prevent future drug therapy problems, and (2) the interventions by the practitioner

and the actions to be taken by the patient to accomplish the objectives of the care plan

caring

the commitment to alleviate another person's vulnerability and suffering

a state of responsiveness to others that entails the willingness to become personally involved

often considered to be the "cornerstone" of the therapeutic relationship

consists of three activities that practitioners should engage in: (1) assess an individual's needs, (2) obtain whatever resources are needed to meet these needs, (3) determine if the help provided has produced positive or negative outcomes. If one or more of these activities is missing, care has not been provided.

causes of drug therapy problems

the most likely explanation for the existence of a drug therapy problem

suggest a means to resolve the drug therapy problem

the common causes of drug therapy problems are as follows:

appropriate indication
1. need for additional drug therapy
   a. an untreated condition
   b. synergistic or potentiating drug therapy required
   c. preventive drug therapy required
2. unnecessary drug therapy
   a. no medical indication present
   b. addictive/recreational drug use
   c. nondrug therapy more appropriate
   d. duplicate drug therapy
   e. the drug is being used to treat an avoidable adverse drug reaction

effective drug therapy
1. wrong drug
   a. dosage form inappropriate
   b. contraindication present
   c. condition refractory to drug

d. drug not indicated for condition

e. more effective drug available

2. dosage too low

  a. wrong dose

  b. frequency inappropriate

  c. duration inappropriate

  d. incorrect storage

  e. incorrect administration

  f. drug interaction

safe drug therapy

1. adverse drug reaction

  a. unsafe drug for patient

  b. allergic reaction

  c. incorrect administration

  d. drug interaction

  e. dosage increase or decrease too fast

  f. undesirable effect

2. dosage too high

  a. wrong dose

  b. frequency inappropriate

  c. duration inappropriate

  d. drug interaction

compliance

  a. drug product not available

  b. drug product not affordable

  c. drug product cannot be swallowed, tolerated, or administered

  d. instructions not understood, remembered, or agreed to by the patient

  e. patient prefers not to take the drug as recommended

clinical pharmacy

a health science specialty which embodies the application, by pharmacists, of the scientific principles of pharmacology, toxicology, pharmacokinetics, and therapeutics to the care of patients

an emphasis in the profession of pharmacy from 1968 to the present

includes services such as individualized (pharmacokinetic) dosing services, nutritional support services, therapeutic drug monitoring, and drug utilization review

the majority of the services are provided to or for physicians and at the request of physicians

this emphasis initially required a Doctor of Pharmacy qualification

occurs in the institutional setting most frequently

cognitive services

a term used by practitioners in the community, independent, retail pharmacy practice setting, refers to those services which require professional knowledge and skills beyond the ones required for the dispensing of a prescription medication

includes services such as counseling, drug information, blood pressure monitoring, etc.

communication

the exchange of information or "message" between a patient and a health care professional

may refer to the content of the message, the manner in which the message is given or received, or the relationship between the communicants

for communication between the patient and the health care professional to be productive and effective, *active listening* must occur

active listening is the skill of understanding what another individual is saying and feeling and, in turn, conveying to that individual what you believe him or her to be saying

compliance

the ability of a patient to adhere to a therapeutic regimen agreed upon between patient and practitioner only after appropriateness, effectiveness and safety have been assessed by the practitioner and determined to be in the patient's best interest

the term *adherence* is often preferred, as it does not connotate an authoritarian posture

concerns, patient

an expression, by the patient, of issues associated with the safety of drug therapy; the patient's fear of what the negative effects of drug therapy can do to him or her

an expression of the impact drug therapy may have on the patient's illness or condition in his or her life

one of three categories of drug-related needs of patients which are addressed by practitioners in the practice of pharmaceutical care (the other two are patient expectations and patient understanding of drug therapy)

contraindications

a reason or explanation, such as a symptom or condition, that makes a particular treatment or procedure inadvisable

curative

restoration of health, a method or course for restoring health, a restorative agent

diagnosis

the process of determining the nature of a disorder by considering the patient's signs and symptoms, medical background, and laboratory tests when necessary

disease

a pathological, objectified condition of the body that presents a group of physiologically and biologically defined symptoms

may be considered as an "event," occurring at a given point or points in time.

a disorder with a specific cause and recognizable signs and symptoms; any bodily abnormality or failure to function properly except that directly resulting from physical injury

disease-state management

an approach to identifying patients and providing services to patients according to disease specifications (e.g., diabetes, hypertension, asthma)

a marketing term used originally by the pharmaceutical industry to identify groups of patients (by specific disease) in order to market drug products on variables beyond unit cost

a cost accounting term accepted by managed care organizations to comparatively assess costs and benefits

drug misadventuring

a term coined by H. Manasse to indicate drug-induced illness

drug-related morbidity

the incidence and prevalence of disease associated with drug therapy

one aspect of the social need addressed in the philosophy of pharmaceutical care

drug-related mortality

the incidence and prevalence of death associated with drug therapy

one aspect of the societal need addressed in the philosophy of pharmaceutical care

drug-related need

those health care needs of a patient which have some relationship to drug therapy (any and all types of drug therapy) and for which the practitioner is able to offer professional assistance

the source of the need could be a prescription drug product, a question from the patient, a request for nonprescription medication or a referral

a need expressed by the patient in terms of his or her understanding, concerns, expectations, or behaviors about drug therapy

a need translated by the practitioner as the absence or presence of drug therapy problems (appropriate indication, optimal effectiveness, maximum safety, and appropriate compliance)

drug therapy problems

any aspect of a patient's drug therapy that is *interfering with* a desired, positive patient (therapeutic) outcome

a translation by the practitioner of a patient's drug-related needs

a problem that can always be categorized in the following way:

1. inappropriate *indication*
   a. requires additional drug therapy
   b. unnecessary drug therapy
2. *ineffective* drug therapy
   a. wrong drug
   b. dosage too low
3. *unsafe* drug therapy
   a. adverse drug reaction
   b. dosage too high
4. inappropriate *compliance* or *adherence*

the major function of a pharmaceutical care practitioner is to identify, resolve and prevent drug therapy problems

the focus of an assessment in the same way a medical diagnosis is the focus of the physician's workup the source can be any and all types of drug therapy (prescription, nonprescription, physician samples, nutritional aids, vitamins, etc.)

effectiveness of drug therapy

ability of the drug therapy to produce the desired or intended beneficial response in a particular patient

one of four responsibilities the practitioner assumes when practicing pharmaceutical care (the other three responsibilities are to ensure that all of a patient's drug therapy is appropriately indicated, safe, and convenient)

efficacy

the power of a drug to produce an effect. The sum of all beneficial biological activities for prevention, alleviation, cure, or diagnosis

epidemiology

the study of epidemic disease, with a view to finding a means of control and future prevention

ethical dilemma

commonly seen as any problem where morality is relevant

the conflict which results from two different resolutions to a situation, both of which are ethical

ethics

the philosophical study of morality

the study of goodness and right action

the moral principles of a particular tradition

etiology

the study or science of the causes of disease

the cause of a specific disease

evaluation

the practitioner's determination, at planned intervals (of follow-up) of the patient's outcome and current status

purpose is to record actual patient outcomes, evaluate progress of the patient toward therapeutic goals, determine if previous drug therapy problems have been resolved, and assess whether new drug therapy problems have developed

the third component of the patient care process in pharmaceutical care practice (the other two are *assessment* and *care plan*)

expectations, patient

an expression by the patient of issues associated with the effectiveness of drug therapy; patient's impression of what their drug therapy can do for him or her

one of three categories of drug-related needs patients have which pharmaceutical care practitioners address (the other two are *patient concerns*, and *patient understanding* of drug therapy)

iatrogenesis

a term describing illness induced by a physician or other health care practitioner

identification of drug therapy problems

one of three functions performed by a pharmaceutical care practitioner when practicing pharmaceutical care (the other two are *resolution* and *prevention* of drug therapy problems)

performed to help meet a patient's drug-related needs

the process used to identify drug therapy problems is the assessment

illness

the subjective experience of a disease or condition

may be considered as a "process," often occurring over a protracted period of time

the experience of illness encompasses social, psychological, and cultural factors

incidence

a measure of morbidity based on the number of new episodes of illness arising in a population over an estimated period of time

indication for drug therapy

circumstances pointing to the cause, pathology, treatment, of disease (or illness), serving as the primary reason for the use of drugs

a sign, symptom, or index to demonstrate or suggest the necessity or advisability to initiate drug therapy

appropriate use of drug therapy for the treatment or prevention of a condition (illness, symptom) in a specific patient

one of four responsibilities the practitioner assumes when practicing pharmaceutical care (the other three responsibilities are to assure— for a patient's total drug therapy—effectiveness, safety, and appropriate compliance)

morality

synonymous with ethics (see *ethics*)

onset of a disease

a beginning, outset, first appearance of the disease

outcomes, desired therapeutic

the *preferred* consequences (results) of interventions made to meet therapeutic goals

can have characteristics that are economic (i.e., cost), social/behavioral (i.e., patient preferences), or physiological and clinical (i.e., laboratory values)

must be measurable, achievable, and have a time frame associated with it

outcomes, actual patient

the *actual* consequences (results) of interventions made to meet therapeutic goals

can have characteristics that are economic (i.e., cost), social/behavioral (i.e., patient preferences), or physiological and clinical (i.e., laboratory values)

palliative

a medicine that gives temporary relief from the symptoms of a disease but does not cure the disease

paternalistic approach to patient care

an approach in which an authority undertakes to regulate conduct of those under its control in matters affecting them as individuals as well as in their relations to authority and to each other

a traditional approach that is inconsistent with the practice of pharmaceutical care

patient

an individual who is the recipient of health care services

a person who possesses a unique set of needs, values, beliefs, and behaviors that are brought to an interaction with a health care professional

increasingly thought of as client, consumer, and even customer

patient advocacy

the willingness to assume an active role and provide resources on behalf of a patient

may require an intervention or confrontation on the part of a health care professional for the benefit of a patient

patient-centered care

care designed in response to a patient's drug-related needs—*all* of a patient's drug-related needs

care that maintains the patient in a "holistic" form and does not fragment the patient into drug categories, disease groups, organ entities, or systems

one of the four dimensions of the philosophy of pharmaceutical care (the other three are *social need*, *caring*, and *practitioner responsibilities*)

patient care process

what actually occurs between the practitioner and the patient when pharmaceutical care is provided

consists of the assessment, care plan, and follow-up evaluation

provided so a patient's drug-related needs are met, ensuring that a patient's drug therapy is indicated, effective, safe, and taken properly

one of three components that make up the practice of pharmaceutical care (the other two are the philosophy of practice and the practice management system)

the descriptive component of the practice; describes what occurs on a patient-specific basis today; applies to one practitioner and one patient

patient concerns

expressed views of the patient related to drug therapy issues, specifically safety issues

the primary concern of the practitioner providing pharmaceutical care

the beginning of the patient care process

pharmaceutical care

a practice in which the practitioner takes responsibility for all of a patient's drug-related needs and is held accountable for this commitment

is delivered when an *assessment is performed*, a *care plan developed*, and a follow-up *evaluation is completed* for a patient

consists of three components; the philosophy of pharmaceutical care, the patient-care process, and the practice management system to support the practice (see individual definitions of each) the responsible provision of drug therapy for the purpose of achieving definite patient outcomes

a health care professional practice designed to meet the patient's drug-related needs by identifying, resolving, and preventing drug therapy problems

the mission of the pharmacy profession since 1990

pharmaceutical process

a series of actions that involve getting the drug into the patient. Includes disintegration of the dosage form and dissolution of the drug— bioavailability. Mainly governed by chemical and physical properties and influenced by dosage forms and methods of administration.

pharmacodynamic process

a series of actions involving what the drug does to the body. The activity of the drug at the site of action. Drug-receptor interaction as well as subsequent events which leading to a pharmacological effect on the cell, tissue, or organ.

pharmacokinetic process

a series of actions involving what the body does to the drug; the time course of drug concentrations in the body. Includes absorption, distribution, metabolism, and elimination.

Pharmacist's Workup of Drug Therapy

a rational, decision-making process for identifying, resolving, and preventing drug therapy problems

the pharmacist's cognitive activities involving the patient's demographic, medical, and drug therapy information for the purpose of making an assessment of the patient's drug-related needs

documentation of the thought processes, decisions made, and problems solved in providing pharmaceutical care

philosophy of pharmaceutical care

caring for a patient's drug-related needs

taking responsibility for the identification, resolution, and prevention of drug therapy problems

includes: meeting a social need, a patient-centered approach, caring for a patient, and prescribed practitioner responsibilities

one of three components of the practice of pharmaceutical care (the other two being the *patient care process* and the *practice management system*)

practice

the creative application of knowledge, guided by a common philosophy, to the resolution of specific problems in a manner and at a standard accepted by society

the experiences a practitioner encounters in the process of caring for someone

repeated performance for the purpose of learning or acquiring proficiency

use of one's knowledge to bring about a particular good for a patient

cooperative human activity exhibiting shared norms and purpose, a unifying set of meanings and inherent goods

practice philosophy

a set of values that guide behaviors associated with a certain act, in this case a professional practice.

how a practitioner practices, day in and day out

the function or purpose of a practice philosophy is to help the practitioner determine what is important and to help set priorities. It also aids the practitioner in making ethical management decisions, and clinical decisions.

one of three components of a professional practice (the other two being the *patient care process* and the *practice management system*).

prescriptive in nature, indicates what "should" be done, is "timeless," and applies to all practitioners in a professional practice

practice management system

the underlying organizational framework to support a practice

includes the mission of the organization, the necessary financial, physical, and human resources, the evaluation system, and the reward mechanisms.

practitioner, health care

an individual who possesses a body of knowledge and/or skill in any one of a number of health care fields and uses this knowledge to meet the health care needs of a patient

subscribes to a philosophy of practice and way of

practicing that is consistent with other members of the profession

prevalence

a measure of morbidity based on current sickness in a population estimated at a particular time

preventive

measures intended to thwart or ward off illness or disease prophylactically

prevention of drug therapy problems

one of three functions performed by a pharmaceutical care practitioner (other two are identification and resolution of drug therapy problems)

performed for the purpose of meeting a patient's drug-related needs

primary health care

a systematic and comprehensive approach to meeting the health care needs of patients at a community level

list of services designed to meet basic (i.e., primary) health care needs of patients

prevention and health promotion receive significant emphasis

is consistent with the philosophy of pharmaceutical care

profession

a vocation in which a professed knowledge of some department of learning or science is used in its application to the affairs of others or in the practice of an art founded upon it

embodies the following attributes: (1) registration or state certification, which embodies standards of training and practice in some statutory form; (2) a fiduciary practitioner-client relationship, (3) an ethical code, (4) a ban on advertising of services, (5) independence from external control, (6) service above self-interest, (7) application of specialized knowledge, and (8) skills in the service of humanity

professional ethics

a set of moral principles and values, defined by a philosophy of practice, that help prescribe appropriate behavior of practitioners

prognosis

an assessment of the future course and outcome of a patient's disease, based on knowledge of the course of the disease in other patients together with the general health, age, and sex of the patient

resolution of drug therapy problems

one of three functions performed by a pharmaceutical care practitioner (other two are identification and prevention of drug therapy problems)

performed for the purpose of meeting a patient's drug-related needs

responsibilities, patient

to present drug-related needs in a timely manner and actively participate in their resolution

to ensure that (1) all concerns, expectations and any lack of understanding about drug therapy are expressed to the practitioner, (2) the information presented the practitioner is accurate and complete, (3) accountability for patient outcomes is shared with the practitioner.

responsibilities, practitioner

to assess a patient's drug-related needs by determining the patient's understanding, concerns, and expectations of his or her drug therapy.

to ensure that a patient's drug therapy is appropriately indicated, the most effective, the safest possible, and to ensure that a patient is able to comply with the therapeutic regimen designed

prescribed by the philosophy of pharmaceutical care (social need, patient-centered care, and caring)

rights, patient

to have all drug-related needs addressed by the practitioner

to receive and benefit from the knowledge, skills, and expertise of the practitioner when and how the patient needs them

safety of drug therapy

the use of drug therapy in a specific patient without harm or risk of adverse effects

preventing harm, injury, or loss (due to drug therapy)

one of four responsibilities the pharmaceutical care practitioner assumes (the other three responsibilities are to ensure that all of a patient's drug therapy is appropriate, effective, and convenient)

severity

the extreme nature of the disease or the extent to which the patient suffers from the disease

social need

the cornerstone of the philosophy of practice; the rationale or justification for a professional practice

for pharmaceutical care, the need is to take responsibility for the drug-related *morbidity and mortality* in society

standards of care

the level of quality at which a practitioner is expected to provide care to a patient

the set of behavior every patient has a right to expect from a practitioner providing care in a particular profession

the set of behavior every practitioner has an obligation to exhibit when claiming to provide care in a particular profession

the set of behavior of a practitioner that is subject to evaluation by peers, regulators, and the public

therapeutic process

the beneficial pharmacological effect (effectiveness) or the detrimental pharmacological effect (safety) of the drug on the pathophysiology of the disease

therapeutic relationship

a partnership or "alliance" between the practitioner and the patient formed for the purpose of identifying the patient's drug-related needs essential for the practice of pharmaceutical care

requires a recognition and assumption of certain responsibilities on the part of the patient and the practitioner

includes the following elements: *trust, empathy, respect, authenticity,* and *responsiveness.*

trust is being confident that one can depend on the character, ability, and truth of another individual. The patient must feel "safe" in sharing his or her thoughts and concerns with the practitioner.

empathy is an active, imaginative understanding of another's feelings. The practitioner must be able to understand the world from the patient's perspective and to communicate this understanding to the patient.

respect is the positive concern and valuing of the patient as a unique individual.

authenticity is the ability of the practitioner to be open and straightforward in a relationship with the patient.

responsiveness is the ability of the practitioner to recognize and accommodate to the unique situation and characteristics of each patient rather than acting on preconceived ideas of what would be best for the patient.

toxicology

the sum of what is known regarding poisons, their actions and detection, and the treatment of the conditions produced by them in humans and animals

understanding, patient

an expression, by the patient, of issues associated with why he or she is taking drug therapy (indications for use)

patient's recognition of the need for drug therapy and of the potential seriousness of his or her medical condition

one of three categories of drug-related needs patients have which pharmaceutical care practitioners address (the other two are patient concerns and patient expectations of drug therapy)

INDEX

Note: Page numbers followed by *t* refer to tables; page numbers followed by *f* refer to figures.

NOTES

NOTES

NOTES

NOTES

NOTES

NOTES

NOTES

NOTES

NOTES

NOTES

NOTES

NOTES

ISBN 0-07-012046-3

90000